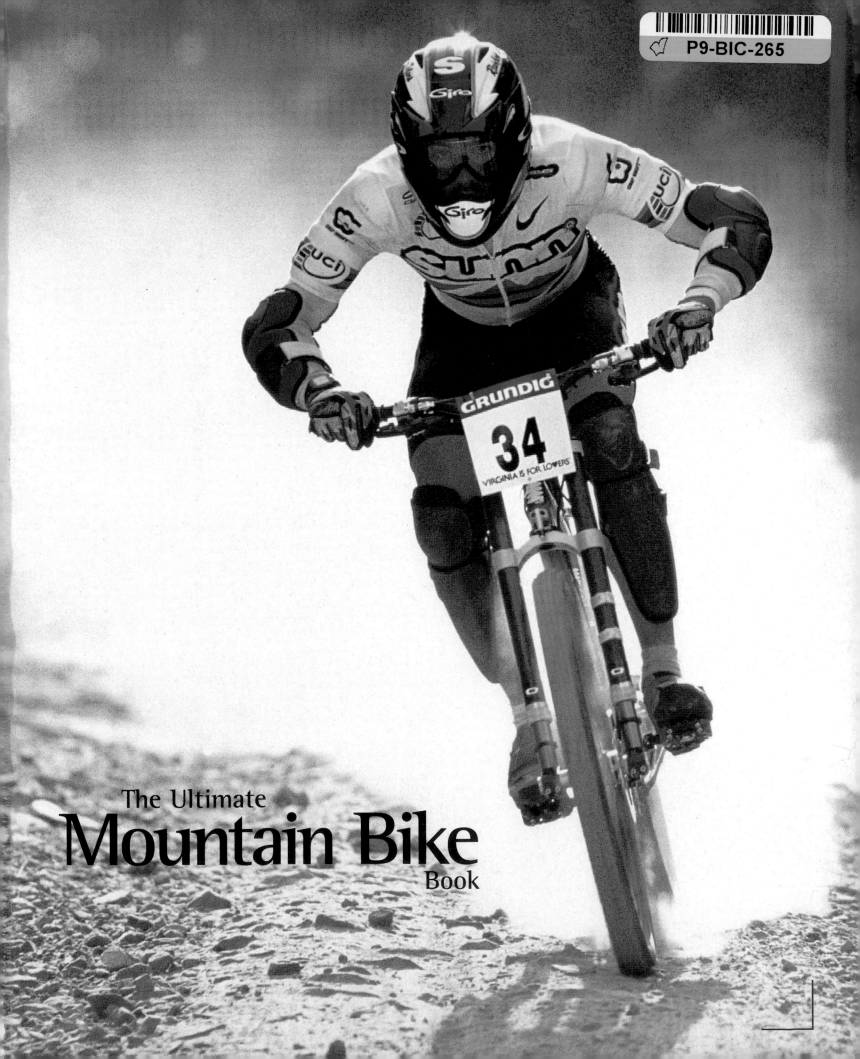

P9-BIC-265

The Ultimate
Mountain Bike
Book

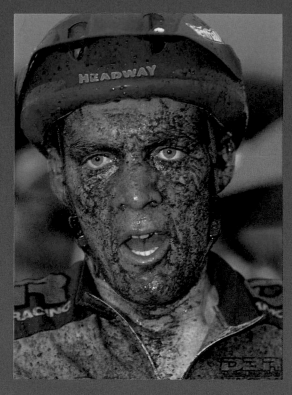

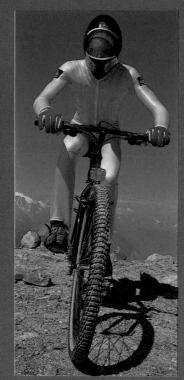

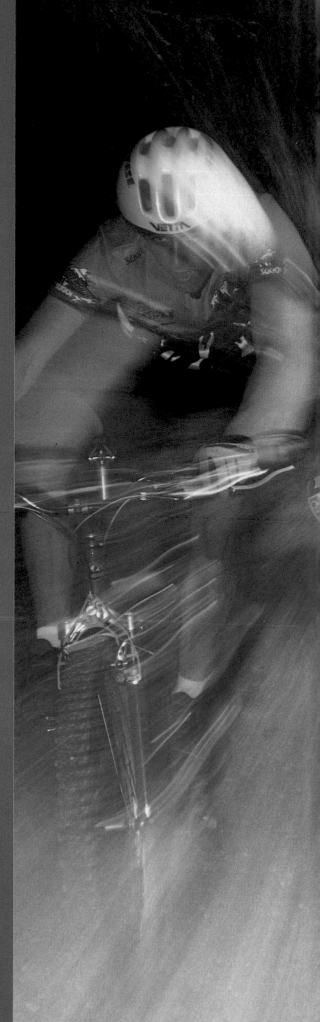

A FIREFLY BOOK

Published by Firefly Books Ltd., 2002

All rights reserved. No part of this publication may be reproduced, stored in a retrieval system or transmitted in any form or by any means, electronic, mechanical, photocopying, recording or otherwise, without the prior written permission of the copyright owners and the publishers.

Text and design copyright © 1996, 1999, 2002 Carlton Books Limited

First printing

National Library of Canada Cataloguing in Publication Data
Crowther, Nicky
  The ultimate mountain bike book: the definitive illustrated guide to bikes, components, techniques, thrills and trails / Nicky Crowther. — Rev. 3rd ed.
Includes index.
ISBN 1-55297-653-X
  1. All terrain cycling. 2. All terrain bicycles. I. Title.
GV1056.C76 2002   796.6'3   C2002-901162-0

Publisher Cataloging-in-Publication Data (U.S.)
Crowther, Nicky.
  The ultimate mountain bike book / Nicky Crowther.—3rd rev. ed.
[192] p. : col. photos. ;   cm.
Includes index.
Summary: A guide to mountain biking including buying a bike, customizing your bike, maintenance and trail riding.
ISBN 1-55297-653-X (pbk.)
1. All terrain cycling. 2. All terrain bicycles. I. Title.
796.6/ 3 21   CIP   GV1056.C76 2002

First published in Canada in 2002 by
Firefly Books Ltd.
3680 Victoria Park Avenue
Toronto, Ontario M2H 3K1

Published in the United States in 2002 by
Firefly Books (U.S.) Inc.
P.O. Box 1338, Ellicott Station
Buffalo, New York 14205

Printed in Italy

While every care has been taken to ensure the accuracy and the completeness of the information in this book, no liability can be accepted by the author, the copyright owners or the publishers for any loss or damage (and where legislation permits injury as well) caused by errors in, or omissions from, the information given.

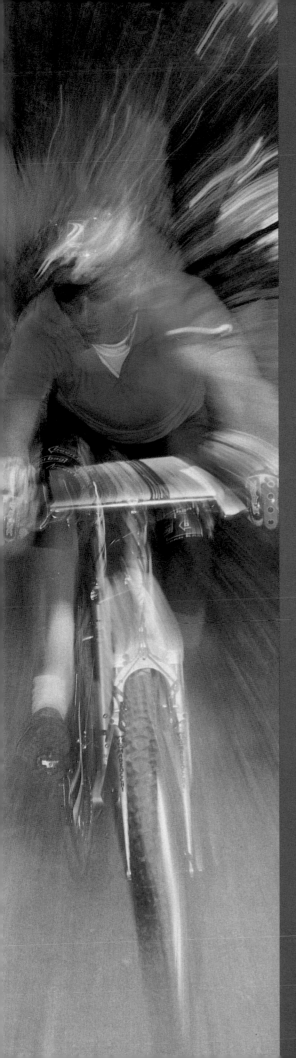

The Ultimate
Mountain Bike
Book

The definitive illustrated guide to bikes, components, techniques, thrills and trails

Nicky Crowther
maintenance section by Melanie Allwood

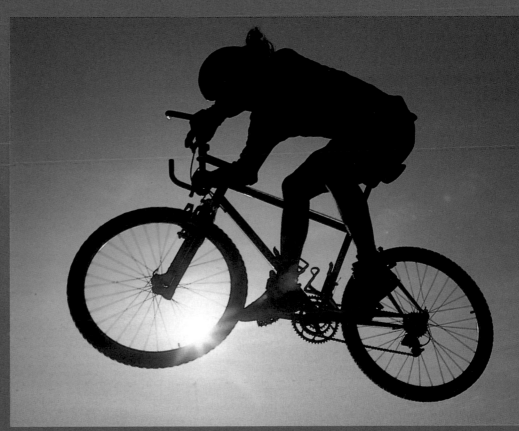

FIREFLY BOOKS

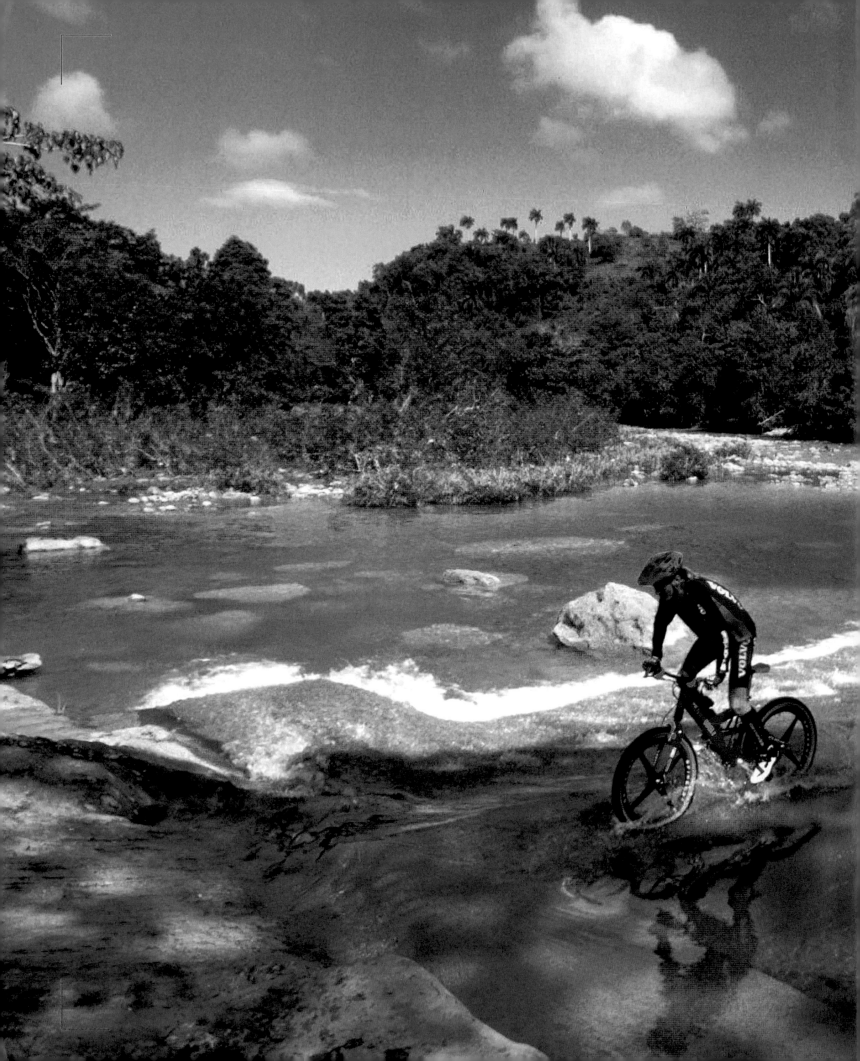

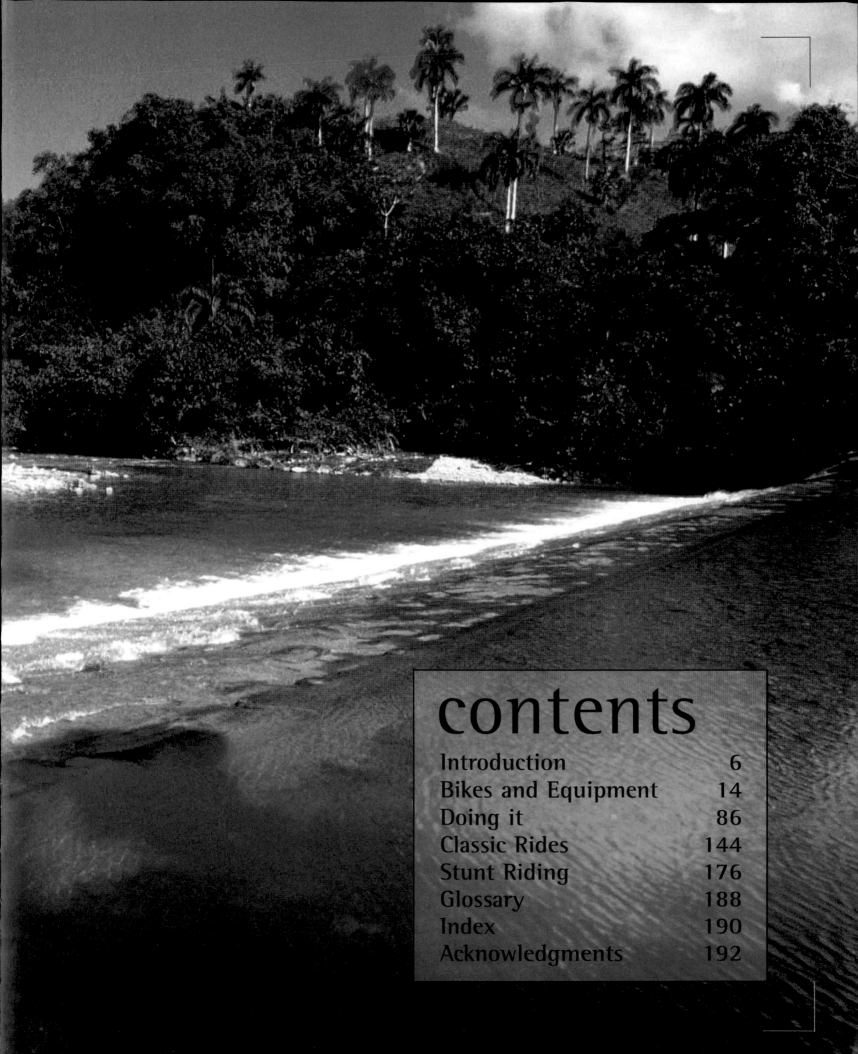

contents

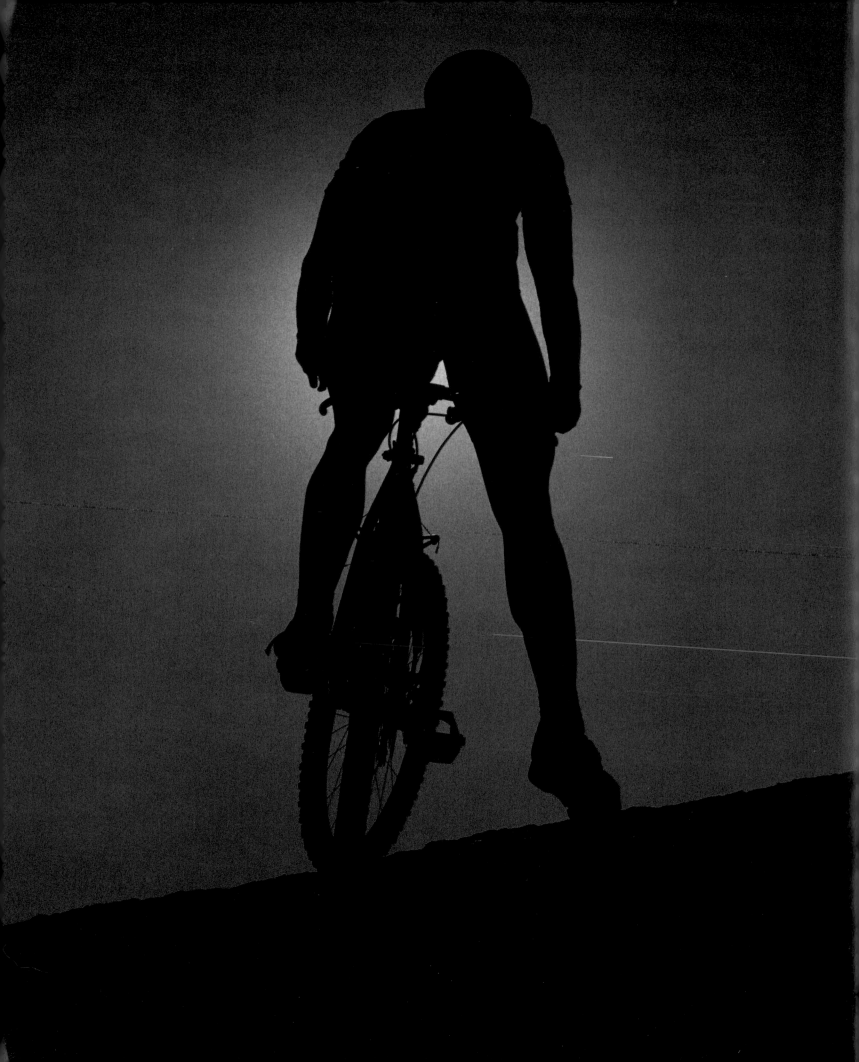

welcome to the world of the
fat tire
bike!

In the late 1970s, after one group of riders climbed a high pass in Colorado and another descended a high-speed fire-road near San Francisco, "mountain" got hitched to "bike" and the sport spread like wildfire. The number of mountain bikes (MTBs) in the world quickly rose from one — Joe Breeze's first Breezer, produced in 1977, to millions. In fact, half the bikes now sold around the world are mountain bike style, of which a third are the genuine off-road article. Anyone who wonders how this is possible has never been in a mountain bike saddle. You can catch off-road fever 10 minutes into a ride, and there is no known cure. Mountain biking can mean different things to different people, but once infected you can't shake it off. For enthusiasts, the sport is more than a game — it rapidly becomes a way of life.

Perhaps the most surprising thing about the mountain bike is that it took so long to invent. It is by far the most versatile of all bikes — bike and rider can go on-road and off-road at speeds of up to 50mph (80km/h) for adventure, commuting, vacationing and training. It is a passport to the alternative pedal-power movement and a guaranteed introduction to the renowned charge of a society of bike lovers. Many people assume that sunshine and dust are the ideal conditions for mountain biking, but when the temperature drops you can adjust your clothing, grit your teeth and keep on riding. Unlike sports such as hockey and tennis, mountain biking is a sport that can be enjoyed all year round.

Today we live in the most mechanized society in history. We need temptations like the mountain bike to keep us active and in touch with the world we live in. On our bikes we abandon passive entertainment of screen and car, saving our legs and hearts from atrophy, keeping our minds sharp and the planet alive. Urbanites can lose themselves in maps and forests, teenage pimples are treated with organic mud-packs, and night-clubbers can find natural highs from exploiting nature's obstacles for the ultimate natural thrill.

Mountain biking is simply the best way to get off your butt and get fit. Cycling will improve your health and increase your energy levels as well as giving you the opportunity to explore and revel in nature's adventure park — you just can't beat it.

in the beginning
– America

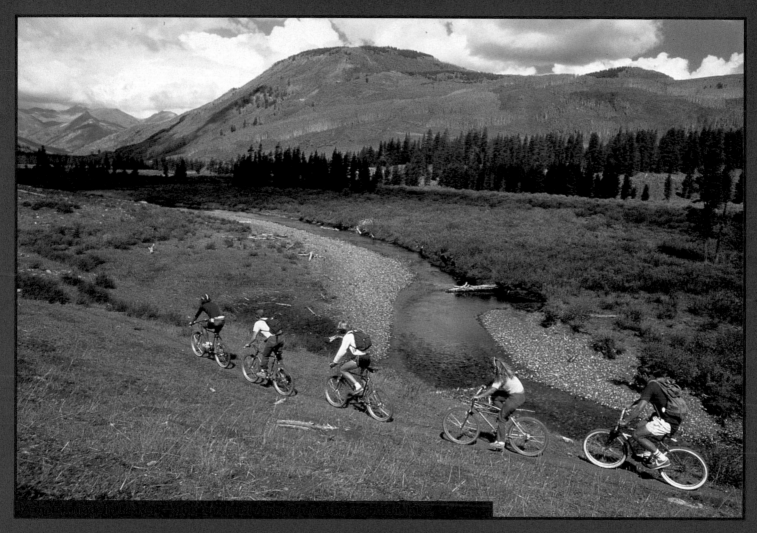

Unlike compact discs and personal computers, two other inventions of the 1970s, the mountain bike owes less to the advance of science than to the pursuit of pleasure. That was how a now legendary bunch of Californian hippie cyclists discovered a great new way to wreck old bikes, and went on to spread the off-road word far and wide.

Of course, cross-country biking is as old as the bicycle itself. Who didn't do it on their local tracks as a kid? However, in 1976, when these guys in Marin County were likewise obeying their natural instincts, they innocently tripped the wire of a new worldwide sport. First, they decided to compete against the clock hurtling down a short, steep piece of track. Then, they beefed up their ancient Schwinn cruiser bikes or "clunkers" with new home-tooled parts.

Daredevil descent

The first Repack Downhill race on Mount Tamalpais above San Francisco was attended by just a fistful of people. The course is 1.8 miles (2.9km) long with a 1,200ft (366m) descent and the record stands at 4 minutes, 22 seconds. It was set, appropriately, by Gary Fisher, whose name has decorated hundreds of thousands of bikes since.

Fisher's Repack rivals included Joe Breeze and Tom Ritchey, who are attributed with designing and building the first mountain bikes. The event's organizer was Fisher's roommate Charlie Kelly, who edited the long-running mountain bike mag *Fat Tire Flyer* from 1980 to 1987 and who wrote the first magazine articles to touch the rest of the world, which were published by *Outside* magazine. Harley-Davidson motorcycle factory rider Mert Lawwill, who was later to collaborate with Fisher in designing the first rear suspension bike, was another Repacker. The event ran intermittently from 1976 until 1984, when riding rights to the trail were lost and the fire track on Repack Hill was closed by the authorities.

Not only does today's bike carry the Repack legacy, but so does the biker's quest for speed. This is officially displayed at the bone-busting big-bucks downhill events of the world series and championships. Unofficially, it is found in the subversive tradition that is relived every time a

grown-up kid survives a white-knuckle descent to ride another day. The bikes the originals used were beasts compared to today's machines. For starters, they were up to 40 years old and weighed up to 50lb (23kg). They had BMX upright handlebars, no gears and a single rear coaster brake, operated by back-pedaling. The speed of the Repack descent was so fast that the grease inside the brake drum would burn off and the brake would begin to seize and had to be repacked for every ride. This gave the event its name and led to the term "smokin'" downhills.

Although incredible fun, the gear-less bikes were too heavy to be much good at climbing — they were only impressive at descending — so pretty soon adaptations that would eventually become standard were flowing quickly out of the backyard workshops and on to the bikes. Along came a front brake and seat post quick release, to make it easier to lower the seat and protect the post from bending. Gary Fisher is

attributed with fixing the first 5-speed gear on a clunker, which also had the first thumb-shifter gear levers. The other major advance was the development of aluminum rims and the improvement of tires, which instantly knocked 4.4lb (2kg) off the bike's weight and a lot more off the rolling resistance. Suddenly, you didn't need to be the Incredible Hulk to go uphill.

The first MTB

The honour of creating the first purpose-built frame for a mountain bike goes to Joe Breeze, who was also the rider to win the most Repack races. Breeze started out as a roadracer; he was a veteran of the local Velo Club Mount Tamalpais and a five-time winner of a 200 mile (320km) tandem race, partnered by off-roader Otis Guy. It was partly to escape the pressures of road racing that he and fellow club members used to truck up Mount Tam with their clunkers.

In 1977, with a little frame-making experience picked up partly from his engineering father and partly from a traditionalist local bike builder, Breeze conceived and constructed the mark one Breezer — the most sophisticated off-road bike then in existence. He followed it up the following year with ten more, built, or so he thought, for his own circle of friends.

The bikes took the best from the clunkers — the fat tires and handlebars — but had different drivetrain geometry for wider clearance, with thumbshifters that operated derailleur gears, and Weinmann cantilevers to replace the old drum brakes, which were operated by Magura levers.

Although the cruiser-style central tube that ran like a bow from the head tube of the bike to the rear hub is long gone, these first bikes forged the path still followed today by hardtail (i.e. suspension-free) mountain bikes.

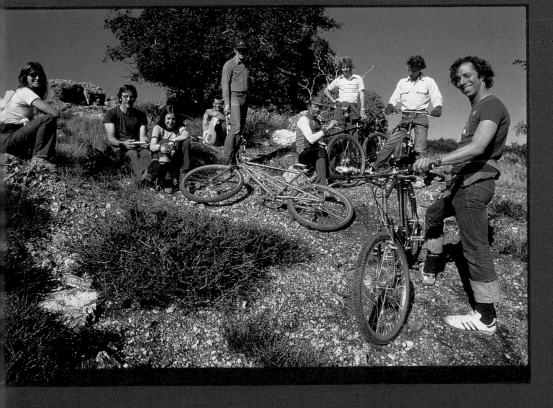

The mountain bike evolves

Then a series of events occured which led to factory production, cheaper prices and high street sales. In 1979, 21-year-old Tom Ritchey, a former US national junior team rider and member of the clunker clan, began to apply Breeze's ideas to his own bikes. Gary Fisher bought one of Ritchey's first three models, and then in 1979 linked up with Charlie Kelly to form the first regular bike-selling company, MountainBikes, which operated until 1983.

The next step from small-town birthplace to the global off-road village came thanks to Mike Sinyard of the then fledgling company Specialized. In 1980, he bought four Ritcheys and took the Californian design across the Pacific Ocean to the factories of

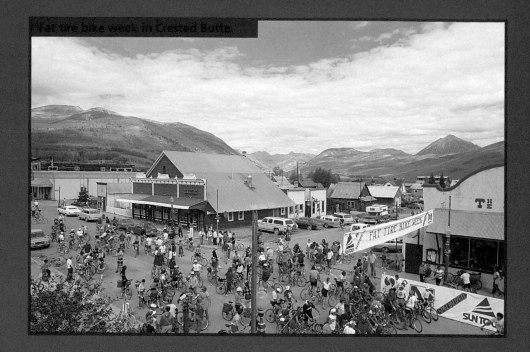

Fat tire bike week in Crested Butte.

Taiwan. In 1981 Sinyard returned with the first model in a line of mass-production mountain bikes — the StumpJumper. Fisher, Ritchey and Sinyard's Specialized have all survived the industry's growing pains and are all still significant players in the market.

Rocky Mountain high

The combination of mechanical curiosity and risk-taking in the Californian riders is what grabs most of the limelight in retrospectives, but no MTB history is complete without mentioning the Rocky Mountain bikers. In 1976, a thousand miles east in the Rockies, a parallel off-road movement was in the making. In Crested Butte, a small isolated mountain town in Colorado with a dirt road for a main street, cyclists tackled the rough ride over the mountains to nearby Aspen.

The cyclists' route, which wound its way about 30 miles (50km) up and over the 12,700ft (3,870m) Pearl Pass, was originally used in the nineteenth century for hauling ore by mule from Aspen to the railway

line at Crested Butte. The inaugural Pearl Pass Clunker Tour took place with 15 riders — seven rode the whole way up, eight took rides in a 4-wheel drive vehicle. In the report of the ride in the *Crested Butte Pilot* of September 17, 1976, it was noted that at the overnight camp 3 miles (4.8km) below the pass the riders "consumed one keg of beer, seven more cases of beer, three bottles of Schnapps, two gallons of wine and three bottles of champagne. Then ... everyone got drunk and passed out on the pass." Richard Ullery, the report continues, became famous on the ride as "the first man in history to cross Pearl Pass in a bathtub." Unlike the fat-tire bike, this variation never caught on.

In 1978 there were 13 riders on the Pearl Pass Tour, several of them invited from California, including Wende Cragg, the only woman who rode regularly in the bunch. Her photographs of the movements in both California and Colorado make up a huge portion of the visual records from that era. The Pass is still open to anyone who wants to ride it, and the Tour has become a highlight of the annual Crested Butte Fat Tire Bike

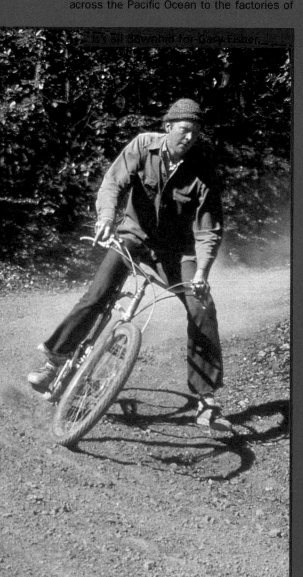

It's all downhill for Gary Fisher.

Week, which was established in 1981. During the 1980s, while the racing scene developed in the USA and Europe, this festival and the Canyonlands bike week in Moab, Utah, enabled hundreds of people to explore those beautiful areas just for the buzz.

Here to stay...

Mountain biking may be young, but it earned its own archive within a decade. In 1988, the Mountain Bike Hall of Fame and Museum was opened in a humble shack in Crested Butte to preserve the history of the sport and recognize its founding parents. Inside the non-profit museum, many retired bikes from the early days grace stands on wooden floors.

There are three Schwinns from 1937, 1949 and 1955, an original 1977 Breezer, a 1979 Lawwill-Knight Pro-Cruiser, a 1982 StumpJumper and the Fisher ridden to US national victory by Joe Murray in 1985. There's also plenty of memorabilia; hand-sewn rosettes, the Repack start sheet and classic photos. By 1995 there were 51 Hall of Fame inductees including bike builders, racers, organizers and trailmakers.

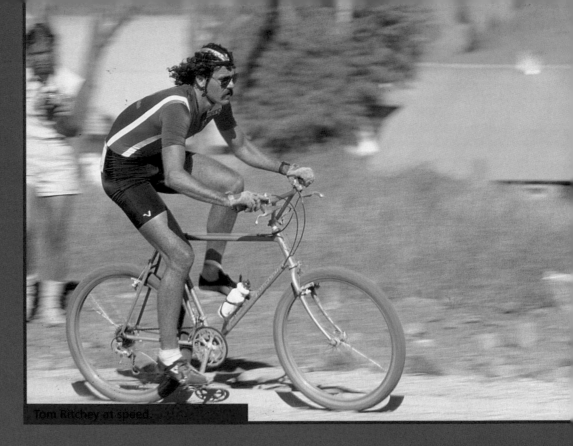

Tom Ritchey at speed.

Honorable members of the Hall of Fame

As well as all of the most-often-mentioned pioneers, the records in Crested Butte include racers Joe Murray and Jaquie Phelan (both inducted in 1988), Cindy Whitehead and Ned Overend (both 1990), and John Tomac (1991) and Sara Ballantyne (1992).

There is trailmapper Chuck Bodfish Elliot (1991), Andean MTB explorer Dr Al Farrell (1991) and a large group of entrepreneurial metalworkers including Chris "Fat" Chance (1990), Ross Shafer (1991), Gary Klein (1992), Gary "Merlin" Helfrich (1993), Keith Bontrager (1994), as well as Ignaz and Frank Schwinn (1994).

Honorable journalists include Zapata Espinoza, the editor (1986–93) of the largest American magazine devoted to the sport, *Mountain Bike Action*.

The curator of the Hall of Fame, Carole Bauer-Romanik, was entered in 1991, and Kay Peterson-Cook, the driving force behind the Crested Butte Fat Tire festival, was added in 1995, as were Steve Ready who has organized the InterBike trade show since 1982 and Junzo Kawai, who brought together Japanese component manufacturers and US backyard designers to create mountain biking equipment.

Although it is based in America, nominations to the Hall of Fame are accepted from bikers anywhere and include key figures in the fat tire world.

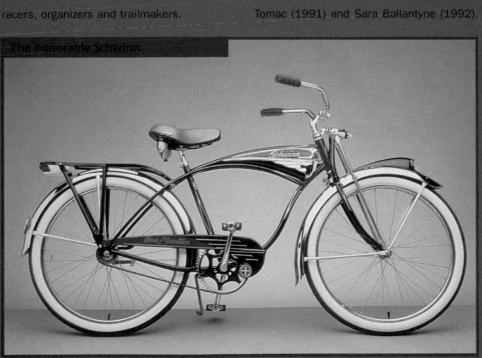

The honorable Schwinn.

British beginnings

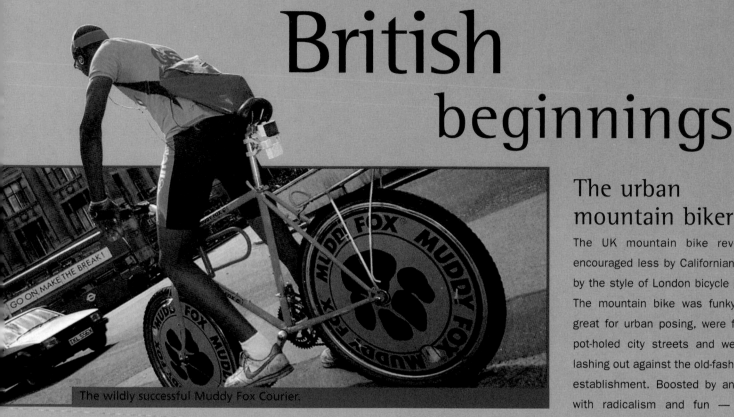

The wildly successful Muddy Fox Courier.

The urban mountain biker

The UK mountain bike revolution was encouraged less by Californian terrain than by the style of London bicycle messengers. The mountain bike was funky. They were great for urban posing, were functional on pot-holed city streets and were great for lashing out against the old-fashioned cycling establishment. Boosted by an association with radicalism and fun — windsurfers apparently turned to mountain biking when there was no breeze — the fashion press helped push the bikes into the limelight. They were aided by Muddy Fox's advertising expertise, which had British boxer Frank Bruno astride one model and showed Jaquie Phelan crouching beside a stream with pawprints up her bare back in another. Sales to bike messengers hit 300,000 annually, the total of today's annual sales of all quality MTBs in the UK — the MTB had taken over.

Until the early 1980s touring was the most popular form of recreational cycling in Britain, with a small group of serious, hardcore road racers. A small off-road movement called the Rough Stuff Fellowship was formed in 1955, but although they preferred single track to pavement, they rode, and still do ride on touring bikes. At the time, most bikes in Britain were made by traditional domestic manufacturers like Claud Butler, Dawes and Raleigh, with custom builders filling the high-end niche. The touring market was buoyant when the first MTBs hit Britain in 1983. The handful of costly Specialized StumpJumpers which made an appearance at the main trade show that year were quickly dismissed by the traditional cycling set as toys.

Fringe builders and the more adventuresome disagreed, and the first dirty dozen were snapped up by stores mainly in Edinburgh and London. The first hand-built British mountain bike also appeared. Geoff Apps' Cleland Range Rider, which sold 20 models, was short and high and had a sloping top tube with extra front end bracing. Then David Wrath-Sharman fitted an extra long head tube and long cross-braces (also for a very strong front end) on his hand-built bike, called the High Path.

From 1984 on, sales of imported mountain bikes increased so fast that suppliers were caught by surprise and new British producers were inspired. While Specialized, going gangbusters with the cheaper RockHopper, sold 600 bikes, Ridgeback put out their first models and Muddy Fox put the wildly popular Courier on the market. Soon, another British touring manufacturer, Saracen, jumped on the bandwagon and launched what would become another early classic British mountain bike, the Tufftrax.

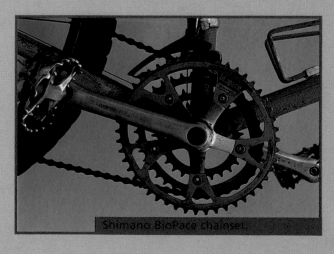

Shimano BioPace chainset.

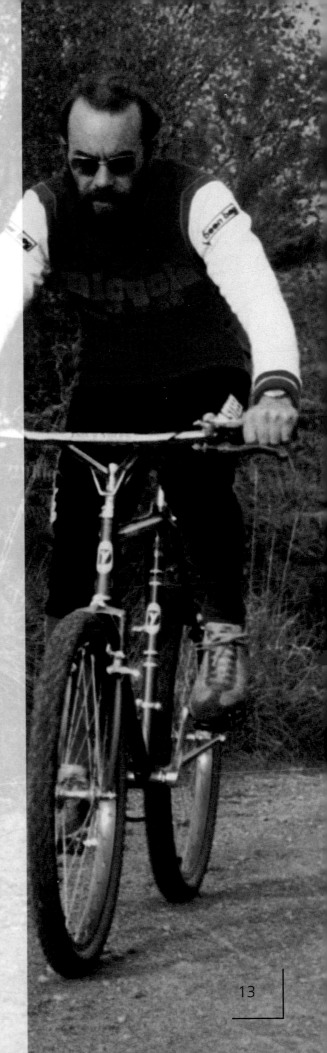

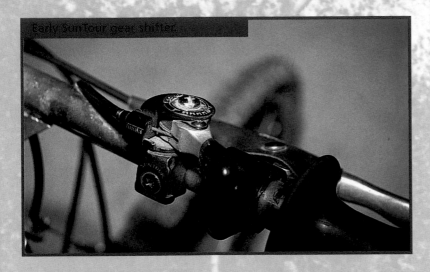

Early SunTour gear shifter.

early components

U-BRAKES

For a couple of years in the late 1980s, the rear brake was fitted underneath the chain stays behind the pedal spindle, not on the seat stays below the saddle. It was called a U-brake because of the long, arcing arms that replaced the cantilever wire triangle, and its design and position supposedly meant more powerful braking. MTB design was obsessed with strength and anything that made them different from road bikes. But the U-brake had a major disadvantage — it was too close to the ground. The calipers and the cable clogged and it was difficult to install. The chainring teeth often gouged knuckles in the process. U-brakes were discontinued in the early 1990s.

BIOPACE CHAINRINGS

The theory of BioPace, tradenamed by Shimano and later emulated by SunTour, said that elliptical chainrings got more power out of the pedalstroke than circular rings. The power of the downpushing leg is strongest at the start of the downstroke at 3 o'clock, so the ring should be flatter there, for increased leverage. At about 8 o'clock, the curve on the ring is sharper, to decrease the leverage and give the leg some help as it pulls back up. BioPace claimed to be efficient and knee-saving for beginners and climbing, and was plugged as a pure-breed mountain bike part. The problem was that riders felt like they were lurching with each rotation and BioPace gradually fell from grace. The road rider's preference for pedaling in smooth rotations came back in style and oval chainrings became uncommon. However, these Shimano chainrings are now tradenamed BioPace Pro.

HITE RITE

Patented by Joe Breeze and his partner Josh Angell this was a sprung clip that was attached to the seat post cluster and gripped the seat post. It allowed the rider to lower the saddle for descents, then reset it automatically at the right height. The gadget sold in the hundreds of thousands in the early days so that riders could get right over the back of the bike. In the end, though, riders got fed up with dismounting and they learned to bow their legs around the saddle to drop behind it for descents, without changing the saddle height. The Hite Rite is now almost never spotted on the trails.

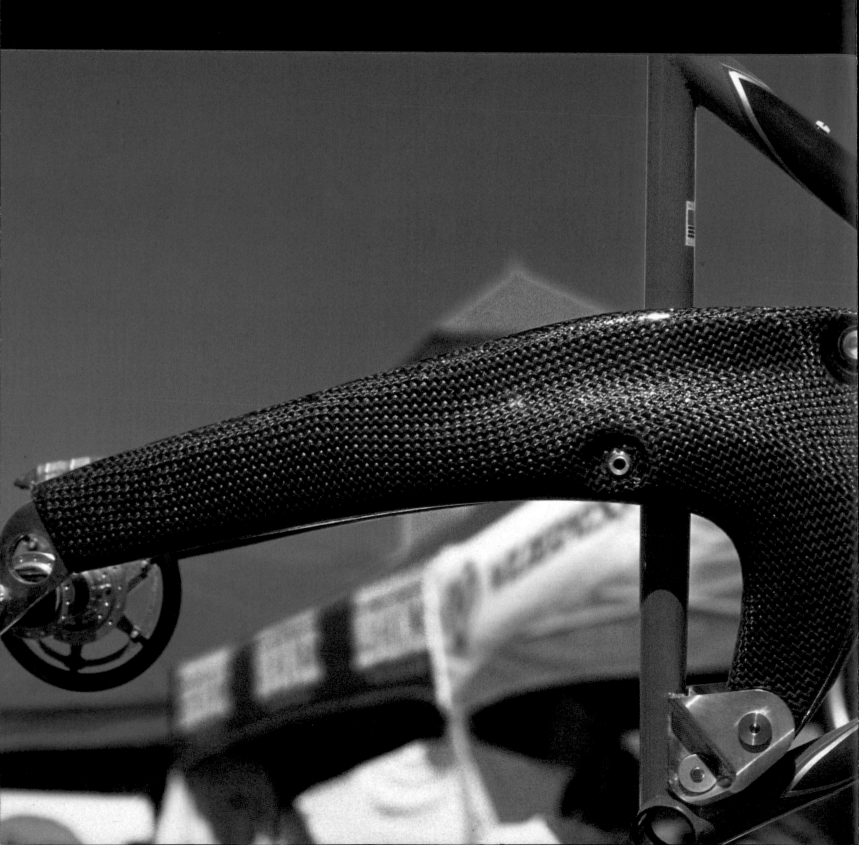

bikes an

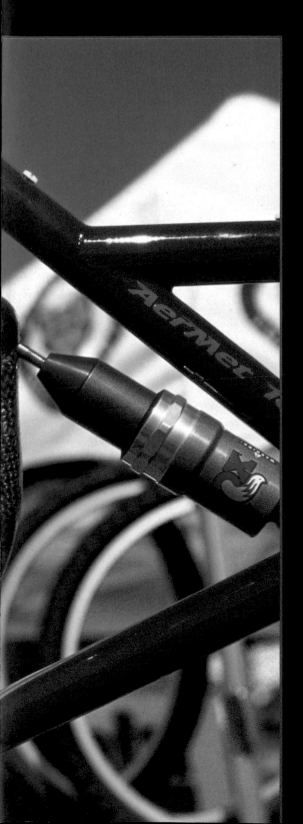

mountain bikers have introduced a new language to cycling — one that takes a little practice to understand. This chapter translates the technical jargon and teaches the principles of the equipment. It will help you to find the right bike, and the ultimate gear to go with it. Once fluent in mountain bike-speak, you should be able to read and assess reviews and pieces of equipment on your own. You should have the confidence to keep the bike and yourself going, and the ability to realize the right time to upgrade. You'll able to avoid the clothing mistakes that can ruin a winter ride, and, with luck, you'll even learn enough about mechanics to save yourself huge maintenance bills.

The idea that mountain bikes are slow in design is long dead. With frames built from high-tech metals such as titanium, aluminum, steel and carbon fiber, and with specialized shock absorbers, the top off-road models can match the speed of the fastest road-racing bikes. But, you don't need to be rich to ride off-road. At the other end of the price scale, even the simplest MTB, with a solid frame, over two dozen gears, powerful brakes and of course the fat tires, is ready for a day's trail action.

A lot of mountain bikers get hooked on the sport after having had a ride on a friend's MTB. They then go on to develop their own taste in equipment. Restricted by cost, most cyclists equip themselves with the basics — a decent bike, helmet, shorts and perhaps SPD pedals, upgrading or customizing when significant advances in materials, safety or mechanics roll off the production lines. After all, riding just once a week will get the bike dirty enough and cause enough breakdowns to keep you busy maintaining it, never mind keeping up with all the upgrades that appear on the market.

It's not necessary to use the latest equipment, but the rate of new production is so high that you could, if you really wanted to, upgrade your gear and the bike's components annually for style, and to take advantage of any small improvements in performance. Bikes and equipment are improving, although not at the speed that advertisers would like us to believe.

Eventually, though, the advances trickle down to even the most basic models and equipment. Watch out for advances in materials and technology that will form the mountain bike of the future. New applications are being obsessively explored as you read this, like the continued use of computer-aided metallurgy, the development of bigger, stronger, lighter suspension and the weaves and dyeing processes in sports textiles.

But without human energy to transform it into an adventure tool, the mountain bike is a lifeless hunk of metal leaning against a wall. It's a cliché, but however flashy the equipment, it's the thighs that count.

what makes a
mountain bike

While the visual differences between a mountain bike and a road bike are obvious, the structural differences are a matter of adaptation rather than radical invention. A mountain bike (MTB) is built to be stronger because its environment constantly subjects it to stresses that would destroy a road bike. Also proportionally smaller than a road bike, a mountain bike is more maneuverable on uneven ground. And there are those tires — chunky, knobby beasts with superb gripping ability — fitted onto smaller wheels with a 26in diameter. A mountain bike is easier to ride too — you can brake, change gear and steer simultaneously — without even taking a hand off the handlebars. You can get astride without being a gymnast and, once on board, you will find a mountain bike more comfortable and upright, so you can laugh at potholes and trafficjams as you sail past them on your way to school, work or the grocery store.

The Mountain Bike Frame

A cyclist's mountain bike is ideally about 3–4in (75–100mm) smaller than their equivalent road bike frame. For a full explanation and details about how to figure the correct frame size see pages 22–23.

FRONT END

The place on a mountain bike frame that takes the most stress is the area where the down tube and the top tube join the head tube. This is a region where a head-on impact can cause damage — either cracking in the welds or a fold showing on the underside of the down tube. Manufacturers reinforce the area with extra jointing material, or with a thicker internal wall or external width in the tube. Be sure to inspect and feel the tubes periodically to check for any damage.

DOWN TUBE

The down tube is the backbone of a bicycle. The longest tube on the frame, it carries more stress than the others and is strengthened accordingly — either by fattening and reinforcing in the case of aluminum, by butting (thickening the wall at stress points) in the case of steel, or by directional layering of the fibers in the case of carbon fiber.

TOP TUBE

Instantly recognizable in an off-road bike is the low and sloping top tube. Good MTBs have longer top tubes to ensure a crouched, aerodynamic position and to balance the bike between the front and back when climbing steep grades. The distance between the top tube and the ground is the standover height, and is the central measurement in sizing (see pp. 22–23).

SEAT CLUSTER

Early MTB frames were weak around the seat cluster because the seat post extends much further from the frame than on road bikes. The extra leverage in the post would cause it to fold, or for cracking to appear around seat cluster joints. These days frame builders reinforce this area with butting and over-sizing.

THE MAIN TRIANGLE AND REAR TRIANGLE

A bike's strength is concentrated in the main triangle. This means that on lower-

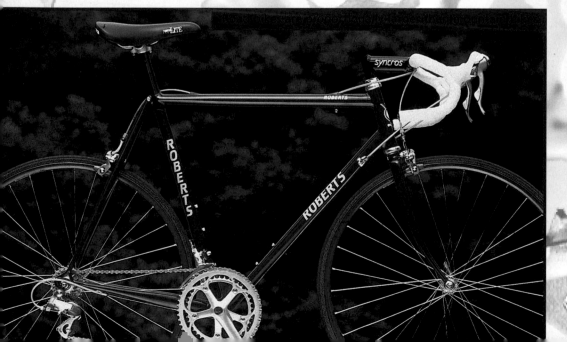

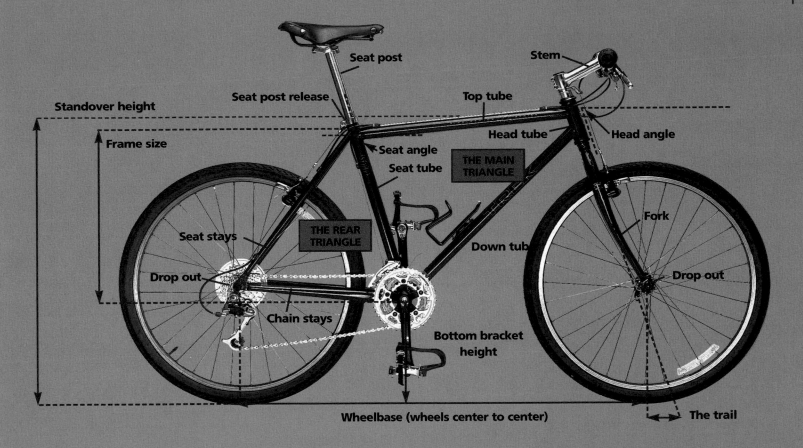

priced bikes the rear triangle may be made from lower-grade tubing than the main triangle. When choosing an MTB, try to get good quality tubing throughout. The rear triangle will be constructed from thinner tubing, because stress is shared between the chain stays and seat stays. This allows room for mud to build up on the tires without clogging.

THE FORK

As the first thing to bend in an impact, MTB forks, both of suspension and rigid design, are incredibly strong. If they break they contribute greatly to the absorption of a crash, but if they become damaged, or you wish to upgrade them, they are easily replaced.

SEAT POST

Easily interchangeable, the seat post should be kept lubricated for easy adjustment. It is measured in diameter to sit flush inside the seat tube.

DROPOUTS

The wheel sockets are part of the fork at the front and the frame at the rear. Safety dropouts are sometimes on the front to stop the wheel falling away if the release comes undone accidentally. On the rear wheel it's better to have a replaceable dropout — if it bends in a crash, the frame is still usable.

STEERING-HEAD ANGLE AND SEAT ANGLE

Both measured against the horizontal, the steering-head angle and the seat angle decide the handling feel of the frame because they influence the relative lengths of the tubes, the rider's angle over the pedals and the steering. The steeper they are, the stiffer and faster the handling. MTB angles for trail bikes are usually 70°–71.5° for steering-head angle and 72°–74° for seat angle. Steering-head angles on downhill bikes are much shallower — at 67.9°–70.5° — to accommodate the "travel"

of big-hit suspension forks. The steering is right when it rides easily with no hands, without flopping about, or holding too firmly in a straight-ahead position. This is governed by the trail (degree from vertical, see diagram) that's optimal at about 2.5–3in (60–80mm).

WHEELBASE

The distance between the centers of the wheels. This increases with the size of the bike, from around 40–43in (102–110cm). Suspension bikes are longer — to allow for movement — and are up to 46in (116cm).

CHAIN STAY LENGTH

The lower stay's average length is 16–17in (40–43cm). Short stays on hardtails make for quicker climbing and bouncier descending.

BOTTOM BRACKET HEIGHT

This is typically 1in (25mm) higher than on a road bike for obstacle clearance.

mountain bike
components

GROUPSET

A complete set of components from one manufacturer, the groupset consists of the brakes, hubs, headset, gearing and levers. Each piece is of a similar grade, compatible with the other pieces, and adapted according to the bike type. Most new bikes, regardless of manufacturer, come ready-specified with one groupset or another. It is an area dominated by Shimano, which has a dozen or so smooth and efficient groupsets for all budgets and types of bike. There are, how-

ever, numerous small parts manufacturers who compete successfully with the market rulers with short lists of high quality pieces.

BRAKES

Brakes, a vital control on any bike, are even more important on mountain bikes because of the more intense nature of off-roading and high downhill speeds. Straight-arm, top-pull rim brakes called V-brakes and hydraulic disc brakes have become standard, stemming from side-pull cantilever rim brakes on road

bikes. A V-brake, unlike side-pull brakes, can straddle the width of MTB tires, providing the stronger braking force necessary for powerful deceleration. In the early days of mountain bikes rear brakes were commonly caliper-type "U-brakes" fixed to the underside of the chain stays. These proved trickier to maintain and, being closer to the dirt, often clogged up and stopped working well.

Rivaling V-brakes are hydraulic disc brakes, in which a fluid-filled cable pushes pads to clamp onto a separate disc at the

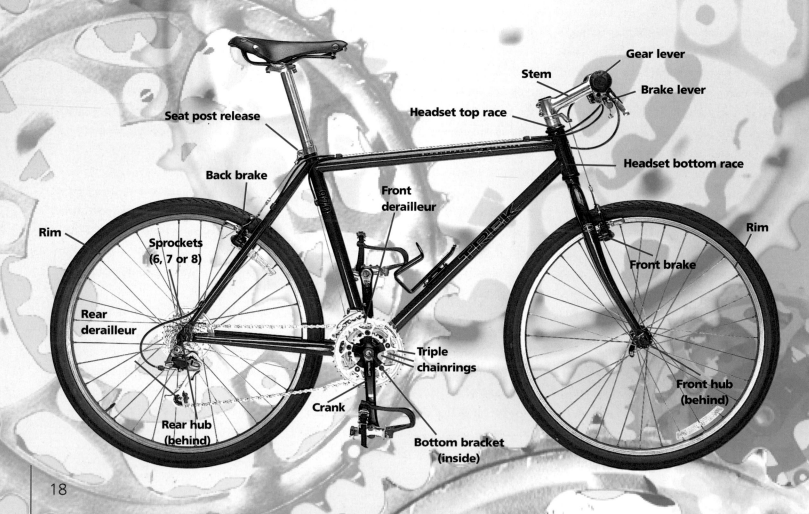

Gear lever

Stem

Brake lever

Headset top race

Seat post release

Headset bottom race

Back brake

Front derailleur

Rim

Rim

Sprockets (6, 7 or 8)

Front brake

Rear derailleur

Triple chainrings

Front hub (behind)

Crank

Rear hub (behind)

Bottom bracket (inside)

Suspension Fork

Adjusting knob

Fork crown

Fork brace

Fork leg

Rocker Arms

Dropout

hub. Adapted from motorbikes, these are exceptionally powerful, more resilient in wet and don't deform the wheel under pressure. They've become universal on downhill bikes, and slimmer versions often appear on high-quality suspension or hardtail cross-country bikes. Another type is the hub brake, where the braking surfaces are sealed inside the hub housing, keeping the mud out.

GEARS

Mountain bikes have 21, 24 or 27 gears, combining three chainrings on the front, and either seven, eight or nine sprockets at the back. They are needed to provide diverse pedaling speeds for variety in terrain. MTB gears also have easier gears than a road bike for slow or steep ground. The gears consist of front and rear derailleurs, which are the arms that move the chain across the rings and sprockets, and which are controlled by gear levers on the handlebars. These are either thumb & finger levers, or gripshifts, where you twist the entire grip (see pp. 68–69).

WHEELS

After the frame, the most important parts are the wheels, which need surprisingly little maintenance thanks to good hubs, rims, spokes and tires. Road wheels are 27in in diameter, mountain bike wheels are 26in — and have fatter tires for off-road handling.

Hubs are relatively simple items; they contain an axle and bearings and should

SUSPENSION

Suspension is extremely helpful off-road, but unnecessary on the road because of asphalt. Shock absorbers allow the wheels to move independently from the rest of the bike and the rider, taking up the bumps for better control and comfort. Much talk concerns the pros and cons of different shock absorption designs, although they all operate in the same basic way. Proper shock absorption, whatever combination of springs, bumpers and hydraulics, swallows the bump in two steps. First, the spring gives way to allow the independent movement; second, the damper soaks up the spring energy and allows a clean return.

never be allowed to come loose. Wheel rims should be a strong, lightweight alloy with good braking surface. The laws of physics behind an efficient wheel mean the tension in the spokes should be evenly maintained, keeping the wheel straight and strong as it rolls over the terrain. Efficiency also comes from keeping the rotating mass, ie. the edge of the wheel — the rim and tire — as light as possible. This is the part that moves most, where weight is hardest for the rider to overcome. Tire width and pattern should minimize rolling resistance and maximize grip.

The best wheels come from specialist wheel-builders, but the factory-assembled wheels found on most bikes sold in stores roll and last well. Some mechanically minded

cyclists even build their own wheels. Maintaining a wheel is mostly about truing it by tightening and loosening the spokes with a spoke wrench. This takes out the minor kinks in the rim and equalizes the tension all the way around the wheel (see pp. 58–59).

STEERING

The head tube contains a stacked pair of steering bearings, called the headset. This is fairly standard across all types of bike, with the threadless version most popular in mountain biking, which stays done up under trail stress and is easier to tighten.

PEDALS AND BOTTOM BRACKET

The pedals turn on axles, which screw into the cranks and turn in the frame on the bottom bracket or pedal spindle. This unit contains a double set of bearings, one on each side of the frame's bottom bracket shell. Developments include lighter axles and sealed "cassettes" of bearings, so you don't have to strip and clean them so regularly.

frame
materials

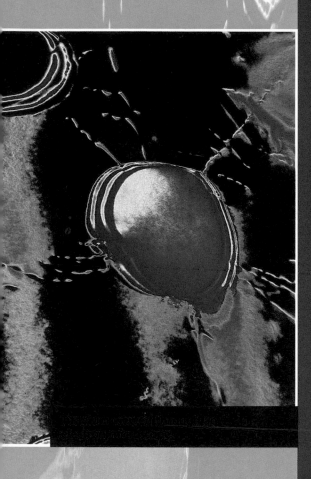

Aluminum has become the most popular frame material for high quality mountain bikes, replacing steel. Carbon fiber has also gained mainstream ground, while titanium, a favorite of the early MTB years, has faded to the fringes of the bicycle world.

ALUMINUM

Aluminum first won a following in the 1980s, with bike manufacturers attracted by its qualities of low weight, good shock absorption and corrosion resistance. Unfortunately, aluminum had poor fatigue resistance, and that made riders cautious. There was also an assumption that an aluminum bike would break much quicker than a steel one — and could not be repaired at the local bike shop either.

The development of specialty welding techniques in the far east, and the hunt for materials to create stronger, longer-lasting alloys — led largely by bike makers such as Giant, Trek and Cannondale — have turned this soft, light metal into the next big thing in frames. Aluminum alloy bikes appear in big-name catalogues by the thousand, almost exclusively dominating the high end range, and often appearing in the frames of cheaper, easy-pedaling bikes.

Aluminum's tensile strength (the point at which it breaks) and yield strength (the point at which it permanently deforms) are both lower than steel. In an alloy, it's mixed with other metals, then heat-treated for strength. A six-figure code, such as 6061-T1, describes the metallurgical processes and indicates which grade of aluminum has been used. The first figure refers to the chief alloy, the following three numbers refer to the added alloys in diminishing proportion, and the letter and number after the hyphen define the heat process. 2XXX has copper as the main strengthening element. 3XXX uses manganese, 4XXX silicon, 5XXX magnesium, 6XXX a mixture of magnesium and silicon and 7XXX zinc. Zirconium is an element used for a high quality alloy. Only the 2, 6 and 7 series alloys can be heat treated. T6 is the most common form of heat treatment, where tubing is given

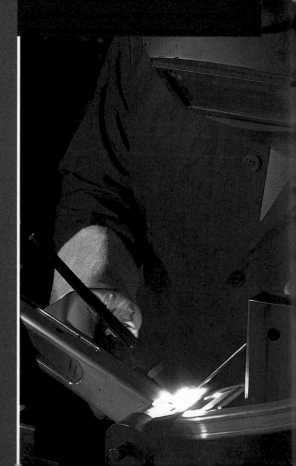

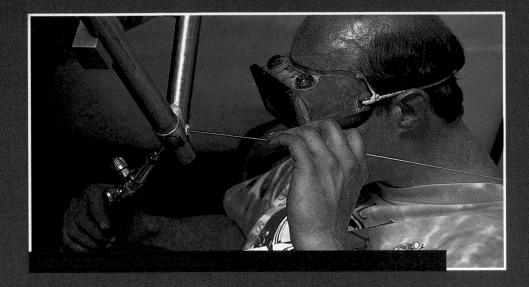

This is accomplished by placing together layers of resin-impregnated carbon fiber, according to the position of the stress points, and curing it to create a rigid, light structure with top fatigue resistance.

Trek has created its own carbon fiber material, called Optimal Compaction Low Void (OCLV), for its best bikes. The material is compressed and the air pockets removed, for low weight and rigidity.

TITANIUM

Briefly the favorite of the performance biker, titanium's high working costs have seen it fall from the most desirable to the least worked-with frame material. A naturally good-looking metal, titanium makes for a light, sharp and at the same time forgiving ride. American bike-builders Merlin and Litespeed remain devoted to the use of titanium, catering to those customers who love swishy bikes.

Titanium is commonly mixed with aluminum to make it more easily welded, and vanadium for tensile strength (eg, titanium coded 3Al/2.5V). It doesn't need painting and is extremely light, two attributes which were discovered in its use in the aerospace and marine industries.

solution heat treatment and artificial aging.

Another way of boosting aluminum's weakness is to make the tubing fatter — the principle being that when you double the tube's diameter, you quadruple its rigidity. The thickness of the tube walls is slimmed down to a couple of millimeters, which keeps the volume of material in line with weight targets.

STEEL

Steel, for a hundred years the leading bike metal, lost its hold in the 1990s. After dominating in both mass-produced and custom-built bike markets, its grip on the industry has been eroded by new manufacturing techniques and materials technology, with factories switching to aluminum. Steel bikes are much heavier but still easy to find. Big manufacturers offer several models (mostly for those riders who've never ridden anything else), but the days when steel ruled are gone forever.

Steel has good yield and tensile strength, for rigidity and durability. It is easy and cheap to work and, when heat-treated, can be used in low enough quantities to match the lighter weight of aluminum.

Lower-quality high-tensile steel tubing is found on cheaper bikes, while the top steel alloy is cromoly. Steel's practical advantage is that broken or dented frames can, unlike other materials, be repaired easily and cheaply.

The main threat to the life of a steel bike is rust. Steel bikes need to be kept well-painted and dry. Water should never be left to sit inside a frame, especially around the bottom bracket, where it can eat away at the structure.

CARBON FIBER

For a while in the 1990s, carbon fiber was the hottest new material. It was a cheap material and there was a lot of experimentation with strengthening and bonding it into a bicycle.

Derived from crude oil, the benefits of carbon fiber include stiffness, low weight and strength. But its number one advantage is that, to create rigidity in the tubes, fibers are layered directionally.

A tube with helical (spiral) fibers will resist bending better than one with lengthways-laid fibers. No extra material is required, which saves extra weight, and fibers can be reduced in areas of the bike where there is less stress.

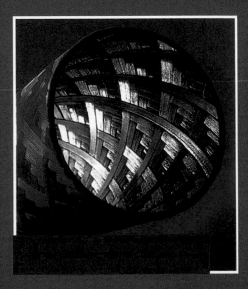

fitting
a mountain bike

Sizing up

Getting the right size bike is easy if you follow a few simple rules.

SIZE

With the exception of a few manufacturers, who use the terms "small, medium and large", bike size is given in inches and is based on leg length. The size of the bike is the distance from the centre of the bottom bracket to the intersection of the seat tube and the top tube, assuming that the top tube is horizontal.

The second most critical dimension is reach. This is the distance from the seat to the handlebars. Manufacturers' sizes vary slightly, but not enough to matter, so this central measurement (bottom bracket to top tube), like shoe sizes, is a reliable estimate of fit that suits the majority of riders. Most suit adults between 4ft 10in (1.47m) and 6ft 4in (1.93m).

SIZING BY EYE

When you stand astride a mountain bike there should be a gap between your crotch and the top tube, of about 2½–5in (7–13cm). Bear in mind that this is more than is necessary on a road bike, where the gap only needs to be minimal.

A larger amount of clearance is needed off-road because MTB frames are smaller for better maneuverability and stability. Rocks and rough terrain throw the rider around too — and the last place you want to

MOUNTAIN BIKE SIZING CHART	
A quick reference guide to MTB frame size	
HEIGHT	**FRAME SIZE**
4ft 10in–5ft	12–15in
(1.47–1.52m)	(33–38cm)
5ft 2in–5ft 4in	14–17in
(1.57–1.62m)	(38–43cm)
5ft 6in–5ft 8in	16–19in
(1.69–1.72m)	(41–48cm)
5ft 10in–6ft	18–21in
(1.77–1.83m)	(46–51cm)
6ft 2in–6ft 4in	20–22in
(1.88–1.93m)	(51–56cm)

unintentionally straddle is an overly intimate top tube. If you know what size suits you in road bikes, calculate your mountain bike size by subtracting four inches from it. As well as the bigger crotch safety net, this takes in the extra 1–2in (2.5–5cm) height a mountain bike bottom bracket is above the ground.

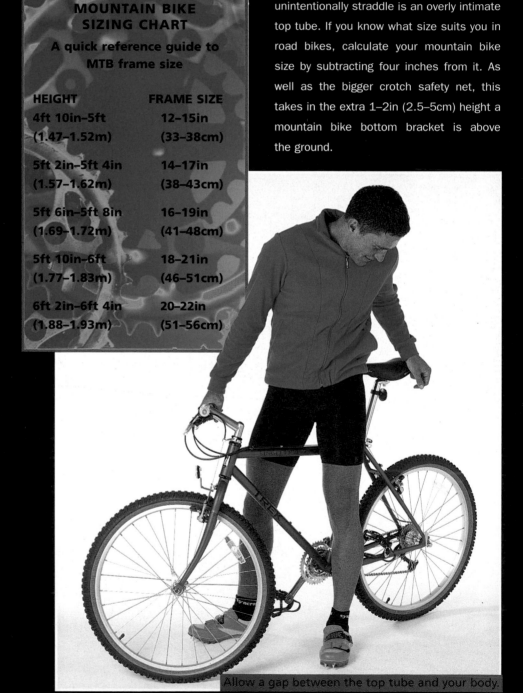

Allow a gap between the top tube and your body.

REACH ▶

One dimension that varies between brands and models is the reach from the saddle to the handlebars. This is determined by the size of the bike and its intended purpose. Cross-country racers prefer a longer, lower and more aerodynamic position, with the handlebars a bit lower than the saddle. Downhillers like a shorter reach with a lowered saddle, which puts them in a position sitting with bent legs (as though in a chair) which is effective for jumping and quick acceleration. For them, aerodynamics are not as important as strength and suspension. Beginners like being more upright than XC racers, for reassurance, so cheaper bikes are also shorter, with handlebars level or slightly higher than the saddle.

Reach is a combination of top tube length, stem, saddle position and the head angle. If you feel overstretched or cramped up, the stem can be changed for a longer or shorter/steeper or shallower model, and the saddle moved backwards or forwards on the rails to fit. Overreaching is a classic

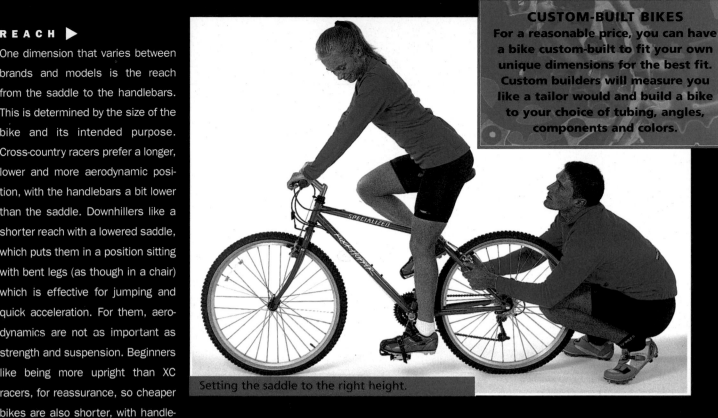

CUSTOM-BUILT BIKES
For a reasonable price, you can have a bike custom-built to fit your own unique dimensions for the best fit. Custom builders will measure you like a tailor would and build a bike to your choice of tubing, angles, components and colors.

Setting the saddle to the right height.

cause of saddle soreness, while other symptoms of misfit in the reach department are bum, shoulder, back and wrist ache. Getting it right can be a little tricky, although the body is good at adapting to different positions.

Getting the saddle position right

SADDLE HEIGHT

For easy pedaling and healthy knees, the saddle height must be right. Your leg should straighten naturally with every stroke, without being stretched (except stunt riders or downhillers who want a low saddle for jump-ready legs).

■ To set the saddle height by eye, get someone to hold the bike for you while you sit on it and pedal, with the ball of your foot over the pedal axle. Hop on and off to adjust the height — do not rush it — until your

foot is horizontal at the bottom of the pedal stroke.

■ Take the saddle adjusting tool on your first few rides, until the height is right — then you can forget about it.

■ If you are new to cycling you may want to keep the saddle low enough to put your feet down on the ground without dismounting when you stop. This is fine for short rides, but you should raise it to the proper straight-leg height once you have gained some balance and confidence.

SADDLE ANGLE AND FORWARD SETTING

For cross-country, the saddle angle should be horizontal, or tilted slightly downward for comfort. Downhillers and jumpers tilt the saddle upward, sometimes steeply. Alter your reach by moving the saddle forwards or backwards along the rails located under the saddle (be cautious, though, as this slightly changes your position over the pedals).

SHE'LL GROW INTO IT!
It's fine to buy a young child a bike at the bigger end of his or her limits but be careful that it isn't uncomfortable to ride. Wheel diameters gradually increase up to the full-sized 26in wheels, to fit people from around 4ft 10in (1.47m). Below that, 24in wheeled bikes with proper off-road componentry are available from Cannondale, Scott and GT, but their expense means you may be happier waiting until the child is big enough for a full-size bike.

the starter bike

The rigid bike, or hardtail

This, the most basic of all the mountain bikes, is the one that is most similar to the traditional road bike. Its simple diamond frame has beefy tubes, enough clearance to allow for fat, muddy tires, plenty of gears and, most importantly, powerful brakes for real off-roading. All the early mountain bikes were this type, and there are still a few traditionalists who will put up with the rougher ride of a rigid (non-suspension) bike for the sake of getting a true feel for the trail.

While some starter bikes are totally rigid without any shock absorption front or rear, the majority now have a simple suspension fork on the front, and are called "hardtails". This is one of the best recent developments in mountain biking: suspension forks used to be a feature found only on the most expensive bikes, but they're now found on bikes for beginners and occasional gentle trail riders.

WHAT WILL I PAY?

The starting price of a real mountain bike is in the region of $350. For this, you get a strong frame, powerful brakes, full gearing and a good warranty. If you're buying the bike from a store, as opposed to by mail order, it will be ready to ride right away (and the store will usually tune it up for you after the first month of riding).

That may seem like a lot of money for a bike, even though it's at the bottom of a ladder of prices that rockets into four figures, but if you pay less you'll be buying an inferior bike.

Imitation mountain bikes may have knobby tires and flat handlebars, but they're not a bargain. They handle badly on trails, weigh a lot and creak and groan when the going gets rough. Most importantly, they aren't safe. The braking of bikes below this price isn't powerful enough to make the bike secure for riding off road. Learning to mountain bike is tricky enough already. Don't limit yourself by starting with inferior equipment.

If you spend above our recommended minimum for a lower-end genuine mountain bike, the models offered are usually good deals. Most of the bikes at this price, regardless of brand, are standard. You get minimal (but decent) components; the price rises as you learn more about bikes and what you want from yours and begin to demand more individual features.

A few hundred dollars guarantees an inspiring, solid bike that'll open a whole new world to you.

Sampling the Trek 4300

Typical of the quality that genuine starter bikes can provide, the Trek 4300 has several features that have trickled down from more expensive bikes. This simple Trekkie is a classic mountain bike and a very good deal.

You get the frame, the tires, the styling of a mountain bike that could have cost a lot more, and a respectable overall weight.

The bike is fitted with 24 gears (three chainrings at the front multiplied by eight sprockets at the back), powerful industry-standard V-brakes and an impressive suspension fork that actually works despite the low price tag. Everything you could need to get started.

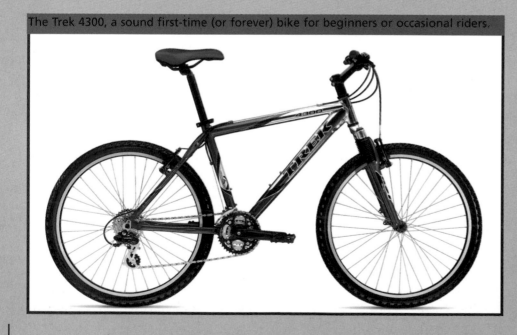
The Trek 4300, a sound first-time (or forever) bike for beginners or occasional riders.

WHO IS IT FOR?

The Trek 4300 is a great bike for anyone who wants to test the water on trails, or who occasionally explores simple, easy-to-ride routes. It's also great as an all-purpose transport machine, for commuting to work and college.

This bike is made to last. Suited to cruising on asphalt as well as technically straightforward paths like forestry fire-roads and rail trails, you'll find it fun, responsive — and safe.

4300 FRAME AND COMPONENTRY

The core of any bike is its frame, and the 4300 has a good tubeset of regular aluminum alloy called Alpha. The alloy is bike-grade low-density lightweight aluminum, formed into oversized tubes, which increases their strength to that of steel and carbon fiber. The tubes are thickened near the joints (the stress points) at the front end and the bottom of the bike. The middle sections are left as thin walled as possible, to save weight. These metalworking adjustments create a frame that is strong enough to carry a rider over bumps and through grinds, and light enough to leave them fighting the trail, not the bike.

The 4300 has two features that evolved on expensive bikes: the suspension fork and the disc brakes. Both of these are signature mountain bike items, guaranteed to impress everyone. The fork gives over 2in (5cm) of travel, for comfort and better control. The disc brakes (which are optional) are standard in millennium-style bikes. Rather than gripping the rim, they grip motorcycle-style rings near the hub of the wheel. Their main advantage is that they work better in bad weather, because they're

further above the track and don't get clogged with dirt.

You get 24 gears (three at the front and eight at the back), which is plenty, as they overlap considerably (27 is the maximum). The Bontrager tires bite well and suit pavement as well as dirt. One reason this bike is so reasonably priced is because it has ordinary pedals, so more experienced riders may want to upgrade to SPD clip-in pedals, for efficiency and security on slopes. Otherwise, the 4300 has a deceptively low price.

WHO ARE TREK?

The Trek Bicycle Corporation is a major player in mountain biking, in terms of numbers of bikes and, most recently, celebrity. Originally a mountain bike-only company, Trek worked hard for acceptance in the road racing scene over the last few years, and this paid off when Lance Armstrong successfully defended the Tour de France title in 2001 on the Trek 5900 Team Superlight bike, becoming an all-American hero on American gear. The Superlight bike is made of Trek's own patent OCLV material (Optimum Compaction Low Void), a sophisticated carbon fiber found in no one else's bikes.

The company is a long-standing pioneer of bike materials technology. Trek was in on the MTB scene at the start as one of the first builders to use aluminum. They rode out the wilderness years as the possibilities of steel were explored and exhausted, to the point where, in 2002, of the 58-strong range of Trek bikes, including MTBs, road bikes and hybrids, only two were made of steel (both hybrids).

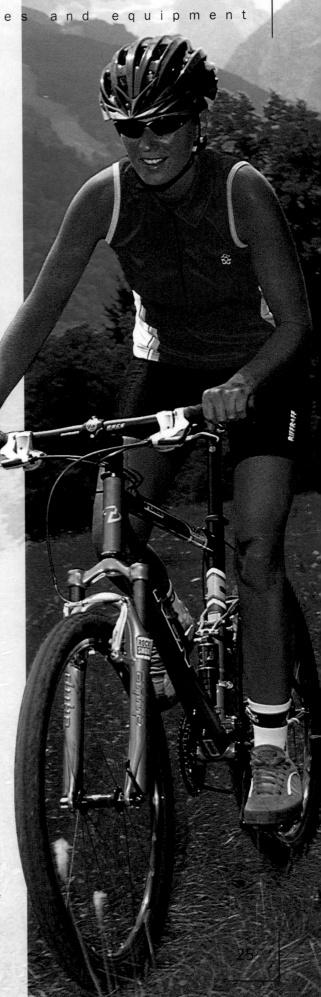

full suspension
bikes

For cross-country racing and trail-jumping junkies

Suspension means speed, and more weight on the bike. Originally, this was taboo for cross-country racers and mountain-biking junkies. Early bikes with big springs went downhill only, because climbing was considered essential to the rest of the sport. To gain universal appeal the developers had to come up with a compromise between shock and weight. Tweaks to downhill shock units and developments in how to make the back wheel move have led to the evolution of fully-suspended lighter weight bikes, where the shock can even be locked off completely for climbing. The new breed of elite cross-country and 24-hour racers have learned the hard-butt way that suspension means less ache and better results, and, now that the bikes have lightened up, have welcomed full suspension with open arms.

Full-suspension trailbikes subdivide into (a) lightweight race models with less suspension like the Foes FXC cross-country bike, and (b) "freerides" or "playbikes" like the Rocky Mountain Pipeline, which has more suspension for dirt monkeys who like to pull stunts as well as cruise up and down trails all day.

One note of warning. Cheap "lookalike" full-suspension bikes don't work and don't last, so don't pay less than $1500 for one. The shock units need to be finely engineered, and the rear wheel cleanly and cleverly bolted to prevent side-to-side play which puts stresses on the equipment. It may only be a bike, but these refinements make the most of your legs.

Sampling the Foes FXC

Take a close look at the Foes FXC and see how fast a full-suspension bike can be when built for speed, and not comfort.

The bike may resemble its downhill cousins, but its main aim is flex-free uphill shifting and climbing for racing and trail mileage. This is tackled through a simple, single-pivot, stiffened-aluminum swingarm that holds the rear wheel. This is supported by a Fox shock that can be totally locked off if desired, turning the bike into a regular hardtail for climbing. Despite the extra metal and features, the frame on its own weighs only 4.4lb (2kg), around 2.2lb (1kg) more than the extreme-lightest cross-country bikes. It's a weight worth paying for in the extra speed given by the free-flowing nature of the suspension — especially in the hands of a cross-country rider who's got downhilling nailed too.

The aim of the FXC is low cross-country weight, which is achieved through the top quality aluminum frame and super reinforced boxwork (monocoque) that holds the saddle in place above the shock unit.

The Fox shock is adjustable: set it harder or softer, and to rider weight, or, as mentioned, turn it off completely.

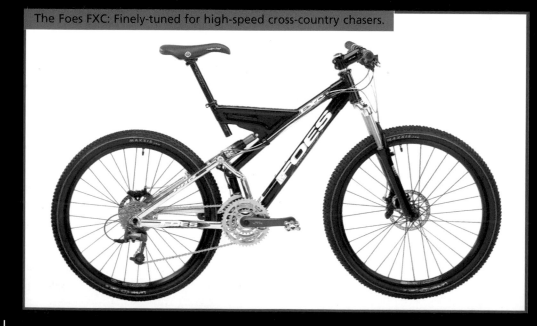
The Foes FXC: Finely-tuned for high-speed cross-country chasers.

The complexity of this racer over a hardtail is held in check by the bike's slimline, minimalistic design, which retains the elegance of a cross-country bike.

Foes sells the bike either as a frame alone, which allows you to fit whatever lightweight, cool componentry you like, or will build up a bike for you, with equipment like a Rockshox suspension fork or something similar (Foes' own forks are too long-travel, from about 4.5in (100mm) travel, for DH and freeriding), as well as powerful wetweather disc brakes, full cross-country 9-speed gearing and SPDs.

WHO ARE FOES?

Based in low-key warehouses in the San Gabriel Mountains bordering Los Angeles, motoring engineer Brent Foes and his crew build aluminum frames by hand. He works alongside Herr Curnutt, a shock specialist with a background in dirt car racing, to bring out new developments every year. Renowned for their downhill bikes, ridden to fame by Missy "the Missile" Giove, Foes has a thrash image, although their cross-country bikes ride with finesse, too.

Sampling the Rocky Mountain Pipeline

Downhill bikes jump and carve, and weigh a ton. Cross-country full-suspension bikes are designed for hard graft on the trails and race results.

What freerides and playbikes do is somewhere in between, appealing to the street kid who first skinned his knees on a BMX as well as a regular trail rider. They are full of the fun of the latest suspension, kick butt on a climb, and win huge points with riders. Freerides are mountain bikes without tears.

The stresses doled out by the jump park, or on the technical trails, are not big enough that the bike needs to be a lumbering fortress of coils, motorcycle-style tires and trampoline-like suspension. The freerider can run all day on the trail, pushing the bike to the limits of its suspension, without pretending he or she wants to subject themselves to an Olympic training schedule.

Freeride bikes like the Rocky Mountain Pipeline sag sweetly when you sit on them, like an old, favorite (but finely-tuned) arm-

chair. The bike is designed around technical riding, its central feature being an NE3 rear shock which boasts the unique quality of being adjustable to 4, 5 or 6in (100, 125 or 150mm) of travel which allows for anything between full-on trail work and burning up the berms. The geometry of the bike, too, can be adjusted using a knob in preparation for the downhill, uphill or ramp ahead.

The Pipeline frame is sleek, with shades of the traditional diamond frame road bike peeking through. The high quality Easton aluminum tubing is boxed up at the head tube, to resist the landings and front-end smacks that the bike begs for.

A nifty elevated motocross mudguard on the front wheel emphasizes the give at the front end that you get from the high grade Marzocchi 5in (125mm) travel Dirt Jumper forks.

Its brakes are the essential disc models, supplied by number one component manufacturer Shimano, and operated in this case by fluid-filled (hydraulic) cables. These are more powerful than rim brakes, and don't clog up in bad conditions because they're positioned higher above any dirt, sand or mud that you may encounter.

WHO ARE ROCKY MOUNTAIN?

Established in 1981, Rocky Mountain is one of the longest-running mountain bike builders. They produce a small range of high-end, mostly full-suspension aluminum bikes.

Most bikes are now built in Taiwan, but Rocky Mountains have always been put together, as you might expect, in the Rocky Mountains, British Columbia, Canada, and still are. It's a region renowned for serious trailriding, hence Rocky Mountain's loyalty to the mountain bike, and only the mountain bike.

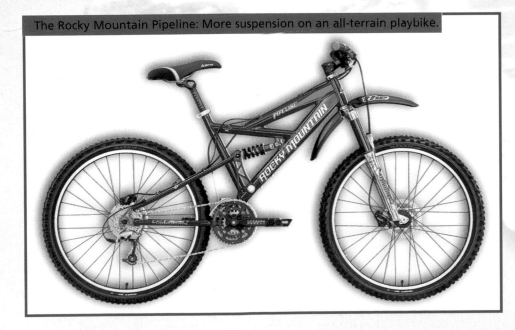

The Rocky Mountain Pipeline: More suspension on an all-terrain playbike.

downhill bikes

Beautiful they ain't, unless you're the type who thinks elephants and rhinos are cute. But the most progress in mountain bikes is being made in downhill models, which continue to mess with unfeasible degrees of suspension travel and to treat nothing behind the handlebars as sacred.

Downhilling is a niche sport within mountain biking, practiced by a small minority of obsessive maniacs for whom a dedicated bike is critical. Preferably a mountain bike which is almost useless for any other cycling activity.

It's not that you can't pedal down to the 7-11 for munchies on a Santa Cruz V10 (10in/250mm rear suspension), a Foes Mono (8.5in/210mm), an Orange 222 (8in/200mm) or a Rocky Mountain DH9 (9in/220mm), it's more that you just wouldn't use a jackhammer to crack open a nut.

In downhilling, stable means better. The longer the suspension travel the bigger and steeper the bouldery slopes you can conquer — preferably faster, and more importantly, still in one piece. Released from the constraints of having to produce lightweight bikes that you can pedal uphill, designers are adding more metal to the rear to allow the wheel more movement and to maximize suspension travel. Bikes are also built to be

bombproof — the forces exerted on them are much higher than on regular trail bikes — so the designers have the rider's blessing to pile on more weight.

For full maneuverability, riders use an upright sitting position with a low saddle and knees bent. Big downhillers often appear to tower over their machines, which are built compact so that when they stand to sprint, jump or corner, the bike is tucked hard beneath them. The head angle of the bike is shallower than on hardtail or trail bikes to take account of the extra length of the shock forks, which boast up to 7in (170mm) of travel, and the way they sag, which steepens the angle back up again. That's what gives downhill bikes their laidback look.

With staggering price tags, from $2000 to $6400, downhill bikes can be the millionaires' toys of mountain biking, but plenty of diehards save up to buy bikes like these. The bikes are often the product of small-scale backyard builders (because they're hard to put into mass factory line production) so the manufacturing process stays close to the rider.

Sampling The Santa Cruz V10

The fact that the Santa Cruz V10 weighs double a good XC bike (43lbs/19kg) is irrelevant. The fact that the Santa Cruz V10 takes you 10in (250mm) into the rear suspension void, to ride bigger obstacles than ever before — now that's the key.

The focal point of the V10 is its monster rear end: a mash of pivots and swingarms designed to let the rear wheel sop up big smacks without throwing the rider off course or splintering into pieces. It's said that 2lbs (1kg) of the weight is saved strictly by having a titanium (not steel) spring on the shock.

One of the weaknesses of downhill bikes is that they swing around during pedaling. Downhillers have to be very strong and fast, with the type of leg-power that accelerates them out of corners at top speed. The trouble is that the bikes are so soft that a good push on the pedals is sometimes enough to activate the suspension and thus waste energy (called "pedal feedback").

The V10 tries to stop that in two ways. The framework that holds the rear wheel is designed as a "virtual pivot point". The wheel doesn't move in a simple arc around the bottom bracket, but is allowed to move forward and backward too, in a slight S shape. When you sit on the bike, the 3–4in (75–100mm) of sag and the tension in the chain places the rear wheel in the middle of the bottom curve. It takes the sharper, harder bumps on the trail to activate the suspension up and down the S shape. That leaves the softer, steady pedaling force strictly going in a forward motion.

The suspension of the V10 is adjustable. In downhill, a bump is no simple thing. It starts, it builds, it climaxes, and then the shock needs to return in time to tackle the next obstacle. So the V10 uses a shock unit called the Fifth Element, which has five separate areas of adjustment; first response (getting the suspension going in the first place), rate of initial stroke compression (the early response/softer hits); high speed compression (the later response/harder hits); the linear/progressive adjustment; and rebound damping (how quickly the shock returns). The idea is to tweak the first response and initial stroke adjustments so that pedaling, which is a relatively low-key movement, doesn't move the suspension.

The V10's other features are customizable to the rider, but you could include Boxxer 7in (170mm) forks, flat-studded Shimano DH platform pedals and hydraulic disc brakes.

The bike is highly specialized. It takes skill and nerve to use this beast like you're supposed to. But wouldn't we all like to try...

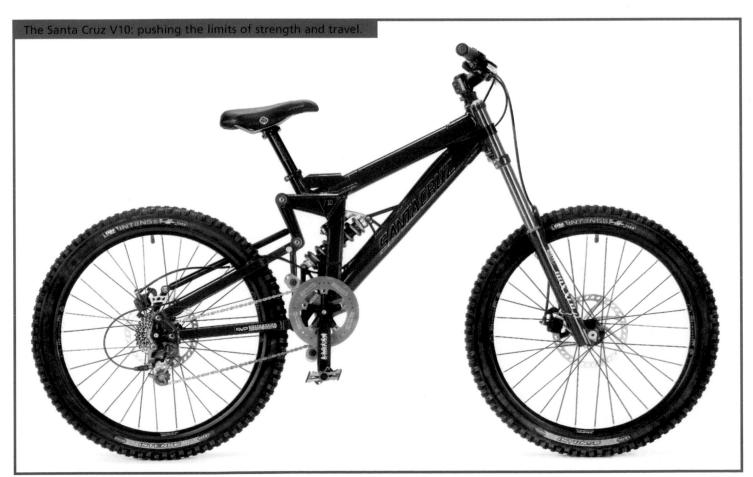

The Santa Cruz V10: pushing the limits of strength and travel.

what to wear

Obsessive cyclists end up with more cycling clothes than day-to-day clothes as they try to find the perfect combination for every condition and trend. It's not hard to see the attraction — cycling clothing can keep you comfortable, warm, looking hip, and riding happily in any weather you may encounter.

There's black, or there are those clashing shades that confirm to the uninitiated that color-blindness is a pre-requisite for cycling. In addition to standard polyester or lycra, new textiles have taken the sports clothing market by storm. The jargon is sometimes overwhelming, but there's no doubt that man-made fibers are great at replicating the warmth and water-repellent qualities of goosedown and wool, and they easily overrule cotton T-shirts, sweatshirts and shorts, which are cold when wet and dry slowly. The advantage of the new textiles is their lightness and their quick-drying and wash-ability — qualities that everyone appreciates!

In the heat you can generally wear any clothes you want, but you may choose to invest in a good cycling jersey that deals with sweat and dries quickly. In 90°F+ (32°C+) temperatures you'll also feel cooler if you wear white.

Water and wind are elements that every cyclist has to fend off, especially in cold temperatures, — these are conditions that carry a high misery-risk. Give up and go home when the suffering increases beyond the charge of cycling in adverse conditions. Getting cold can be painful and unpleasant, and, in a worst case scenario, can lead to life-threatening hypothermia, where the core body temperature drops and the victim will need the correct kind of warming-up.

HOT/DRY/COOL WEATHER
Short- or long-sleeved cycling jersey
Shorts
Fleece shirt
SPD shoes
Waist pack or backpack
Dark shades
Lightweight, water repellent

CHILLING OUT
■ **On a day with temperatures around 50°F (10°C), a 10–20mph (16–32km/h) breeze drops the temperature to between 41°F (5°C) and 32°F (0°C). When it hovers around freezing, a wind of 10–20mph (16–32km/h) drops the temperature to between 14°F (-10°C) and -4°F (-20°C) (and that's only while you're standing still!)**
■ **The temperature drops 1.8°F (1°C) for every 300ft (100m) climbed.**

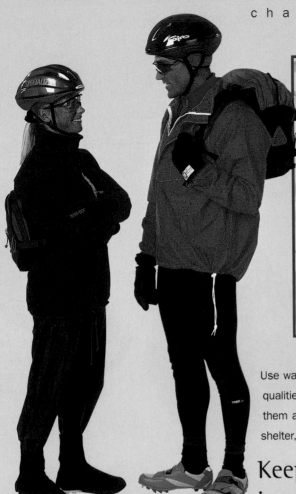

COLD/WET WEATHER
Gore-tex, or other
waterproof jacket
Shell pants
Winter tights
Fleece jacket
Silk underwear
Boots
Overboots
Winter gloves
Clear shades
Headband
Gloves

Use waterproofs as much for their windproof qualities as their waterproof ability. Remove them as soon as you've stopped and found shelter, to let your body and clothing air.

Keeping warm in winter

Avoid drafts. Plug gaps at the neck with a scarf, use those wriststraps that come with your long-wristed gloves. Don't pack layers too tightly, otherwise you'll get too hot, then too cold if they become soaked in sweat and are exposed to cold air.

A large percentage of body heat is lost through the top of your head. Keep your head warm by wearing a bandana in cool temperatures and a thick fleece headband in very cold weather; use one that covers your ears as well as blocking the gap between your helmet and head. Wear a vest to keep the chill off your torso.

The challenge of battling the elements can be a big thrill in cycling, but the chill of wind on wet flesh and clothes needs to be understood if you're going to safely enjoy the ride, especially in remote, exposed areas. Winds are chilling enough, but a

cyclist's speed increases the chill-factor, and feet, which are moving faster than the rest of the body and are closer to wet or icy ground, can be kept from going numb with a pair of waterproof overboots.

Shorts

An essential part of every cyclist's wardrobe, shorts are available in many styles. Some are padded for comfort and to prevent chafing on the inner thigh. Baggy styles are available for occasional riders, downhillers and street bikers alike.

Love your layers

Cycling is hot work, so the correct clothing needs to be a balance between insulation and evaporation. Go for layers that you can remove or add easily. Use thin sports underwear next to the skin for core insulation, then as many mid-layers as you're comfortable with. Add shirts made of fleece, polyester, lycra, or any of the brand-name equivalents. Finish your layering with a wind and waterproof shell on the outside. Think of the outer layer as a window, providing a seal from the elements.

Dry – dream on!

Staying completely dry is impossible: nothing, not even the best breathable material, can release perspiration at the rate at which it pours out of an energetic cyclist.

TEXTILES

FLEECE

A textile that miraculously combines coziness with sportiness, fleece comes in different densities for warmth and wind-proofness. In warm and cool conditions go for a lightweight, windproof fleece sweatshirt as an outer layer; in cold and wet conditions, wear lighter weight fleece beneath a shell for insulation without bulk. Your options are:

ECO-FLEECE

A textile made from recycled non-biodegradable plastic soda bottles.

POLARTEC

Providing warmth and windproofness, Polartec comes in different thicknesses of fleece. Some Polartec is recycled.

SILK

Underwear made from silk is not only warm and light, it feels nice on the skin. One turtleneck on the inside does the job of an extra thick, wool sweater on the outside.

PERTEX

A great material for wind and water-proof shells, Pertex is a super lightweight, densely woven polyester that dries incredibly quickly.

GORE-TEX

The original breathable waterproof fabric invented by Mr WL Gore, now with a dozen competitors of varying brand names.

essential accessories

Helmets

An essential piece of equipment for all cyclists. They're well-ventilated, light and hip enough for any cyclist to wear, wherever and how ever they ride. For mountain biking, where· falling off is part of the game, helmets have become part of the furniture.

The skull is the brain's natural helmet, but it needs help to protect it from falls that happen at high speeds. The skull puts up a good defence against external damage, but most athletic head injuries are not caused by skull fractures. They're caused by the soft tissue of the brain hitting hard against the *inside* of the skull, as well as a twisting and tearing of the covering membrane.

Helmets are constructed with a collapsible ½–¾in (10–20mm) wall of expanded polystyrene that absorbs impact, slowing down the brain's internal momentum and reducing damage. Most helmets on sale are molded shells, and they should conform to either of these safety standards; ANSI Z90 or the Snell Foundation B84 or B90.

Hard-headed hints

■ Get a helmet that fits. The basic sizes, from "extra small" to "extra large", will not necessarily conform to the clothing sizes you wear. Try a range of sizes to see which fits best.
■ Ensure the helmet sits securely on the top of your head. Use the adjustable pads to make the fit firm and comfortable.
■ Adjust the side straps by pulling or pushing them through the sliders below your ears

to keep the helmet in place. Then adjust the front anchor straps, which prevent the helmet from getting pushed backward while you're riding. Pull or push the chin-strap through the buckle clip for a snug jaw fit. You can tape the chin-strap in place if it slips, which they tend to do as the strap gets worn in.

■ Because of the way they are constructed, helmets should be replaced after a hard fall, to ensure your safety. Specialized and Giro have a "new-for-bashed" policy and will send you a replacement helmet for the mere cost of postage and packaging, which justifies their higher initial cost.

MTB footwear

From pedal-locking sandals to knee-length mountaineering gaiters, cycling footwear covers a spectrum of styles and terrain. How much you invest on footwear depends on your experience and how extreme your riding style is.

All cycling shoes have stiff soles, which stop your feet from forming themselves around the pedals. Trail riders and cross-country racers, whose goal is eating up the miles, wear trim racing shoes that clip into bindings in the pedals for secure descending

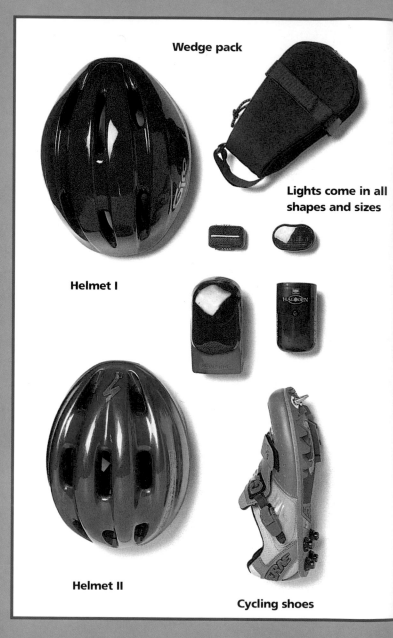

Wedge pack

Lights come in all shapes and sizes

Helmet I

Helmet II

Cycling shoes

and sheer on-the-flat efficiency. Downhillers and jumpers use flat, chunky BMX-style shoes, and then choose whether to clip in or

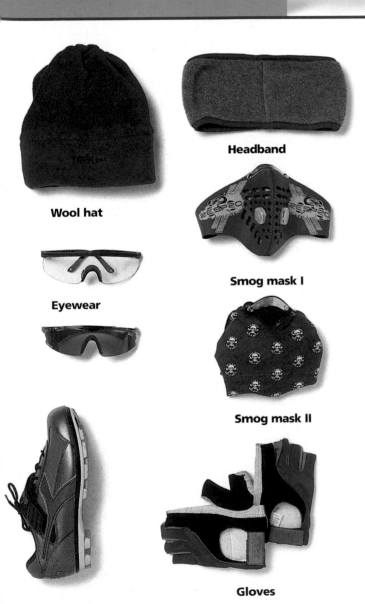

Wool hat

Headband

Eyewear

Smog mask I

Smog mask II

Gloves

to use plain pedals (with grippy pegs) to leave their legs free for scooting round corners and counter-balancing.

The SPD pedal (an acronym for Shimano Pedaling Dynamics) is now a universal

design that houses a mechanism that a cleat in the sole of the shoe clips into. It's also confusingly known as the clipless pedal, because it superseded the toeclip-and-strap design that dominated cycling for most of the 20th century. The quick-release cleat in the sole of the shoe locks the ball of the foot into the pedal at the flick of an ankle, and it releases easily and automatically if necessary. Once clipped in, even beginners can do impressive bunny-hops. The design has been adapted from road racing, but off-road shoes are comfortable enough to walk in, because the cleat is flush with the sole.

A minor drawback of SPDs is that the pedal and cleat can get clogged in bad mud and temporarily stop working. It's not always easy to clip in, especially with cold feet, and the cleat's steel surface doesn't grip wet rock well, if you have to cover a lot of ground on foot. Cleated shoes, boots and even sandals are available for riding in different conditions.

Traditional toe clips and straps are simple and cheap, not quite as efficient, but do have some advantages. They're not as com-

mon as they used to be, but they let you ride in ordinary shoes or runners, or even hiking boots. If you're doing some off-road touring where you may be wet for days, or don't want to carry more footwear than you need to, toeclips may be a good choice. But, you'll need patience in flicking the pedal when you try to get your foot into the clips.

Don't forget that wearing waterproof overboots will keep your toes warm when it's cold, and when it's wet full-length gaiters will keep mud and water thrown up by the wheels off your shins.

Handy Hints

As well as keeping your hands warm, gloves can prevent scrapes and bruises when you fall. If you don't wear mitts or gloves, your hands will eventually toughen up enough to hold the handlebars without blisters or pain from the cold — but who wants to be masochistic? Gloves with terry cloth on the back are nice for wiping away sweat and a runny nose, while padding and rubber on the palms and fingers mean comfort and grip.

When it comes to protecting your hands from the cold, don't be cheap. Every penny spent on a pair of gloves pays itself back in warmth and durability and adds mileage to your riding. The best cold-weather gloves have a kind of mini-layering, with a windproof shell on the outside and a warm lining. Look for a long wrist covering to tuck up inside your sleeves for extra warmth. If you can find waterproof hiking or skiing gloves with fingers that are slim enough to allow you to work the controls, go for them.

The ultimate in warmth and luxury is to have thin silk gloves under your tougher outer gloves.

the maintenance of a mountain bike

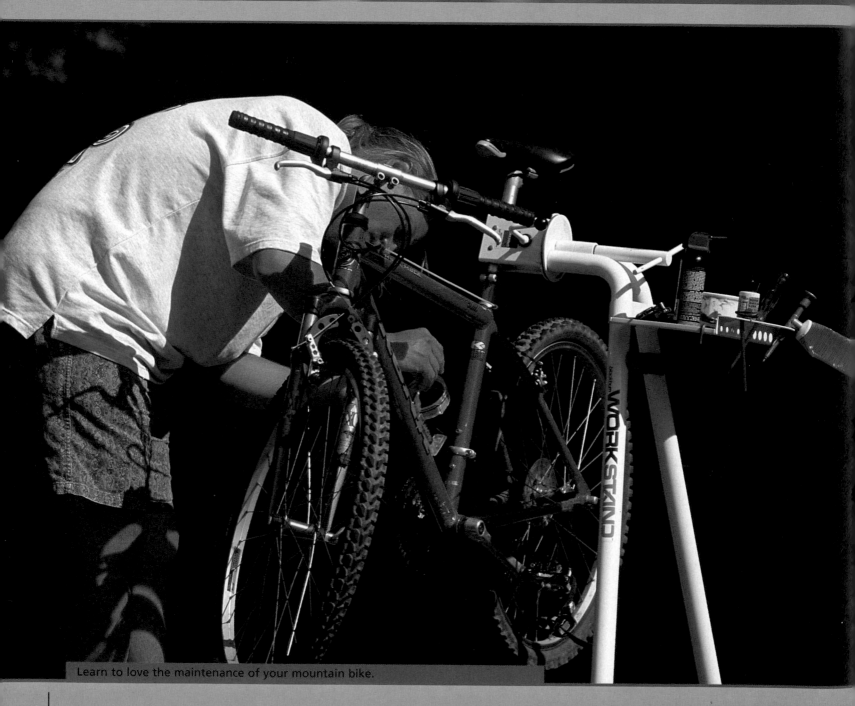

Learn to love the maintenance of your mountain bike.

'You cannot be at ease on your bicycle if you are at its mercy.'

Bridgestone mountain bikes.

Tips and principles for efficient maintenance

Maintaining your bike can give you great satisfaction. Mountain biking often involves cycling in remote areas, so it's important to be as self-sufficient as possible. Knowing your way around your machine will help you to keep it in good shape, allow you to spot problems before they become serious and get you moving after crashes or breakdowns.

At the very least, every cyclist should be able to fix a flat and figure out if their brakes are working properly. Small, simple adjustments to your gears and brakes will also make a lot of difference, and it's incredible how much better your bike will feel after an hour of tweaking here and there.

For more complicated repairs, there comes a point where it will cost you more to buy the tools than to pay a mechanic to do the job for you, and who can also get you back on the trail faster than if you tackle it yourself! The more familiar you become with your bike, though, the more confident you'll feel, and the number of jobs you'll be willing to tackle will increase.

■ If you're really not mechanically-minded, you can still enjoy your biking, but you should remember that regular maintenance by an expert will be necessary.

■ Look at each component of your mountain bike carefully, to see how it works. All the components are visible — there aren't many hidden parts.

■ Every time you buy a new component for your mountain bike it should have clear, comprehensive instructions that tell you how the part should be installed and adjusted; keep them, because you never know when you may need them.

■ New mountain bikes usually come with a whole bunch of instructional brochures, which should be kept and used as step-by-step guides to maintenance.

■ Keep some old rags on hand for cleaning: towels, sheets and t-shirts all work well. You can cut off the sleeves and cut the body into horizontal strips to make loops to hang on hooks on the wall.

■ Work in a warm, comfortable and well-lit environment. You can do most adjustments with an emergency toolkit (see pp. 38–41), although you'll find that a larger toolkit kept at home will make things easier.

■ For most of the gear and brake adjustments, a stand is useful. Something simple will do the job, as long as it holds the back wheel off the ground and the bike upright.

■ When you take each component apart, lay the pieces face up on newspaper in the order that they come off the bike. That way you'll know what order to put things back together in. Clean each part, then wash your hands before reassembling the component or touching clean parts, especially if you're working with bearing surfaces and cables.

■ Never get violent with a part. If something doesn't budge, clean all around it, apply oil (if appropriate) and work at it gently. Excessive force can shear parts or, in a worst case scenario, twist a wheel or frame.

■ Take care of your tools. Clean them every single time you use them and remember to oil them, if and when necessary.

■ Be systematic — always check your work before riding away. Don't half-fit anything, thinking that you'll come back to it at the end of your maintenance session. It's easy to become distracted and forget all about it. Poorly-fitted components are potentially dangerous, for you and other riders.

■ Stop working if you get frustrated — you're more likely to break something than fix it. Take a break for a while, and return to your bike when you feel calm and composed. Don't even begin a maintenance session if you don't have enough time.

the pre-ride check

Every time you take your bike for a ride, give it a quick check before you pedal away. These simple checks should only take about 30 seconds, and might save you a long walk home!

1 PICK UP THE BIKE AND DROP IT

Lift the bike 4in (10cm) off the ground by the handlebars and saddle, and let it drop to the ground, catching it before it falls over. Listen carefully to how it sounds, and learn to become familiar with that sound. You'll be able to detect anything loose that may be about to fall off because it will sound different from the way it normally does. If something sounds downright weird, check it out.

2 CHECK THE BRAKES

The front and rear brakes should be checked independently. Stand beside the bike, and push it forward by the handlebars. When you pull the front brake only, the rear wheel should lift up as the front wheel locks. When you pull the rear brake only, the rear wheel should lock and slide across the ground.

3 CHECK THE QUICK-RELEASE LEVERS

Check the quick-release levers on both wheels and on the seat-post. Ensure that they're holding the component in place. If you're unsure of how quick-releases work, get someone who does know to show you the workings.

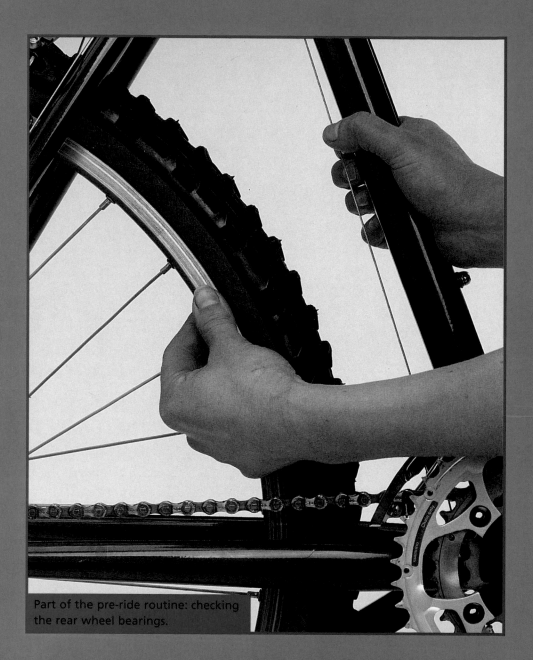

Part of the pre-ride routine: checking the rear wheel bearings.

4 CHECK THE BEARINGS

Bearings are made so that the component can rotate freely around its own axle, without any movement (play) at all across the axle. It's important to check that the adjustment is correct, since they'll wear quickly if they're too tight or too loose. If the wheel bearings are too tight, the wheel will not

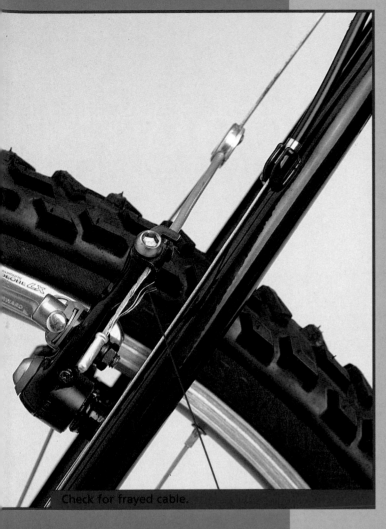

Check for frayed cable.

spin freely. If they're too loose, you'll be able to feel the play.

To check the rear wheel (rear hub), bearings, squat down by the right-hand side of the bike. Hold the seat tube about halfway down with your right hand. Hold the rim of the rear wheel between your thumb and the first finger of your left hand. Rock the wheel gently towards you and away from you, as in the photo to the left. If there is play in the hub bearings, you'll feel a slight clunking and probably also hear a little click.

To feel play is to know it, so if you're still unsure but happen to meet another cyclist whose bike has loose bearings, ask them to let you feel the wobble before they get it fixed.

Check the front hub bearings the same way.

5 CHECK THE BOTTOM BRACKET

Hold the seat tube and line the crank arm up with it. Grab one of the crank arms (not the pedal because play in the pedal bearings might be mistaken for bottom bracket movement) and rock it gently. A loose bottom bracket will click. Repeat on the other crank arm. If you can feel play in only one crank, that crank may be loose on the bottom bracket axle. If that is the case, tighten it immediately — riding on a loose crank is a surefire way of destroying it, fast.

6 CHECK THE HEADSET

Headset bearings are tricky to check — if there's play, it can be hard to know whether it's coming from the headset, or whether there's movement between the parts of your suspension forks. To eliminate any fork play, turn the handlebars sideways, so that the front wheel is perpendicular to the bike. Apply the front brake, and rock the bars gently backwards and forwards. If you can feel a clunking or hear a clicking, you have loose headset bearings.

7 CHECK THE WHEEL ALIGNMENT

Lift each wheel off the ground and spin it. Watch the rim as it passes between the brake pads. Check that the brakes pads hit the rim centrally; too high on the rim and they'll bite into the tire, causing a blow-out; too low and they'll jam in the spokes, bringing you to an abrupt halt. See pages 50–51 for further details about brakes.

8 CHECK THE TIRES

Check that the tire pressure is acceptable, and not below 35psi. Check the tread for excessive wear and cuts in the sidewall and pick out anything that's lodged in the tread. Sharp objects can take a while to work their way through the tire casing into the inner tube, and sometimes you have a chance to catch them before they do any damage.

9 CABLE CHECK

Check all cables for kinks, fraying or breaks in the housing. Cables usually break a strand at a time, either where they make sharp turns or where they're held in place.

10 CHECK THE HANDLEBARS

Stand in front of the bike, hold the front wheel between your knees and twist the bars firmly (but not too hard because you could bend the front wheel). The stem should not move. Check the saddle the same way. It should not twist sideways at all.

preparing for breakdowns

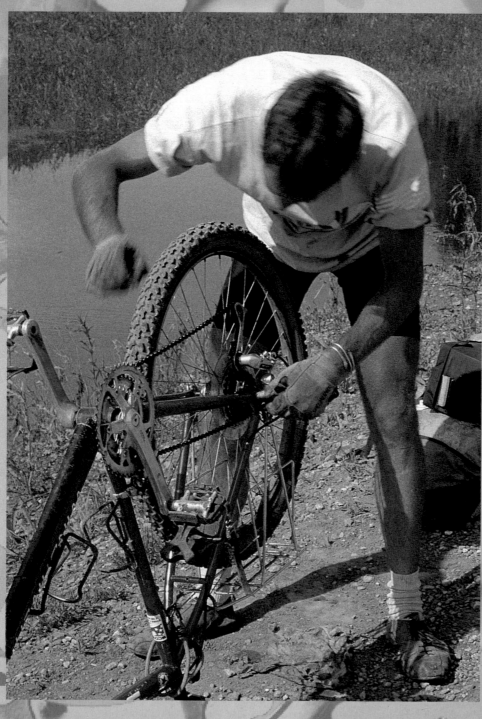

Proactive maintenance reduces the chances of trailside breakdown, but everybody's luck runs out sometime. The simplicity of bicycles can become a disadvantage, because almost nothing about them is superfluous. You can't get away with breaking any part of a bike, because every part is in use. The priority, if you're in the middle of nowhere, is to be able to get yourself home.

As soon as you realize something is wrong, stop and get off the bike. Think about the problem. There aren't many problems that fix themselves. Problems will compound themselves into more problems if you decide to fix them at the end of a ride instead of immediately. You'll also have a shorter walk back to where you heard pieces fall off.

Every day brings a new way to break a bicycle and a new way to fix it. These are general repairs that cover most breakdowns. They sound obvious, but they work.

Tips and principles

■ Stay calm — panic doesn't mix with effective, safe repair.

■ After a crash, first check yourself for damage. Excessive blood, unusual visual effects or nausea may mean that you need to be taken care of before your bike does!

■ You'll be able to work out what's gone wrong much more quickly if you remember what your bike looked like before you broke it! Work out the difference between how it's supposed to look, and how it looks now.

CREATIVE TOOLS AND SPARES

■ Zip-ties are very useful, so carry them wherever you go. Use them to temporarily repair pedals, flat tires, bags, lights and even to keep long hair out of your eyes.

■ Anything you're wearing or carrying on you can be turned into a tool — shoelaces come in handy in the strangest places.

■ Include a spare rear brake cable in your emergency repair kit. They don't weigh anything and can be used on either front or rear brake — just secure any excess cable so that it doesn't get caught in your wheel.

■ It doesn't make sense to carry spares if you don't have the corresponding tools, or conversely, to carry tools for spares that you're leaving at home.

■ Make sure your spare inner tubes fit your rims. Schraeder valves are fatter than Presta and will not fit through the holes drilled for Presta valves.

■ Some duct tape wrapped around a wrench may come in handy.

■ Whenever you buy additional components, revise your tool-kit.

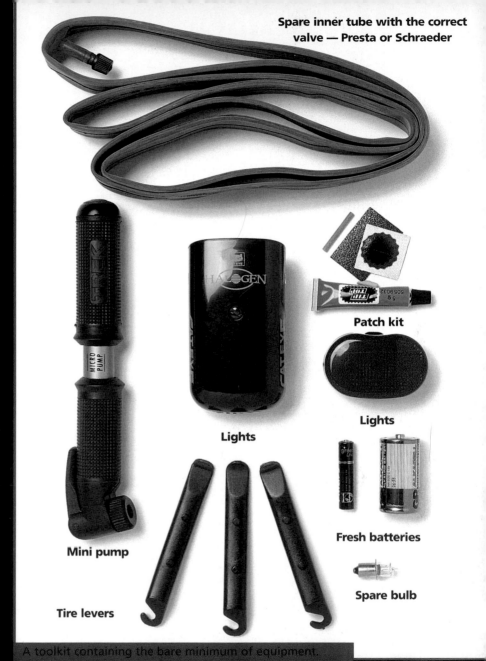

Spare inner tube with the correct valve — Presta or Schraeder

Patch kit

Lights

Lights

Fresh batteries

Mini pump

Spare bulb

Tire levers

A toolkit containing the bare minimum of equipment.

Figure out how serious the problem is. After your own health, the primary objective is to get the bike rideable, for which you need to have two brakes and one gear functioning. You may have to settle for less than perfect performance, but salvaging a bike so that it stops and starts is enough

■ Remove as much of the dirt around any broken part as possible, and take a good look at it. Make sure you haven't thrown away any loose pieces.

■ Find a clear patch of ground to work on, or place all loose parts on your bag or jacket, so that you don't risk losing anything.

■ Be creative with tools. Rocks, locks and SPD shoes all make good hammers.

■ After completing the obvious repair, check the bike for related damage before riding away. Did the crash take out anything else?

■ Repack all your tools, and any broken parts so that you can look at them more closely when you get home, if necesary.

■ Is the repaired bike trailworthy? Would it be better to walk home than to risk further injury to it or yourself?

tools for trails

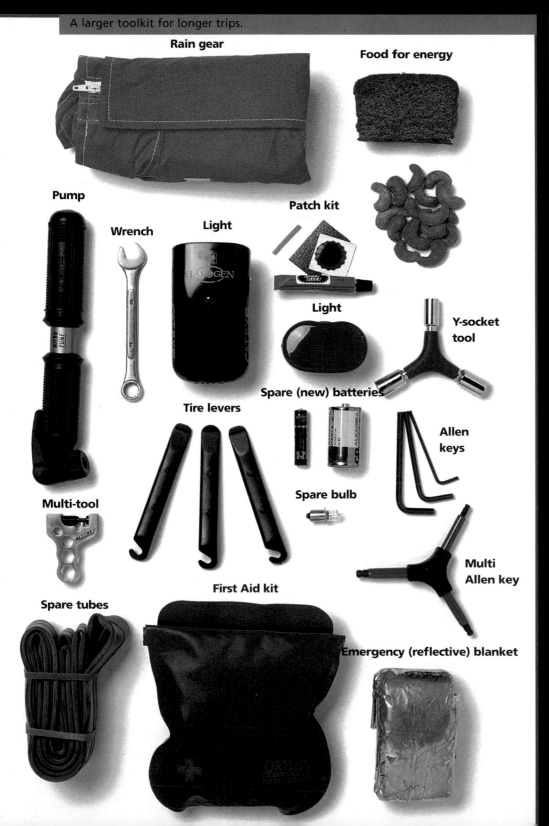

A larger toolkit for longer trips.

Rain gear

Food for energy

Pump

Patch kit

Wrench

Light

Light

Y-socket tool

Spare (new) batteries

Tire levers

Allen keys

Spare bulb

Multi-tool

Multi Allen key

First Aid kit

Spare tubes

Emergency (reflective) blanket

Here's a list of the tools most experienced mountain bikers carry to cover all of the usual emergencies. Add to them based on your own experience and check out what other riders carry. The range of your trailside toolkit depends on where you're riding. Discovering that your patch kit glue has dried out is fine on a summer afternoon when there's still lots of daylight left to walk home in. Discovering the same problem at the top of a mountain at dusk in December is a lot more dangerous.

Essentials for fixing flats

- Patch kit
- Pump
- Tire levers

Never leave home without a spare inner tube and recently inspected patch kit, which should contain some patches and glue that is still liquid — once opened, a tube of glue lasts about six months, even with the lid screwed on tight.

There are also a number of glueless patch kits currently on the market. It's rumoured that these were developed by the army as emergency bullet wound patches, but there's never been any evidence of that application. The most common brand is the Park glueless patch kit, which comes in a re-sealable, plastic box.

A glueless patch kit is fine for emergencies, and makes fixing a flat easier, but the seal is not as reliable as it is on a

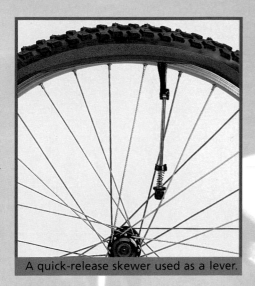

A quick-release skewer used as a lever.

regular patch, especially if the patch is placed over the seam of the inner tube. A patch will also stick better if you clean the surface of the inner tube before applying the patch to it. Ask your bike store for suitable cleaning swabs.

PUMP IT UP

All this is useless without a pump to re-inflate the tire once you've patched the tube. There are lots of different kinds of hand pumps on the market. Try to test different brands and models before you buy one. Metal pumps are stronger, but heavier. Short pumps are harder to use, but easier to carry around.

If possible, get a pump that adapts to both shapes of inner tube valve: Presta (long and thin) and Schraeder (like on car tires, short and broad), because you never know who you might be riding with or who you might meet sitting forlornly by the trail. Mountain bikers seem to think that there will always be someone else carrying a pump — a dangerous assumption to make.

TIRE LEVERS

You can get away with carrying only one tire lever, but you're better off with two. A stick or a screwdriver or even the handle of a fork or spoon can be used as a substitute — but

that's a little drastic. A better alternative is to use your quick-release skewers. Be careful using them because it's easy to damage rims and pinch the new inner tube as you're refitting it, which will only mean another flat tire, fast.

Fixing a broken chain

The next essential tool to have on the trail is the chain tool. It's a good idea to practice with it at home before you need to use it for real.

Also, before you leave for a ride, find out if your chain needs special replacement rivets or pins. For example, the rivets in Shimano chains are not designed to be re-used. Instead, the special rivet must be located and replaced with a new special rivet. This is not an easy task if the light is fading or if you are immersed in deep mud or cold weather, so practicing at home first is a good idea. Different pins are needed for 7-, 8- and 9-speed chains.

Some of the handy multitools come with an integral chain tool. The Park CT-5 Mini Chain Tool is excellent and easy to use even while wearing gloves, and comes with comprehensive instructions on the box.

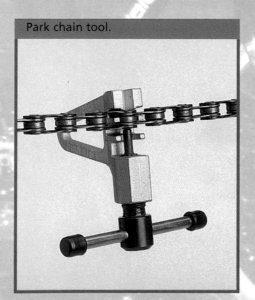

Park chain tool.

Which wrenches?

Almost nothing on a new mountain bike needs a wrench, but check, just in case! If you have an older bike, wrenches between ⅜in to ¾in (8mm and 18mm) will cover most of your needs.

You should also bring along a small adjustable wrench. Many people manage fine with just one but before you throw away that spare, make sure that you have no parts that need two wrenches simultaneously tightening or loosening anything.

Which Allen keys?

The Allen keys you carry also depends on your bike; the sizes needed for most models is shown below. Allen keys are measured in metric sizes.

6mm — for saddles, stems and some brake systems.

5mm — for headsets, chainring bolts and some brakes.

4mm — for some leverless skewers and some brake levers.

3mm — for some SRAM grip shifters, SPD pedals.

2.5mm — for some SRAM grip shifters, some brake-centering bolts.

Loose Allen keys are fine, but those that fold up like a pocket knife are more convenient because the body of the tool acts as a handle and gives more leverage.

SCREWDRIVERS

Screwdrivers with Phillips and flat heads are always useful. Some of the multi-Allen key tools also come with screwdrivers. They're needed for adjusting gear end stop screws and brake centering bolts.

The packaging

Choose a sturdy tool bag that you can strap under the seat or to the frame of the bike.

fixing trail breakdowns

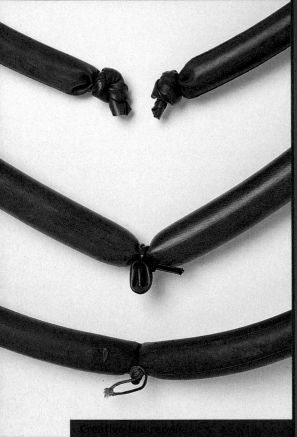

Creative tire repair

Emergency tire repairs

■ String and zip-ties isolate the punctured area of the tube.

■ A knot tied in the tube works, but it needs to be pulled very tightly to stop the air from escaping. This makes the tube shorter and harder to get between the tire and the rim and the knot makes a noticeable lump in the tire that will make for an uncomfortable ride.

■ Anything that sticks to the surface of the tube may keep the air in long enough to get you home.

■ If the hole in the tube is too big to isolate or patch, forget the tube and stuff the tire with something else. Grass is a traditional substitute (if you can find some), but it's hard to get enough inside the tire to protect the rim from rough terrain, and rims damage quickly if you ride them with a soft tire. The tires don't like it much either. If you have to, ride gently — and remember that you'll lose steering power on the front wheel and traction on the back. It's usually quicker (and better for the bike) to walk.

■ Any large cuts in the tire will cause another flat as soon as the inner tube bulges into the hole — the edges of the hole in the tire will simply cut into the tube. Find something to wrap around the tube, to stop it from bulging out. Paper is usually strong enough, so try to improvise with money, bits of map or candy wrappers.

Gear repairs

If either derailleur cable snaps, the spring in the mechanism will pull it back into its resting position, leaving the chain in one cog (the easiet on the front derailleur, or the hardest on the rear). Only that derailleur will be affected so you should still be able to change gears with the other shifter.

FRONT DERAILLEUR

If the front derailleur cable snaps, screw in the end-stop screw (see p. 55) so that the chain sits in the middle ring. Alternatively, a lump of wood wedged between the seat stay and the derailleur can keep the chain in the middle or largest ring. If the front derailleur is broken beyond repair, remove it. Run the chain over whichever ring you want, usually the middle. With practice, you can change down gear with your heel as you cycle along!

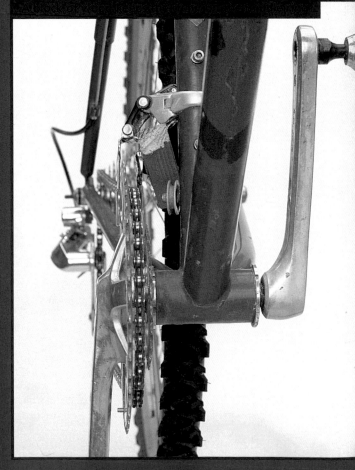

A block of wood keeps the chain in the middle ring

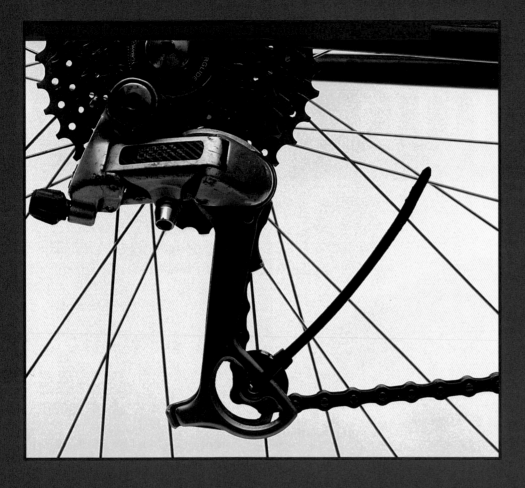

brake and remove the wheel from the frame. Hold it up and spin it. If the warp is nice and even, with the top and bottom bent one way and the front and back bent the other, there is hope that it can be fixed. Remove the quick-release skewer from the hub of the wheel, and lay the wheel on the ground.

Step onto one high point, then ease your weight gently onto the other. Bounce gently up and down. If you're in luck, the wheel will suddenly pop back into its previous shape — which is, hopefully, fairly round. Make sure you jump off the wheel quickly, though, before you start to warp it the other way.

Fine tune the wheel with a spoke wrench (see pp. 58–59), if you have one. Replace the quick release, wheel and brakes, and ride on.

REAR DERAILLEUR

Screw in the end-stop screw so that the chain sits in a comfortable gear. If the rear derailleur itself breaks or falls apart, it's sometimes possible to jury-rig it. Zip-ties can be the answer. Above, a jockey wheel bolt has been replaced with a zip-tie and the jockey wheel bearing.

If you can't fix the derailleur, you may have to remove it. Because the rear derailleur extends the chain beyond the sprockets in order to move it across them, if you remove it you'll also have to shorten the chain to make it tight enough to just run around one sprocket. Take out as many links as you need to run the chain in a comfortable gear. If you have rear suspension, make sure you leave enough chain slack for the rear end of the bike to move.

Turn the pedals backwards to make sure the chain runs freely, with a little bit of slack. It's tricky to get the length right and without the rear derailleur to keep the chain tensioned it'll still have a tendency to skip around on the rear sprockets and you may have to stop regularly to readjust. Don't throw away the extra section of chain because you'll need it again when you replace the rear derailleur.

Fixing wheels

It is possible to salvage a wheel that resembles a potato chip. Release the

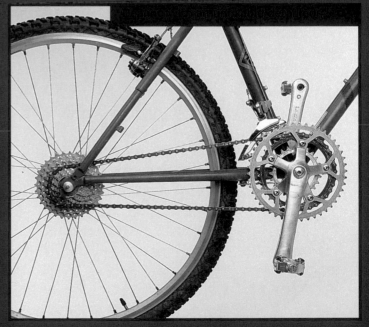

cleaning a muddy bike

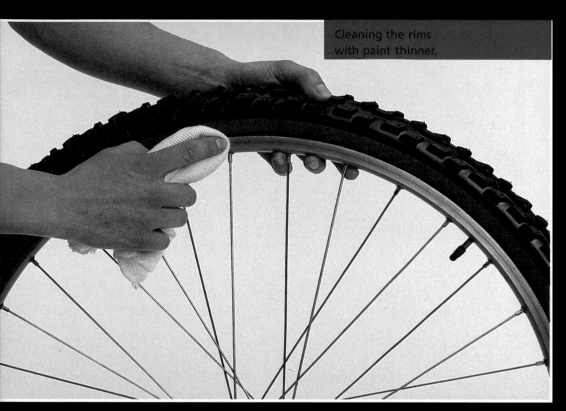

Cleaning the rims with paint thinner.

Cleaning your bike is either considered something to be put off as long as possible, or a way to inspect and bond with your bike! Regularly cleaned parts last longer; for example, clean rims will not wear brake pads out so quickly, and vice versa. Surface dirt needs to be washed off before it works its way into hidden parts, like the inside of a cable housing and into bearings. It's also a good time to check the condition of your bike.

A CLEAN FRAME

Brush off any dry, loose mud. Remove the wheels to make it easier to get in between the stays. If you can, hang the bike up to make it easier to work on. Use a pail of warm, soapy water to clean the frame and components. Rinse the bike off afterwards with fresh water. Polish the frame after you've cleaned it. Mud doesn't stick as well to a smooth, polished surface, so the bike will stay cleaner longer. Check for cracks in the frame — they show up as fine lines that dirt gets stuck into.

CLEAN WHEELS

Keep the braking surface of the rims as clean as possible. Brake pad residue accumulates on wheel rims, and limits the effectiveness of braking. If necessary, wipe the rims down with paint thinner. Riding down a paved road at a good speed clears most of the mud from the tires — scrub off the rest with warm soapy water. When the tires are clean, check them for deep cuts or sharp things and remove anything embedded in the tire.

A CLEAN DRIVETRAIN

The chain, cassette (sprockets), front chainrings and jockey wheels are the elements that constitute the drivetrain. Sprockets wear very quickly if they aren't clean. Chains can last as little as a week in bad conditions if they're neglected; the dirt they pick up gets carried around the drivetrain and forced into the holes between the chain plates. When you put pressure on the pedals, those particles of dirt get ground up by the chain, and wear down the metal surfaces. Try to wipe your chain down once for every six hours of riding time; it sounds frequent, but it only takes a few seconds and will leave your bike running smoother. How often you wipe down the chain will also depend on the riding conditions.

BRUSHING YOUR BIKE

Keep a selection of soft brushes, scrub brushes and toothbrushes. Pot scrubbing brushes with an angled head are perfect for getting into gaps behind brakes and gears.

chain tool. Hang the chain up, and spray it with a specialist bike chain cleaner, like Pedro's Oranj Peel or Finish Line 'Eco-Tech Degreaser'.

Use a toothbrush to scrub each link, then rinse the chain off with clean water. Dry the chain and lubricate it again immediately (see p. 46).

wheels will put all your work to waste, so clean these too. Hold a cloth against each jockey wheel while pedaling backward. A stiff brush will be fine for cleaning the cassette (sprockets) and chainrings. If you have the tools and the time, remove the chainrings from the chainset and clean them separately; this makes it easier to get into the gaps.

seeping into other components and bearings, and driving out the grease they need to keep them running smoothly. It's a good idea to remove your cassette for cleaning, to protect the bearings in your rear hub.

Always follow the manufacturer's instructions — if they recommend washing off the degreaser, then do it. Otherwise, it might react with whatever lubricant you put on. Depending on the degreaser, water also activates emulsifiers, which help lift grease off components. Dry off the degreased part, and lubricate it immediately to prevent the unprotected surface from corroding.

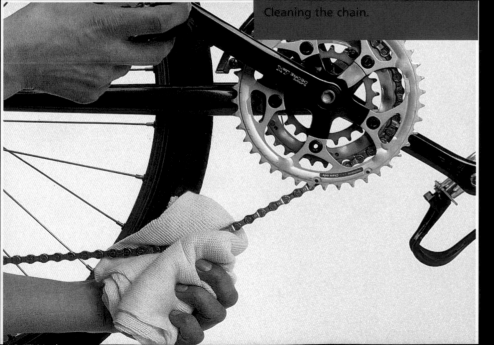

Cleaning the chain.

FLAMMABLE PRODUCTS
Many cleaning and lubricating products ignite if exposed to a flame, so handle them with care.

45

lubricants and lubrication

The golden rule with lubrication is little and often. It's much better to give your bike a small regular oiling than to wait until it's really desperate and then smother it in oil.

Like cleaning, lubrication should be part of your essential regular relationship with your bike.

What does a lubricant do?

Lubricant does three things.

First, it lets two surfaces to pass over each other with a minimum amount of friction. Energy wasted when rough surfaces grind over each other is energy that could have been used to push you forward — getting you where you're going faster and sooner, or with less effort!

Friction also generates heat and hot parts are more at risk of being damaged, as well as seizing up or shearing.

So, a lubricant's second job is to reduce wear on a bike's components. Surfaces that rub together should be as smooth as possible, and lubricated to form a tough protective film between them, reducing the amount they wear each other down.

Third, a thin film of oil or grease on metal surfaces will also prevent corrosion by preventing the lethal combination of water and air attacking the fabric of the bike. Bike components should always be greased when assembled.

WHICH LUBRICANTS TO USE

Grease is for bearings. Don't contaminate it — it should always be clean and applied to clean surfaces. If it's worth getting to bearings to grease them, then it's worth using a more expensive bicycle grease so that you won't have to repeat the job in a hurry. Waterproof grease is recommended. Oil, which is thinner, is used in more exposed places on the bike. While grease doesn't move, oil gets sucked into cracks and crevices by capillary action.

LUBRICATING PLASTICS AND TITANIUM

Gripshift gears are a plastic-on-plastic friction, and need a special lubricant. Although the plastic won't corrode, it will wear without

lubrication, leading to sloppy shifting. Similarly, titanium parts need an anti-galling compound to prevent them corroding — one brand is Ti-Prep Anti-Seize.

LUBRICATING CHAINS

The main reason for oiling chains is to get lubricant in between the plates, and

HOW OFTEN?
How often you need to lubricate your bike depends on:
- **How often you use your bike**
- **How often you clean your bike**
- **The weather and conditions that you ride your bike in**
- **How much abuse you put your bike through**

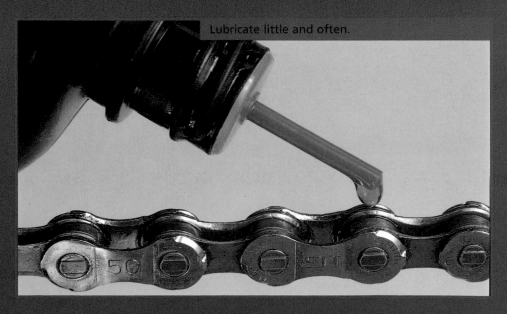
Lubricate little and often.

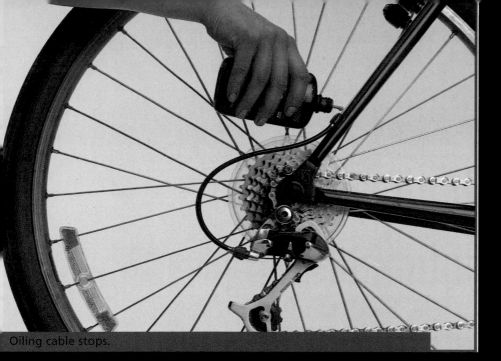

Oiling cable stops.

derailleurs are in the firing line of crud thrown up from the back wheel. A drop of oil on all four pivots in the rear mechanism can make an amazing difference in shifting. The back inside pivot is the most awkward to get to, and is probably most easily oiled when the wheel is off. Oil the jockey wheel pivots too. Wipe off any excess.

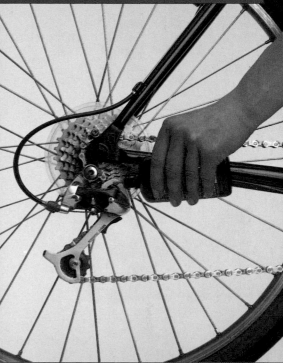

Oiling the pivot points in the rear derailleur.

between the pins and the rollers. Once the chain is clean (see p. 45), drip a small drop of oil onto each link on either side of the top of the roller. Leave it for several minutes to soak in, then wipe off any excess oil with a cloth.

Using a lubricant

Lubricant works best when applied to clean surfaces because it will flow more easily and there is no danger that it will flush dirt into cracks. Give the oil a few minutes to soak in, then wipe off the excess — excess oil attracts fresh dirt and defeats the purpose of cleaning and lubricating in the first place.

LUBRICATING CABLES

The most common place for the cables to break is at the nipple end, inside the brake and gear levers. The nipple should be kept greased so that it can turn in its seat. If it can't, the rest of the cable becomes twisted and over-stressed. Be forewarned — pre-break fraying can be difficult to see because it might be on the inside of either the lever or cable housings.

Good cables are lined with Teflon, which is very smooth. Without oil, however, the cable will still corrodes and become rough

so you should still oil Teflon-lined cables. Oil them at all cable stops, the places where they attach to the frame, and where the inner cable emerges from the outer casing. Lubricating will help repel water and stop it from collecting inside the cable. Gore-Tex cables should never be lubricated at all.

LUBRICATING DERAILLEURS

Derailleurs work more smoothly when the pivots are oiled. Lubrication should be frequent, because both the front and rear

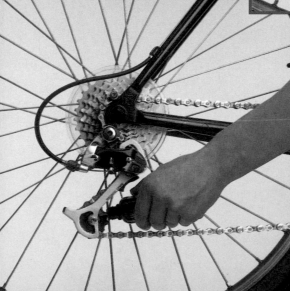

Oiling the jockey wheels.

LUBRICATING THE HANDLEBAR AREA

Oil the brake lever pivots. Turn the barrel adjusters so that the slots point upward and you can see the cable. Drop a little bit of oil into the slots.

The part closest to the end of the cable needs the most oil and from there the oil will seep into the rest of the cable. Turn the slots so that they face down again, to protect them from dirt and rain.

fixing a flat

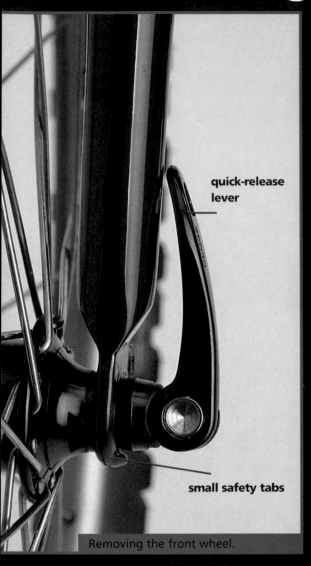

quick-release lever

small safety tabs

Removing the front wheel.

You can get a flat tire at any time during a ride, so it's essential that you know how to fix one. This is a step-by-step guide to flat tire repair. It's a good idea to get used to removing and replacing wheels and tires at home first.

REMOVING THE ▲ FRONT WHEEL

1 Release the front brake cable (see p. 51 if you're not sure how). This lets the brake pads move away from the wheel rim so that the wheel can be easily removed and replaced.

2 Flip open the quick-release lever.

3 Front wheels have small tabs at the bottom of the dropouts, to prevent the wheel from dropping out if your quick release lever accidentally opens. The tabs are there to give you time to notice that your front wheel is banging around and to refit it correctly. Release the front quick release then unwind the lever a few turns while holding the nut on the other side. This enables you to remove the wheel.

REMOVING THE REAR WHEEL ▼

Rear wheels are just as easy to remove, once you've learned how.

1 While turning the pedals, lift the back wheel off the ground and change gear into the smallest cogs at the front and back (for maximum chain slack).

2 Turn the bike upside down and rest it on its bars and saddle.

3 Undo the quick-release lever.

4 Stand behind the bike and put the first finger of your left hand in front of the guide jockey wheel (the one nearest the body of the derailleur) and your thumb behind the tension jockey wheel (the one that normally hangs down, see picture 1, below). With your left hand, push your finger backward and your thumb forward to tighten the chain and pull the derailleur out of the way (see picture 2, below). With your right hand, pull the wheel up and forward. Lift the wheel upward to the right, so that it pulls away from the chain.

STRIPPING THE TIRE ▶

The next step is to remove the tire. Press the valve to remove any air left in the tube. Now pinch the top of the tire in ward so that the tire bead facing you moves toward the centre of the rim. Do this around the whole rim so that the tire is looser on the rim,

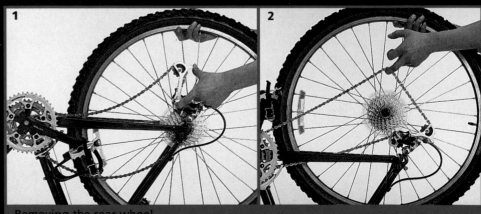

Removing the rear wheel.

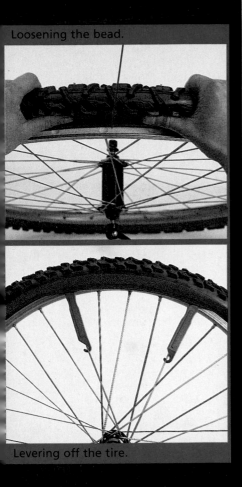

Loosening the bead.

Levering off the tire.

making it easier to remove. Pop the flat end of a tire lever under the bead, flick it down and hook the other end around a spoke. Repeat with another tire lever until the tire is loose enough to pop over the rim. Do this on one side only and then remove the inner tube. Leave the tire on the same place in the rim, so that once you have located the hole in the tube you can match the position to the tire and find out what caused it.

LOCATING THE PUNCTURE

Pump up the inner tube to medium pressure. Squeeze it gently and pass it slowly in front of your lips — they are very sensitive — so you can feel any air coming out of the tube — you may even hear it. If the hole is very small, you may have to pass the tube across your face a few times and at different angles to find it.

Once the hole is found, let out the air again and patch it. Remember to let the patch kit glue dry completely before putting the patch on top. This usually takes about five minutes. Or, you can just put a new inner tube in and take the punctured tube home to fix some other time (but before your next ride!)

TYPES OF PUNCTURE

Try to figure out what caused the puncture. Two common causes are "snakebite" punctures and sharp-object punctures.

Snakebite punctures occur when you hit a bump or rock with a lot of force, squashing the tire against the rim and pinching the inner tube on both sides of the rim. There will be two holes to patch, though they will be close together. If you get snakebite punctures often, increase your tire pressure.

Sharp object punctures happen on the outside of the inner tube. To locate this kind of flat, run a finger gently around the inside of the tire, but take care, because sharp objects on the inside of the tire can rip your fingers. Match the position of the hole in the tube to the tire, using the valve hole as a reference. The object that caused the puncture may be very small, or it may have dropped out already. You may also want to check the rim, for sharp-ended spokes or shifted rim tape. Another type of puncture is when the brake pad rubs against the tire — it can slice open the sidewall of the tire, causing the tube to bulge out and blow.

REMOVING THE CAUSE

Remove whatever caused the puncture. Try not to make the hole bigger when you do so. Make sure that there's nothing else poking through to the inner tube.

REFITTING THE TIRE

Once the glue on the repair is dry, pump a little air into the tube. A patch is not strong

until it's trapped between the tube and the inside of the tire, so you can't pump a repaired tube up too hard when it's off the wheel in case it blows the patch off. A slightly inflated tube is also easier to fit, as it won't get trapped under the tire bead so easily. Put the valve in place first, then tuck the rest of the tube into the tire. Pop as much as possible of the tire back onto the rim with your hands, massaging the bead into the centre of the rim as you do. If possible, refit the whole tire with your hands, although you may have to use tire levers.

WHEEL REPLACEMENT

Replacing the front wheel is the reverse of removing it. To replace the rear wheel hold the bike upside down and hold the derailleur out of the way like you did before, with your left hand. Insert the wheel between the stays, and maneuver it until the cassette sits between the upper and lower parts of the chain. Rest the smallest cog on the lower part of the chain, then push the wheel's axle into the dropouts. Check that the wheel is sitting centrally between the stays, and close the quick-release lever flat along the stay, so that there's no chance of it getting caught on anything.

Refit the brakes, pump up the tire and you're ready to go!

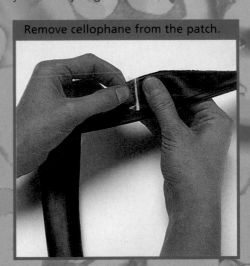

Remove cellophane from the patch.

brake replacement and adjustment

V-brakes and disc brakes have pretty much replaced the cantilever brakes that were universal on mountain bikes a few years ago. V-brakes are light and easy to adjust. They're also much more powerful, and need less strength to depress the levers. Disc brakes offer powerful, controlled braking. The images on these pages are of an Avid V-brake unit, but other V-brake models are adjusted the same way.

It's vital that your brakes are adjusted regularly and properly, for your own safety. If you undertand how they work, you can adjust them to your own preference. If you're in any doubt about how to do it, ask your bike store.

BRAKE LEVERS

Make sure that the levers are comfortable to use. Adjust the angle that the levers are fixed to the handlebars at so that your hands fall naturally onto the levers. You should be able to move your fingers onto them without dropping your wrists. If you have small hands, use the reach adjust screws to move the lever blade inward, so that you don't have to stretch for it.

CABLES

Brake cables work best if they're not kinked or forced around tight bends. However, as excessive cable creates extra friction and is more likely to get snagged on things, find a balance between too long and too short. Cables in graceful curves work best.

For best results, use the best cables you can find. Exposed cables should be Teflon-lined, for smoothness. For extra performance try Gore-Tex cables, which come fully enclosed. Similar products are produced by Avid, who make Flak Jacket cables, and Venhill, who make Thinline. All three products seal the outer casing, to prevent dirt from getting in between cable and casing.

Clean and oil your cables regularly, to keep them moving smoothly. Grease the nipple where it fits into the lever, to allow it to rotate. If the nipple can't turn as you pull the lever, the cable will soon snap from fatigue. Wherever possible, put endcpas on the ends of the housing or outer casing. This prevents the ends of the casings from splaying, and helps keep the brakes feeling sharp. The section of casing that fits into the brake noodle won't need an endcap because it's already built into the noodle.

V-BRAKES

V-brakes are simple to set up and adjust, but since they pull so strongly on the rim, they will wear out brake pads relatively quickly. Check the wear on your pads frequently, since worn pads won't brake effectively. If you don't change them when they're worn, the pad will wear even further through its metal support, and braking will damage your rims.

Brake components consist of several parts. The brake cable housing fits into a noodle, which acts as a cable stop and directs the cable into the hanger on one of the brake arms. The cable then passes through a gaiter, which helps keep dirt out of the casing and off the cable. The cable is clamped onto the opposite brake arm by a pinch bolt. The brake unit rotates around the brake post (part of the frame of the bike), and the two brake pads are bolted to the brake arm with a series of curved washers.

QUICK-RELEASING BRAKES

These brakes are very easy to quick release, so that you can take a wheel off without

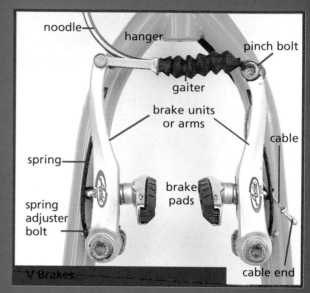

noodle — hanger — pinch bolt
gaiter
brake units or arms
cable
spring
brake pads
spring adjuster bolt
V Brakes.
cable end

Adjusting brake lever reach.

large hands   small hands

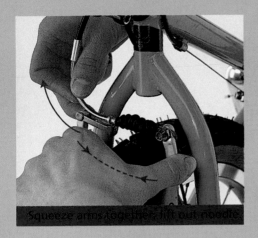
Squeeze arms together; lift out noodle.

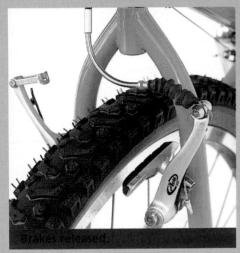
Brakes released.

letting all the air out of the tire to get it past the brake pads. Squeeze the brake arms together with one hand to create some slack in the cable. Then pull the noodle gently but firmly away from the pinch bolt, releasing it from the hanger. Lift the noodle up and away. Let go of the arms, which will then fall away to either side.

To refit the brakes, reverse the procedure. Squeeze the arms firmly together, then pull back the gaiter and ease the end of the noodle back into the hanger. Make sure it's seated firmly — check what it's like on your other brake if you're unsure of what it should look like.

Pull the end of the gaiter back over the end of the noodle, to keep dirt out of the casing. Check that the brakes are operating by firmly squeezing the lever.

BRAKE PAD ADJUSTMENT

Brake pads need very frequent maintenance. Inspect them for wear on a regular basis. Release the noodle so that the arms spring apart and check that the surfaces of each pad haven't picked up pieces of metal or grit. If you find any, pick them out carefully with a sharp knife, otherwise they'll damage the rim surface when you brake. If the brake pad surface has become shiny, scour it lightly with clean sandpaper, to improve grip. Most pads will have a wear line imprinted on the side. Replace the pads as soon as that wear line is reached.

You'll need an Allen key to fit and adjust these pads — usually a 5mm (¼in). The pads need to be set up to maximize the contact between the brake and the rim, to make the brakes as effective as possible. V-brake pads have a series of curved washers on the fixing bolt, which let you alter the angle

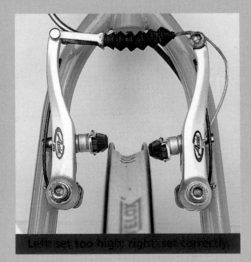
Left set too high; right set correctly.

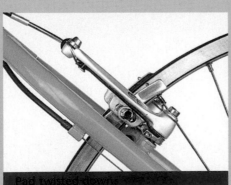
Pad twisted down.

at which the pad approaches the rim. The bolt fits through a slot, rather than a round hole, so that you can also adjust the height. The pads should be parallel to the rim, with the bottom edge of the pad aligned with the bottom edge of the rim.

The photo on the bottom left shows the pad at an angle to the rim, with the back of the pad too low and the front too high. Make sure the whole pad isn't set so high that it touches the tire during braking — you'll wear through the tire and puncture the tube very quickly. The center photo shows the left hand pad set too high, with the right hand pad at the correct height. Check that the pads are tightly fitted after you've adjusted them — try twisting them with your hands. If they move at all, they're not tight enough.

CENTERING ADJUSTMENT

The brakes need to be adjusted so that both sides operate evenly. If one brake pad rubs on the rim, or sits too close to it, you can use the spring adjustment to equalize spring tension. Either one or both of the arms will have a small screw with an Allen or a slot head. Screw in to increase the preload on the spring and move the pad away from the rim. Or, you can undo the screw on the opposite side, to release some preload, so that that side sits closer to the rim.

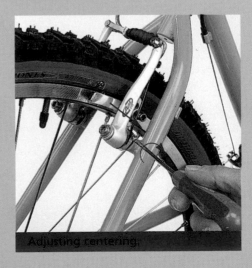
Adjusting centering.

gear
maintenance

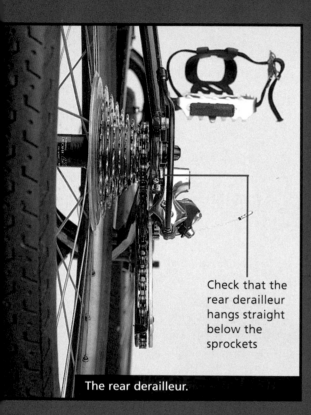

Check that the
rear derailleur
hangs straight
below the
sprockets

The rear derailleur.

Gear levers may all look different, but they all work the same way — one click of the lever pulls the cable enough to move the chain over exactly one sprocket. Since the cable can only pull, and not push, both derailleurs have springs. When you click the lever in the other direction, it releases enough cable so that the spring can pull the cable back exactly one sprocket.

If you're replacing components make sure that all parts are compatible. The levers will only work if they have the same number of "clicks" as your bike has sprockets. Check the components before you buy them, even if they're from the same manufacturer.

Derailleur differences

The rear derailleur shifts the chain across the sprockets and regulates the amount of chain needed for each gear. Each jockey wheel does a different job. The top one is a guide pulley, marked "G". It often has a little side-to-side movement to help the gear change. The bottom jockey is marked "T" (tension) and is sprung, so that it always tries to move backward, taking up slack in the chain. If you take the jockey wheels off to clean them, make sure you put them back in the same places or they won't work.

Are the derailleurs bent?

Check that the rear derailleur hangs straight and vertical below the sprockets. Put the chain on the middle ring at the front, and look at the rear derailleur from behind. If it's not straight and vertical, take it to your bike shop. This is the cause of most persistent gear-changing problems and you shouldn't try to straighten it yourself — the hanger needs to be treated with care. A lot of frames have a separate hangar, which can be unbolted and replaced if it gets bent.

When you look at it from above, the outer plate of the front derailleur should appear parallel to the outer chainring.

ADJUSTING DERAILLEURS

It helps to have your bicycle up on a stand that will keep the back wheel off the ground and allow you to turn the pedals. If you don't have one, ask a friend to lift the saddle at critical moments.

REPLACING THE REAR DERAILLEUR CABLE

1 Remove the old cable. Watch where the cable routing goes and where it comes out so that you can refit it later. With Shimano RapidFire gears you may need to unscrew the cover of the shifter. Don't lose the little screw — it's an unusual size.

2 Put the chain on the middle ring at the front, and check that the rear derailleur hangs vertically. If it doesn't you won't be able to adjust the indexing later.

3 Set the end-stop screws. It's easier to do this now than later after the cable is fitted. Then, if you find, for example, that the chain won't drop into the small ring, you'll know that it's because the cable is sticking, or the lever is broken.

4 Screw in the "H" end-stop screw five or six turns (or as far as possible) and turn the pedals. You'll find that the chain won't drop down into the smallest ring, because you've deliberately screwed the end-stop in a long way. Keep pedaling, unscrewing the "H" screw as you go. Gradually, you'll see the derailleur moving and dragging the chain toward the smallest sprocket. This is a slow motion version of what happens when you change gear. Whenever the chain is midway between the sprockets, it'll clatter noisily,

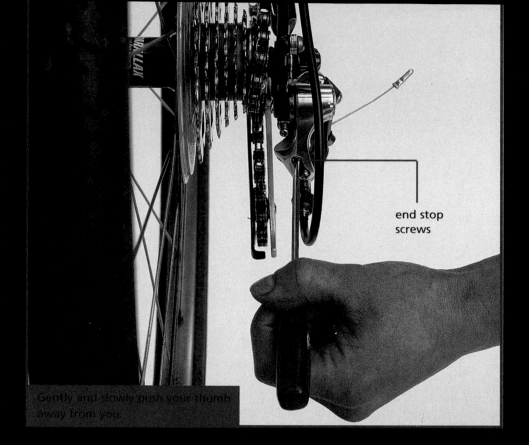

end stop
screws

Gently and slowly push your thumb
away from you.

the same sound you hear when you ride with badly adjusted gears. When you unscrew further, the chain will drop into the smallest sprocket. Continue unscrewing until the chain sits evenly across the smallest sprocket, then unscrew a tiny bit further — less than a quarter of a turn.

5 Next, set the "L" end-stop screw, which prevents the chain from jumping over the largest sprocket into the spokes. This is a little trickier. Setting the "H" screw is easy, because the spring always pulls the cable back toward the smallest sprocket. However, shifting toward the largest sprocket, it's the cable that does the work, but, because you've removed the cable, you'll have to shift the derailleur by hand.

Turn the pedals with your right hand, and hold the derailleur with your left hand, as shown; first finger behind the barrel adjuster, thumb at the front of the derailleur, ahead of the forward pivot points. Curl your other fingers into your palm, to keep them out of the way of the chain and sprockets. Push your thumb away from you, gently and slowly. As you pedal, the chain will lift toward the largest sprocket imitating the action of the cable. Play with it, find out what happens. Don't push too far, or the chain may jump over the last sprocket.

Give the "L" screw five or six turns, then try to push the chain on to the largest ring, while pedaling. If it will not go, unscrew it a little. Keep testing and unscrewing until the chain drops easily on to the largest ring, then unscrew it a little bit — less than a quarter of a turn.

6 Now you're ready to fit and adjust the gear cable. Grease the end of the cable and its nipple. The cable should be oiled before being pushed into the housing to keep it running smoothly. The housing should

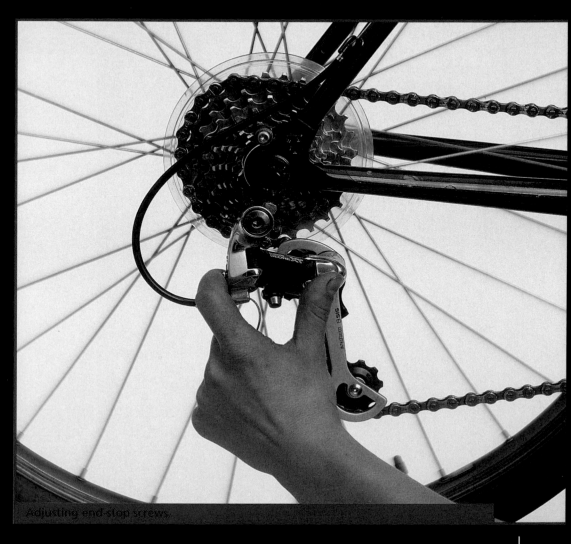

Adjusting end-stop screws.

always be Teflon-lined. Gore-Tex cables are also smooth, and don't need lubrication.

7 Once you've fitted the cable into the lever, put gentle pressure on the end of the cable and test the action of the lever by clicking up and down through the gears. This can save some head-scratching later on, because if the lever doesn't work properly now, it won't be any better when the cable's attached to the derailleur! Place some tension on the cable by pulling it out of the lever — when you shift, you should distinctly feel each click. Leave the lever in the highest gear position, ready for tightening.

8 Fit all the sections of cable housing together, with an endcap on each end, and oil as you go. Make sure all the sections of cable housing are just long enough so that the cable is not forced around any tight corners, and so that the bars can turn easily, but without excess. One way of doing this is to cut new housing to the same length as the old housing, assuming it was the right length. Check the cable as you slide it into each section of housing. If, once the cable is tightened, it doesn't work, you'll have to go back and check each piece of housing anyway. The last section of housing, at the rear derailleur, is the most exposed and needs replacing most often. Cracks in the old housing where it inserts into the derailleur mean it wasn't quite long enough.

9 Take up any slack in the cable by feeding it into the cable clamp bolt on the bottom of the derailleur, making use of the little groove either in the washer or on the derailleur. Tighten the bolt. Turn the pedals and change gears up to the largest sprocket — or the largest sprocket it will reach — and then change them back down again to the smallest sprocket. You haven't adjusted the cable tension yet, so the indexing won't work properly, but the cable is settled into

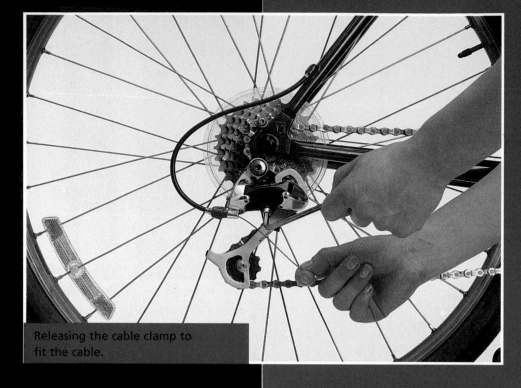

Releasing the cable clamp to fit the cable.

place. Or, pull the cable through the derailleur with pliers, which may fray the cable end.

10 Test how the gears work. Moving the lever or rotating the barrel adjuster at the back of the derailleur one way pulls the cable, moving it the other way releases it, folding and unfolding the derailleur, shifting the jockey wheels and moving the chain over the sprockets.

ADJUSTING THE INDEXING

To test the gears, move the lever one click; the chain should move exactly one sprocket, but it probably won't the first time. If it doesn't move far enough, the cable is too slack, so

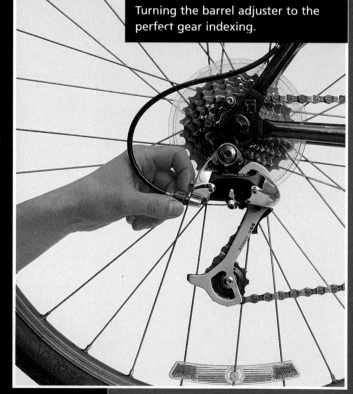

Turning the barrel adjuster to the perfect gear indexing.

tighten it with the barrel adjuster. Fine tune the derailleur by putting your thumb on the barrel adjuster, then roll the barrel with your thumb moving in the direction you want the chain to go. If the cable shifts more than one sprocket when you move the lever one click, release the cable tension by rotating the barrel adjuster back in. If you reach the limit that the barrel adjuster will turn, return it to its center position and adjust the cable tension using the clamp bolt. Then fine tune again with the barrel adjuster. Once you're done, the chain should move quickly and precisely between sprockets when you click the gear levers. Experiment with adjusting the barrel position until shifting is perfect.

THE FRONT DERAILLEUR

1 Check if the front derailleur is parallel to the outer chainring. Check that there is sufficient clearance between it and the chainrings — a couple of millimetres is perfect.
2 To set the cable tension, put the lever in the smallest ring position. Take up the slack by unclamping the cable bolt on the derailleur, pulling the cable through, and reclamping the bolt. Change up to the largest ring, then back down to the smallest to settle the cable. Pull the cable through the clamp bolt again to take up any slack. At its slackest the cable should be just taut.
3 Check your end-stop adjustment by changing onto the largest and smallest rings. If the chain can't move as far out as the largest ring, undo the "H" end-stop screw. If the chain falls off the outside of the chainset, screw the H screw in a little bit. Adjust the "L" end-stop screw the same way.
4 If the front derailleur is indexed you'll have to set that, too. Put the rear gear into the smallest sprocket, then shift the front lever from the smallest ring position to the middle ring. If the chain won't lift, there isn't

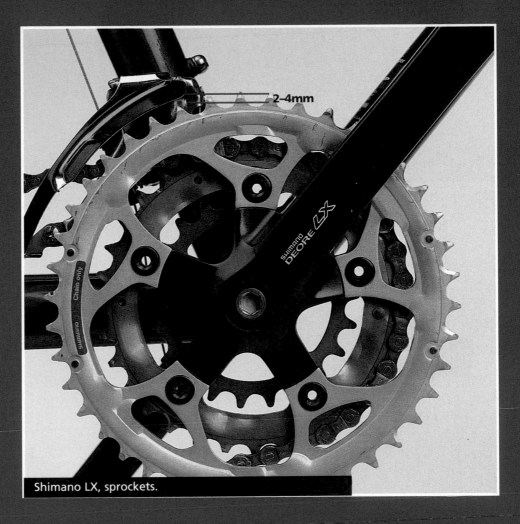

Shimano LX, sprockets.

enough tension in the front gear cable. Undo the barrel adjuster on the lever to increase tension. Test until the chain lifts easily on to the middle ring. Put the chain on a middle sprocket at the back and the middle ring at the front. Adjust the barrel until the ring sits evenly between the plates on the chain.

NEW CABLES

A new cable stretches slightly and the cable housing settles into the cable stops, so, after you a while, you'll need to adjust the cable again. Repeat for setting the indexing. Put cable ends on the end of all your cables to avoid fraying, and test before going riding.

ROAD TESTING

Gears always work differently when you actually ride the bike than when the bike is on the stand. It may take several test runs before your gears are perfectly adjusted.

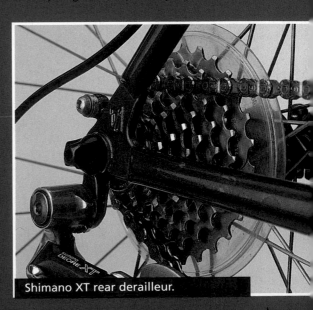

Shimano XT rear derailleur.

maintaining bearings

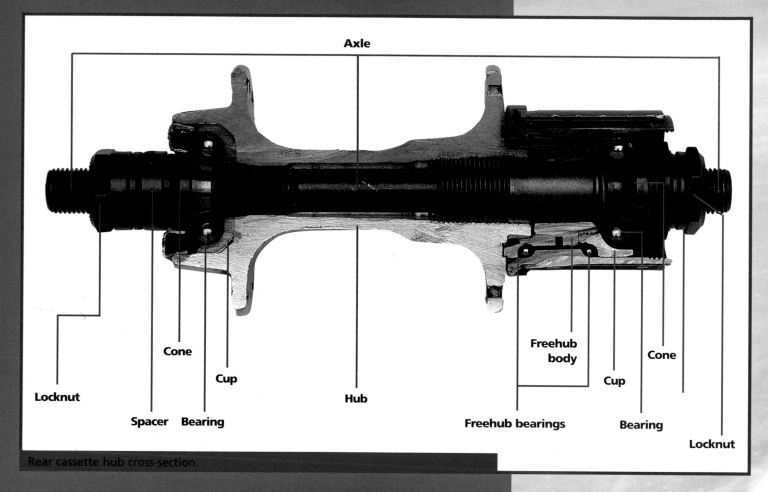

Axle

Cone

Cup

Freehub
body

Cone

Locknut

Hub

Cup

Spacer   Bearing

Freehub bearings

Bearing

Locknut

Rear cassette hub cross-section.

There are four major sets of bearings on your bike — front wheel, back wheel, headset and bottom bracket. Each allows a part of the bike to rotate freely. The wheels and bottom bracket have to be able to spin, but without side-to-side movement. Headsets need to turn easily without rocking back and forth. All bearing units work on the same principles; the cone is adjusted to hold the ball bearings in place and is prevented from slipping out of place by a locknut.

The cups and cones should provide as friction-less a surface as possible for the bearings. If the cones come even slightly loose, they rub against the bearing surfaces every time they come into play, making little pits. Once a tiny pit has formed, each ball falls into it every time it goes around, and the pits grow bigger. Loose cones wear all the bearing surfaces very quickly.

REAR CASSETTE HUB

The cutaway image of a rear cassette hub (above) shows how cones work. The two sets of larger bearings support the wheel, each sitting in a little cup with visible outward-facing edges. The two cones are screwed onto opposite ends of the axle, so that they come to rest against the balls. The balls are trapped between the cup and the cone, able only to run around and around in

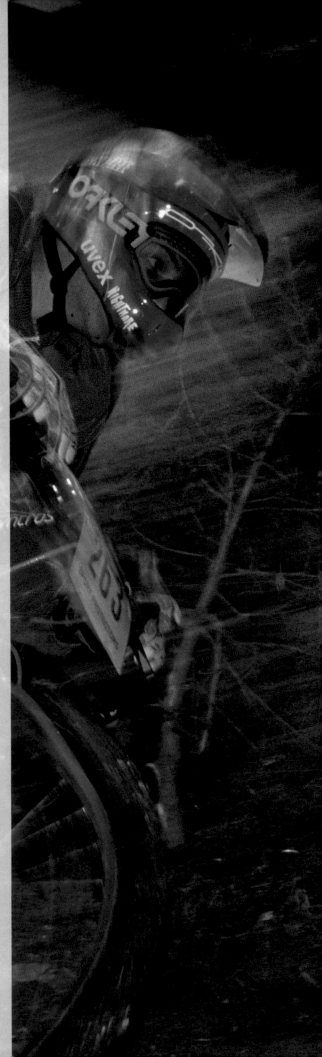

CONE WRENCHES
Take your bike with you to the bike shop when you buy cone wrenches to make sure you get the right size. Front cones are usually smaller than back cones.

their allotted space. Once the cone spins freely without play, a locknut is wedged against it to hold it in place.

CLEANING AND REFITTING THE FRONT HUB BEARING

This is the most accessible example of how to clean and refit bearings, and the principles can be applied to all the other bearing units.

1 Remove the front wheel, and the quick-release skewer if there is one. The cone and locknut are wedged together, so firstly you need to release them. The cone is the section nearest the wheel, and will probably have two flat surfaces. It's very thin, so use cone wrenches instead of regular wrenches.

2 Fit the cone wrench firmly on to the cone. With another wrench, grip the locknut (the outer-most nut on the axle). Keep the cone wrench still, unscrew the locknut. Watch you don't scrape your knuckles on the spokes.

3 Once the first locknut has been released, transfer the cone wrench to the second cone — this will keep the axle steady. Wind off the loosened first locknut. Remove any washers and lay them beside the locknut. Now transfer the wrench to the opposite locknut and hold the axle steady that way. Use the cone wrench to remove the loose cone. You can now gently pull the axle out of the hub, with one cone, washer and locknut still firmly attached.

4 Hold the wheel flat, with a jar under the hub. Knock the bearings into the jar — a small screwdriver is useful for this.

5 Clean the cups and cones and inspect them. There should be no pits at all in either cup or cone. The track of the ball bearings should not be more than $\frac{1}{8}$in (2mm) wide. Replace worn or pitted cones or bearings. If the cone attached to the axle is not worn, there's no need to remove it. If you need to get parts, take an old bearing to the bike store, so you know its size. Grease the cups, ensuring you cover the bearing tracks. Put the same number of new bearings on each side — up to their middles in grease.

6 Slide the axle back through the hub, ensuring you don't dislodge any bearings. Screw the loose cone carefully back on to the axle. Start it off by hand, then, holding the loose cone with the cone wrench, wind the axle through, using the ring wrench on the fixed locknut. Don't push the cone, let it rest against the bearings. Slide the washers on and, still holding the axle with the cone wrench on the fixed cone, wind on the loose locknut until it rests against the washers.

7 Adjust the cone carefully, aiming for no play from a freely spinning wheel. Lock the cone by wedging the locknut against it. This must be done carefully, as the cone tends to move when the locknut becomes wedged against it. When you think the setting is about right, replace the wheel in the frame and spin it. There may be play at the rim that can't be felt at the axle. If so, try again!

wheel maintenance

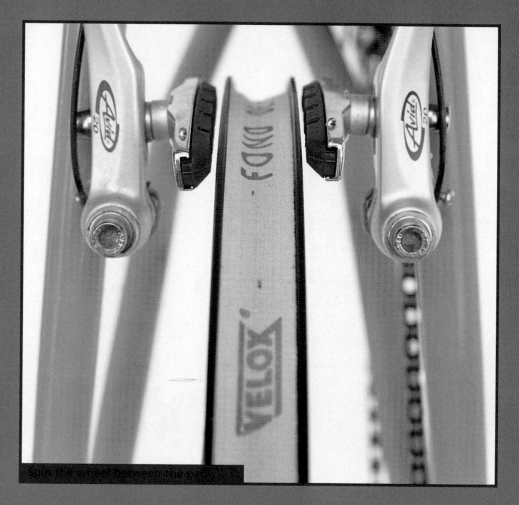
Spin the wheel between the pads

The best wheels are those you don't even have to think about — and if the attention they do get is high-quality, then they shouldn't need much of it. Wheels need slow and gentle work, working in small adjustments. Don't rush the job — more wheels are destroyed through misplaced enthusiasm than misunderstanding the technique. Deal with your wheel as soon as it becomes a bit wobbly. That way you should only have to adjust one or two spokes. The longer you

ride on an out-of-shape wheel, the more resistant it becomes to returning to a circle.

TRUING A WHEEL

There are three steps in truing wheels:

1 True

A true wheel has no side-to-side wobble as you spin it.

2 Hop

A round wheel has no up-and-down movement as you spin it.

3 Dish

A dished wheel sits centrally in the frame, equidistant between the two stays.

TRUING

Truing the wheels means balancing the tension of the spokes so that the rim sits in the middle. It's a little like a tug-of-war, with half the spokes pulling to the right and half pulling to the left. When the two teams are evenly matched, the rim will stay still even though both sides are pulling hard.

Truing is best done on a truing stand. However, most people don't have one kicking around at home, so here's how to do it with the wheel on the bike.

1 Start with the rear wheel. Remove the tire and tube and replace the wheel on the bike. Suspend the bike so that you can spin the wheel. Sit behind it, so that you have a view similar to the one shown here. Spin the wheel, to get an idea of its condition. Concentrate on the part of the rim that you can see between the brake pads and use the pads as reference points. You'll see some side-to-side movement and some up-and-down movement. The wheel may not sit centrally, either.

2 Deal with the trueness of the wheel first. Find the section of the rim with the biggest wobble. Pull it toward you, and look at a section of the rim about five spokes long. Look past the rim at the hub. You will see spokes falling away from the rim, toward the hub. Half fall to one side, half to the other. As you

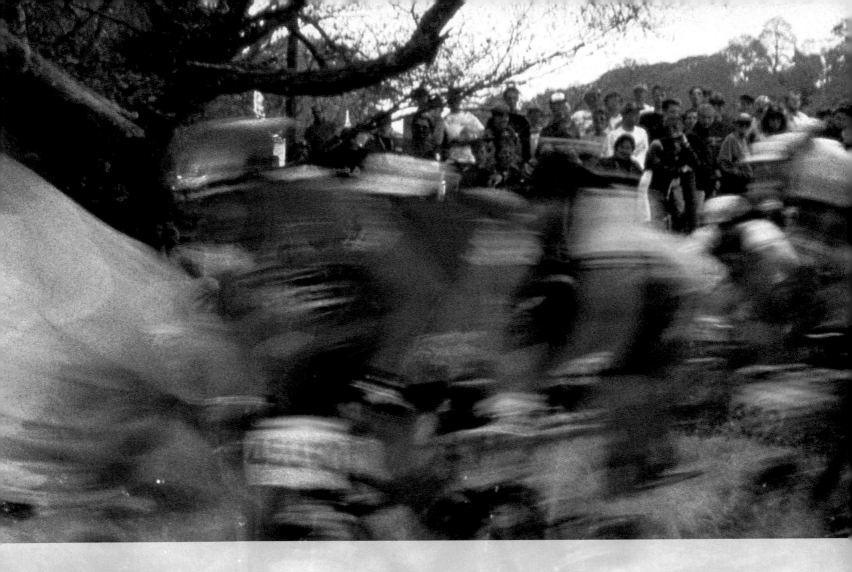

look at the wheel from this angle, it's clear that tightening (shortening) the spokes that go to the right-hand side of the hub and loosening those that go to the left will pull that portion of the rim to the right, and vice versa.

3 Spin the wheel again to get an indication of how true the wheel is. Just observe at first. Isolate the largest side-to-side wobble. Work in quarter turns of the spoke key and, with a spoke wrench, loosen the spoke on the outside of the bulge, then tighten the two on the inside.

4 The spoke is essentially a long screw. It's attached to a funny-shaped nut, the nipple, which has a normal thread that tightens and loosens in the same direction as any other. Choose a spoke wrench that fits firmly on the nipple. A loose one will round it off, making it harder to turn. Don't be surprised if you get confused at first about which way the nipple should be turned.

5 Always work on the largest wobble first. Then spin the wheel and work on wherever the largest wobble is again. It may be in the same place.

HOPPING

When you've removed the worst side-to-side wobble, work on the hop in the wheel. Spin and watch how the wheel passes above the brake pads. Isolate the areas where the rim is most oval. You'll have to spin and watch several times to get an idea of the normal position of the rim. Concentrate on the largest bumps and tighten about four adjacent spokes in that area. Spin the wheel again and repeat the process. When you've smoothed the worst of the hops, work on the truing again.

DISHING

Finally, have a look at the dishing. The wheel has to sit centrally in the frame. To test it, remove the wheel and place it in the dropout the other way around. A dished wheel will sit in the same place whichever way it's fitted. If it sits too far to one side, you'll have to loosen all the spokes on that side and tighten all the spokes on the other, as if it was one big wobble. You may have to test the wheel several times. Remember that it's much better to work in quarter turns of the spoke wrench, and go around the wheel many times — putting less strain on the rim.

Once you've dished the wheel you'll probably find you have to work on the truing and the hop again. When all is said and done, you'll have to go over the whole wheel three or four times. Repeat the process until you're satisfied and finish with a true.

long life for chains, sprockets & chainrings

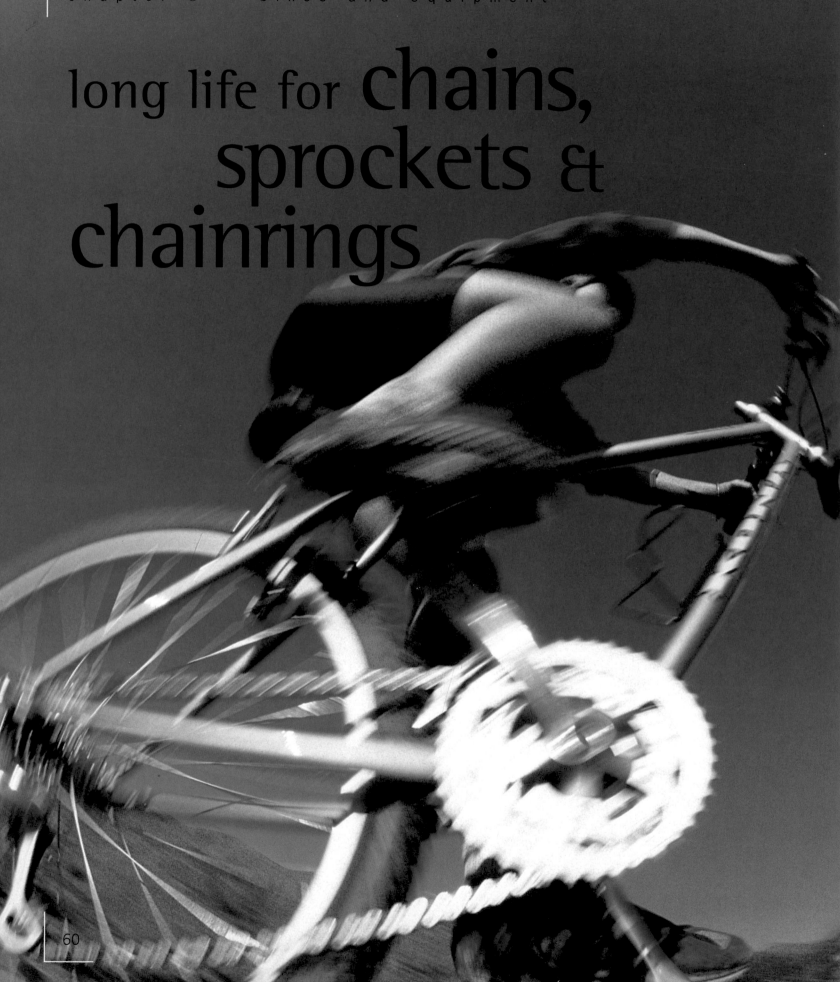

Like any bicycle components, chains, sprockets and cassettes will need regular attention. The amount of time you spend looking after them will pay for itself in performance and lifespan.

THE CHAIN DILEMMA

There is a problem with chains. You need oil on them, because it reduces friction, which wears down both the bike's surfaces and your legs. The flip side of this is that lubricants attract the abrasive dirt that's thrown up by the wheels, which only makes things worse. However, you can minimize the problem if you follow these three steps.

1 Clean
2 Lubricate
3 Wipe off excess lubricant.

The facts of friction

Look closely at the chain. Sit beside the bike and rotate the pedals backward. Watch a couple of links as they pass over the sprockets. Notice how each chain roller drops into a valley between two teeth and remains in there as the sprocket rotates. The roller can rotate independently around the pin. You can see this if you roll one over the end of a screwdriver — the chain doesn't need to slide over the surface of the sprocket. It just drops into the valley at the top of the cassette, and drops out at the bottom. The roller pushes against the tooth, which forces the sprocket and the wheel around — it doesn't slide. No sliding, no friction.

Friction plays a role elsewhere. Watch a section of chain again, but this time watch two adjoining chain plates. As they approach the sprocket, they're in line. As they move around the block, they twist and then return to a straight line.

EXPERIMENTAL FRICTION

Now, place your palms together. Push gently, then twist your hands against each other, as if they were two links of chain. They soon become warm because of the friction that develops between them. However, now try repeating the experiment with soapy hands. The soap acts in a similar way to a lubricant, so your hands don't get as warm as they would without it. Friction not only occurs in the chain plates, but between the pin and the roller as well, when it turns to accommodate the valley between the sprocket teeth.

The parts of the chain that are really exposed to dirt — where the rollers touch the sprockets — don't slide over each other, so there's no need for the sprockets to be covered in dirt-attracting oil. The places where most friction occurs, in between the plates and inside the rollers, are relatively protected. Big pieces of dirt can't get into the small gaps between plates, which are, fortunately, perfect size for sucking oil to where it's most needed, by capillary action.

That explains the instructions that come with good oil — the ones that everybody ignores — about wiping off the excess. Most of the oil is needed inside the rollers and between the plates. Oil left on the outside attracts dirt, and only increases wear. If you wipe the oil off after applying it, the chain is left with a thin layer of oil that's enough to prevent corrosion, but not enough for dirt to stick to. Cleaning the chain primarily stops too much oil sticking to it, and helps the oil to slide between the plates. Better quality oil is designed to be sucked into small gaps.

CHAIN AND SPROCKET COMPATIBILITY

To work properly, the chain and sprocket have to have a precise, matching shape.

Nevertheless, they will wear, especially as the chain stretches. Once the chain and sprocket have lost their complimentary shapes, the wear accelerates. The stretched chain wears the sprockets and the worn sprockets stretch the chain. The chain becomes less efficient and eventually will have stretched too much to grip the teeth of the sprocket. So it'll skip over them. If this happens, a new, unstretched chain won't fit old worn sprockets, and vice versa, so sprockets and chains should always be replaced at the same time.

MEASURING WEAR AND TEAR

There are ways of measuring the wear in a chain, so that you can change it before it wears the sprockets. Each link is 1 inch (approximately 25mm) long. Like many other bicycle components, the links are conventionally measured in inches. So, when it's new, twelve links will measure exactly 12in (30.5cm). When a chain has stretched enough that it measures 12⅛in (30.8cm), both the chain and cassette should be replaced.

Measuring gauges that check chain wear are available from Park and Rohloff — Rohloff's appears to be a piece of modern art that can be used for measuring chain wear on the side!

CARE OF SPROCKETS AND CHAINRINGS

The best thing you can do for sprockets and chainrings is to keep them clean. Remove as much of the dirt in the valleys between the teeth as possible. To get them really clean, take the rings off the chainset. Some sprocket cassettes will separate into individual sprockets, which makes it a lot easier to remove the crud.

the principle of upgrading

A standard mountain bike is a naturally sophisticated thing, but you can replace some parts with better ones, as often as you want. You can upgrade components when they wear out; or earlier if the replacements are more efficient, comfortable, easier to use or even prettier. The beauty of the bicycle is its alterability. With a few tools and a little experience, a bike can be stripped to the frame and rebuilt with different parts in a few hours. Once a bike can perform the full quota of off-road tasks to a high standard, the return from upgrading diminishes and then it's down to looks.

Saving weight

Lightweight equipment is always preferable: the lighter the bike, the faster you go and the less energy you use, which is particularly helpful when climbing. Because the mountain bike has much more rolling resistance than a road bike — its average speed is only around 10mph (16km/h) as opposed to around 16mph (25km/h) — every little bit counts off-road. You can feel the difference between an 25lb (11kg) and a 30lb (13.5kg) MTB bike.

The better the bike, the more difficult it is to save significant amounts of weight with individual parts, especially if you take the total weight of the bike and rider into account. Women benefit slightly more from weight-saving than men.

In cross-country bikes it's become acceptable to sacrifice a little weight to gain the speed and control advantages of suspension, to make you go faster overall. The best practical advice when buying lightweight equipment is to fit components from manufacturers with a good reputation. Heavier riders in particular should avoid the lightest parts, especially handlebars. In downhilling, the aims are greater strength — in the frame, brakes and wheels — to handle longer suspension, without much concern for weight.

Priority upgrades

The lower the quality of the bike you start with, the greater the improvement if you upgrade it. The converse is also true; the higher the quality of the part you start with, the smaller the improvement will be.

CHEAPER BIKES

Priorities for upgrading mountain bikes below the $800 mark should be tires (for lighter weight), pedals (to SPD clipless), brake type and brake pads (for more power), and wheel rims (to reduce rolling mass).

PERFORMANCE TRAIL BIKES

Upgrading bikes over the $800 benchmark will produce a significantly better working machine in a number of ways. Upgrade the suspension fork, to save weight. Fit disc brakes, for more power and better wet-weather braking. Fit a stronger, lighter handlebar and stem.

Then there's slimmer, lighter SPD pedals, lighter tires, wheels with narrow gauge spokes and slim rims. The cranks can be beefed up and lightened, and so can the seat post. The variety of high-quality saddles is excellent, with lightweight rails and padded genital areas, or gaps. Or how about a new paint job and some fresh logos?

DOWNHILL BIKES

Visual strength and suspension travel are what the downhill bike's about, and there are a number of changes you can make to their componentry. Starting at the front, try the latest longer-travel suspension fork, or a beefier stem and handlebar. Put a fatter hub on the wheel to handle the awesome disc brakes and heavy twist exerted by the fork. Switch pedals to bigger, flatter platforms. Or move up to a long slim jump saddle, etc…

Customizing and experimentation

Upgrading means customizing, so what starts out as a model number on an

> **UPGRADE YOURSELF!**
> Being in shape is the single greatest improvement you can make to your riding efficiency; think of it in terms of strength, and weighing less yourself — this is known as your power-to-weight ratio.

assembly line becomes unique to you. A lot of it is about creating an identity for your own bike. At first, off-road groupsets followed the aerodynamic looks of Campagnolo's traditional road-racing components. Cross-country equipment may still look little different but downhill componentry takes its cues from the world of motocross bikes, not the Tour de France. Improving your bike yourself does require a bit of mechanical experience. Don't make mistakes on expensive pieces of equipment. For example, don't strip the threads on CNC-cut aluminum cranks. Learn on a basic bike, and move on to high quality parts only when you're confident you can do the job right.

A lot of upgrading has to do with experimentation. For every lasting mechanical improvement that comes out of MTB development there are dozens of dead ends. Trick equipment is made using new materials and/or new manufacturing methods. It can be practical, decorative or both, but it may not be essential. The parts seller is making a small contribution to the development process, but they're making a much larger contribution to the national economy.

When is it time for a new bike?

The price of better quality frames and parts is continually dropping. So, over time, it's not really worth spending more than a half or two-thirds of the original price of a bike on improving it — even to keep it up-to-date and on par with its original quality. If the parts become too good for the frame, it's time for a new bike. You may even decide to build your own bike — most manufacturers sell the frames of their best-selling models separately. This lets you choose your own individual components, right down to the last bolt. But it's never cheaper than buying a complete bike.

SAMPLE WEIGHT SAVINGS
AVERAGE WEIGHTS

Woman		132lb	(60kg)
Average bike	+	28lb	(12.5kg)
Woman on bike total	=	160lb	(72.5kg)
Man		154lb	(70kg)
Average bike	+	28lb	(12.5kg)
Man on bike total	=	183lb	(82.5kg)

SUSPENSION FORK

Average weight	3¼lb	(1.5kg)
Lightest/heaviest	2½–4lb	(1.1–1.8kg)
WOMAN		
% total bike/rider weight:	2%	
% bike weight:	11.3%	
Maximum % total rider/bike variation:	+/- 0.5%	
MAN		
% total bike/rider weight:	1.8%	
% bike weight:	11.3%	
Maximum % total rider/bike variation:	+/- 0.4%	

SINGLE TIRE

Average weight:	3¼lb	(1.5kg)
Lightest/heaviest:	1lb–1lb 12oz	(450g–800g)
WOMAN		
% total bike/rider weight:	0.9%	
% bike weight:	4.8%	
Maximum % total rider/bike variation:	+/- 0.3%	
MAN		
% total bike/rider weight:	0.8%	
% bike weight:	4.8%	
Maximum % total rider/bike variation:	+/- 0.2%	

HEADSET

Average weight:	1lb 7oz	(625g)
Lightest/heaviest:	1lb–1lb 12oz	(450g–800g)
WOMAN		
% Total bike/rider weight:	0.2%	
% Bike weight:	1.2%	
Maximum % total rider/bike variation:	+/- 0.06%	
MAN		
% total bike/rider weight:	0.18%	
% bike weight:	1.2%	
Maximum % total rider/bike variation:	+/- 0.06%	

upgrading tires

Mountain bikers would argue that in terms of evolutionary importance the creation of the knobby tire runs a close second behind the first fish that dragged itself on to dry land. The 26-in (650C) tire is the signature of the sport. Its deep, grippy tread carries you faithfully through slime and over rock. The tires you choose affect the bike's handling and your comfort, because the rubber provides a mountain bike with built-in suspension.

Cheap and easy to change, tires are the easiest thing to upgrade for performance and versatility — especially if your MTB leads a double life as a working vehicle on the road, and a rugged off-road warrior.

Mountain biking has witnessed the rise of the humble tire from a grubby basic into a big-business accessory. It's a lot of fun poring over catalogues and touching new rubber in the bike shop. But most knobbies do the off-road job fine. For fine-tuning, what counts is the overall tread pattern, tire compound and the air pressure.

WEAR AND TEAR

The bite of a brand-new knobby tire adds excitement and confidence to the ride. Like new balls in a tennis game, the best racers will put on new tires way before the old ones wear out.

If you're strapped for cash, choose a long-life tire with a good, hard compound, designed for muddy conditions, and change to slick tires when you ride the bike on pavement. Don't be deceived by the treads, which tend to outlive the trendiness of their pattern and the sidewalls. Although there is no law that requires you to replace tires regularly, the inner tubes will squeeze through threadbare sidewalls long before the tread wears out, and will explode, giving you an unexpected shock.

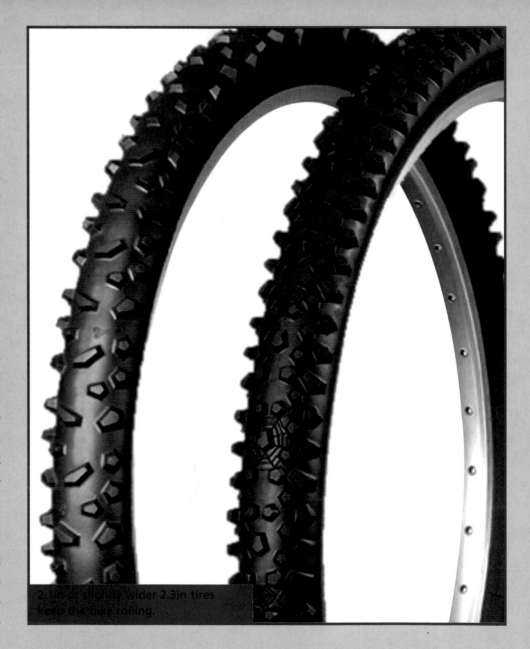

2.1in or slightly wider 2.3in tires keep the bike rolling.

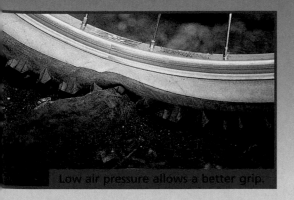
Low air pressure allows a better grip.

WEIGHT

Tires weigh 18–28oz (500–800g) and it's worth paying for lighter ones. It's a simple ratio of weight to force or effort. The force (effort) needed to accelerate anything is proportional to its mass. On a bike, the rider is constantly trying to accelerate the wheel to overpower his or her weight, gravity, rolling resistance and air resistance.

Since the tire is on the outside of the wheel it has to be moved further than the rim and requires greater acceleration; so this is a really important place to consider getting lightweight replacements. The forces in a spinning wheel create a strong and rigid structure, and this is what makes moving downhill at high speeds over rocks and rough ground possible.

ROLLING RESISTANCE

Tires are designed with the objective of minimizing the area of contact with the ground to keep down the rolling resistance while maintaining grip. That's why tires vary

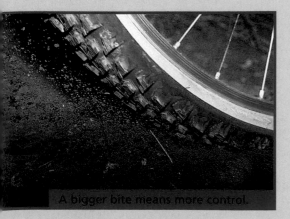
A bigger bite means more control.

according to the surface they're tackling. Road tires are thin and smooth for a small area of contact and low rolling resistance. Off-road tires need to be much more versatile, to dig into soft ground, bridge gaps and cushion the rider against bumps. The idea of minimizing rolling resistance still applies, but as the roughness slows a mountain bike down to half the speed of a road bike, it plays a less important role in off-road tire design than grip.

When conditions are slippery, higher rolling resistance is actually what you want! So we have the 3in (75mm) tractor tire, which is designed with a deep tread to dig in to soft mud and to protect the bike and rider from some of the roughness of the tracks.

AIR PRESSURE

The simplest, quickest way to alter the way your bike handles is to change the air pressure in the tires. In road racing, high performance tires are pumped up as high as 80–100psi, which means minimal rolling resistance and a sore butt. But, off-road riding needs softer tires to handle rougher terrain and the jolts, especially if the bike has no suspension.

Keep within the recommended pressure limits; you'll find them written on the side of the tire. The lower pressure limit is as soft as a car tire, around 35psi, which is best for slippery conditions.

The upper limit should be around 55psi — which is suitable for hard, dry riding. Tradition says the rear tire should be harder than the front to account for the rider's weight: it's a rule worth observing.

TIRE FEATURES

■ For fewer flats, lighter weight and less twisting, choose a tire with a layer of Kevlar beading. It's a carbon-based barrier material that's also used in the construction of

bulletproof vests. Kevlar tires are easier to put on and they fold easily, so that they can be strapped to a pannier if you're out for a longer ride.

■ Directional tires have an asymmetric pattern, which is similar in design to a chevron. These tires are designed to roll in one direction only. The direction usually depends on whether the tire is placed on the front or rear wheel. Follow the arrow on the sidewall, and expect to think twice to get it right.

■ Some tires are sold in co-ordinated pairs with different characteristics for the front and rear. The best combination is a narrower front tire with a round profile for smooth, controlled cornering, and a chunky square rear tire for stability and deeper grip.

■ Downhill competition tires are the monsters of the family, and have the deep tread and wide print of motocross tires. Their purpose is to be flat-resistant and super grippy. Because of that, they're deeper, broader and heavier than other tires.

MUD-CLEARING
Centrifugal force flings mud off the tires when the ground slaps it on, which is handy. Some designers say that more widely-spaced knobs mean better self-cleaning, but it's probably the terrain and speed which decide how much mud gets left behind on your rubber. No tire, however wide its tread, can perform the impossible. When terrain is drying out, dirt is at its stickiest and the most aggressive tread may become a smooth, skidding slick. If this happens, it's time to stop and get scraping with your fingers.

which brake?

RIM V-BRAKES AND CANTILEVERS ▶

Brakes that grip the rim of the wheel are standard on mountain bikes, although the disc brake, which was adapted from motocross bikes, is essential on downhill bikes and also makes regular appearances on trail and cross-country bikes.

Road bike rim brakes with arms that straddle the tire are lighter, but they're too weak over the double-width of a mountain bike tire to be effective for off-road riding. Disc brakes work better than rim brakes in wet conditions, but nevertheless the humble rim brake remains the best design in terms of cost, power and easy maintenance.

By upgrading to models made from better materials, it's possible to save a bit of weight and increase the rigidity for stronger braking. If you're switching from older can-

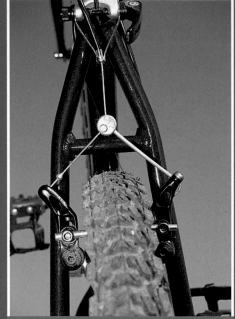

The old-style cantilever brake.

tilever brakes to newer V-brakes, you'll also have to switch your brake levers to a compatible model.

Despite all the efforts of the bike industry, no one has defeated Mother Nature's obstacle to good rim braking — wet weather. Braking distances triple in rain and this means that a lot of bikers in the world's temperate climates are affected for a lot of the time. It's dangerous on the road, and means spicy handling off it.

You can make a slight improvement in your wet-weather braking performance by increasing the area of contact with the rim, by using a longer brake pad or softer compound in the pads; but the trade-off is that the pad wears down quickly, even in a single day if the conditions are very wet and gritty.

ANTI-SKID IDEAS
When wheels lock up and go into a skid, the rider loses control. Designers have tried different ways of slowing down the force on the brake pad as it nears maximum clench to prevent the problem. This has been done mostly by increasing the leverage both at the lever and the V-brake arms to enable more gradual braking, but none of the designs have become standard. Outside the design studio, on the trail, it's up to the rider to use the brakes with skill.

DISC BRAKES ▶

Disc brakes are the most powerful of all brake types. They have a center-wheel disc with enclosed brake pads and mechanism, attached by an extra boss at the frame or fork dropout. They aren't affected by wheels that are out of true, and they fit unconventional downhill and playbike frames that don't have back stays that can be mounted on.

Disc brakes fall into two types, The first is designed for general trail riding, with a smaller disc and a lighter sub-14oz (400g) weight. They release immediately so you can remove the wheel as you normally would to fix a flat or load the bike into a car in minutes.

The second, heavier type is for hardcore downhilling. The disc is much larger in diameter, for greater leverage, and the hub

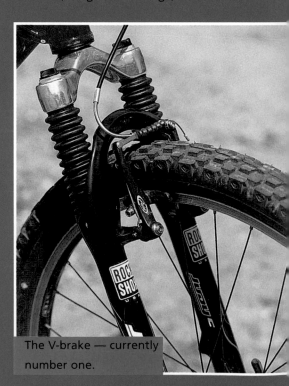

The V-brake — currently number one.

will be up to ⅝in (20mm) in diameter. You need a wrench to undo them and remove the wheel. A number of manufacturers now supply their bikes with disc brakes, and many more construct bikes with mounts so you can install them yourself.

STYLES THAT DIDN'T MAKE IT

The mountain bike brake has evolved a lot during its relatively short life. The brakes that the first mountain bikers relied on when hurtling downhill were coaster drum brakes. The mechanism was housed internally at the center of the wheels and riders had to back-pedal to push plates out to slow the wheel down. In use all of the way down the mountain, they became burning hot and had to be repacked with grease every run. Coasters never made it near a manufactured mountain bike. They were impossible to maintain and inefficient. Can you imagine World Cup downhillers in the start gate not being able to press forward on the pedals with the brakes on, ready to spring out onto the course?

The earliest Cannondale MTBs had rim brakes operated by a pair of small rollers, but they were replaced almost immediately by cantilevers, which have now been taken over by V-brakes.

Shimano spent some time in the R&D department with drum rollerbrakes, which were similar to those on cars. The design had a few advantages: the mechanism was housed inside a drum, which protected it from mud or water. Braking was still perfect when other riders slipped and it was touted as maintenance-free (theoretically). But, ultimately, the drum brakes were too heavy, and the rollers were inaccessible when something did go wrong. So the design never made it big.

A better brake

The poor braking of an imitation mountain bike alone is a good enough reason to save up for the real thing. The steel rims and flexing arms of the brakes on cheap bikes weaken the braking to the point where safety can't be guaranteed when you are riding off-road.

Most good mountain bikes on the market have functional, conventional Shimano V-brakes. An upgrade simply means installing a pair from the next groupset up in the line.

CABLES OR HYDRAULICS?

There are two ways to get the power from the brake lever to the braking mechanism: it can be mediated by regular cable or by funky hydraulic tubing.

Cables are simpler, with high grade wire and housing now also available. However, they're still likely to fray and rust. They have be kept clean for the brakes to work properly.

The hydraulic method uses oil-filled tubes and, even though it's more complex, it gives better braking. It's unaffected by mud, but the oil pressure in the tubes has to be kept high, and this needs to be done at home, and not while you're on the trail. Hydraulic cabling is generally more expensive as well.

A small number of hydraulic rim brakes are still kicking around, but almost all rim V-brakes (see previous page) are cable-operated now.

BRAKE TIPS
■ The best brake levers have a short, kinked design for two-, or even one-finger braking and require a smooth-running cable or hydraulics.

■ The rear brake is not as efficient as the front brake, because the force from your hand on the lever has to travel along three times as much cable before it reaches the pads, and through twice as much grit and kinking. Make sure the cable routing is as direct as possible and change to a housing with a low-friction liner, made from PTFE or Gore-Tex.

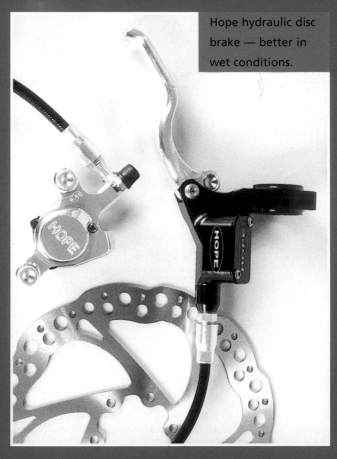

Hope hydraulic disc brake — better in wet conditions.

upgrading
gear shifters

The choice of three styles

There are three different styles of mountain bike gear lever. They all use slightly different finger and wrist movements for the same end result. Levers come in pairs, one to activate the front derailleur and one for the rear derailleur and it's standard for them to be "indexed". That means the lever "clicks" into the right position every time you change gear.

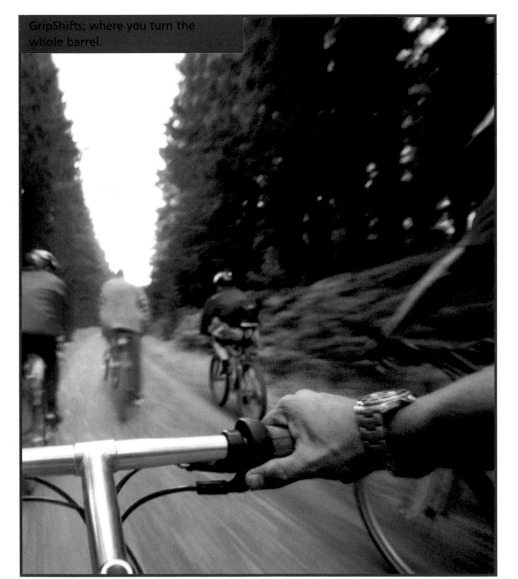

GripShifts; where you turn the whole barrel.

Mountain bike gear levers are mounted on the handlebars. It makes the bikes easier to ride, and is a development that has now spread to road and hybrid bikes. The levers sit within reach of your fingers and thumbs when they rest on the grips, so that, in theory, you can hang on, change gear and brake all at once, without moving your hand position at all.

Besides slight differences in price and availability, the type of gear lever you choose is a matter of taste because each has its own strong points. If you don't have a preference, there is no need to change the version that comes with your new bike.

◀ GRIPSHIFT

Your thumb and forefinger revolve a barrel that fits around the handlebar positioned between the grips and the stem. The best-selling gripshifter is the SRAM Twistshifter, a design installed on some high-end bikes and several hybrids. Gripshifters don't have much ergonomic advantage over the other two types of shifter, but they are light and simple to maintain because they have few moving parts.

For a couple of years they were the favourite style of shifter and were installed on most new MTBs, but they do have two weaknesses. First, simultaneous braking and changing is difficult to do; second, you can't always get enough grip on the barrel to change gear when conditions are slimy and things are clogging up. To try and solve this,

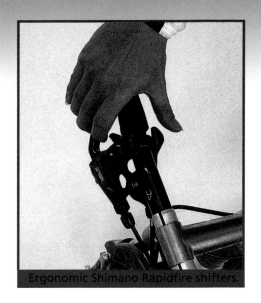

Ergonomic Shimano Rapidfire shifters.

the actual grip has been roughened and sharpened, so that it now resembles the tread of an MTB tire, with chunky protrusions to grab and force.

Upgraded models have stronger, lighter parts, but, ultimately, severe mud will clog even the best shifting system.

TOP-MOUNTED ▶ SHIFTERS

The original design, but not the best, these top-mounted shifters were the first specially made for mountain bikes. Within a couple of years, they were overshadowed by the under-bar shifter, but remain popular with old-school bikers. They're still found in some lower grade groupsets, and on second-hand bikes.

The reason for their enduring appeal is a bit mysterious; you have to lift your hand from the handlebar to reach them, so you can't brake at the same time. The attraction is probably rooted in their simplicity.

With one simple trigger and no ratchet return movement, top-mount thumblevers don't take up much space on the bars.

Cable changing is quick and simple and the shifters are light and sturdy. It takes practice to figure out which gear you're in, but they're really easy to keep working when the gears get clogged in muddy conditions. When your fingers are too cold or tired to shift the lever after a long day's riding, you can use the full force of the heel of your hand instead.

◀ UNDER-BAR SHIFTERS

The most naturally positioned, complex and expensive gear lever is also the most common, the under-bar type, known by the Shimano trade-name "Rapidfire".

There are two levers per changer, one for shifting up with your thumb and one for shifting down with your forefinger. Unfortunately, the whole system is complicated by selling them on the same handlebar mounting as the brake levers. It's possible to get under-bar levers separately from the brake levers, but you don't see it all that

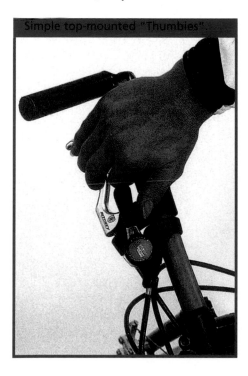

Simple top-mounted "Thumbies".

often on new bikes. Some equipment freaks prefer not to use "Rapidfire", because it limits their freedom to install non-Shimano brake levers.

Putting the gear and brake lever on the same mounting has a small weight and space advantage, but replacing them can be expensive. Break the shifting unit and you have to replace the whole thing — including the brake lever. Under-bar levers are most susceptible to crash damage and, of the three lever types, are both the easiest to break and have the most to go wrong. Their complex internal mechanisms include ratchets and springs, because the lever returns to its position every time.

For beginners, under-bar shifters have the clearest indicators, but getting used to which lever you need to push takes a while.

PROS AND CONS OF UNDER-BAR SHIFTERS

So why bother with under-bar shifters? Although riders have complained of skinning their knees on them, when you have got used to them, they are the most natural shifters to use.

You can simultaneously hold the handlebar tightly, press either lever with your first fingers or thumb and at the same time pull on the brakes with your middle fingers. It's possible, for example, when you're about to climb up the far side of a ditch, to use all the controls at the same time — you can (with practice) change from a high to a low gear both at the front and back, brake hard with both wheels and also keep the steering under control.

Because of that advantage alone Rapidfire levers are the most widely used gear levers in the MTB industry.

upgrading bearings

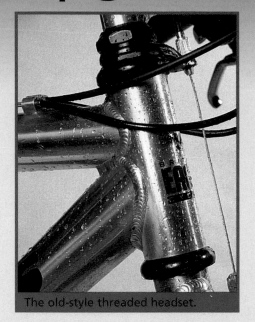
The old-style threaded headset.

Bicycles have bearings in five places: the wheel hubs, the freehub or freewheel, the bottom bracket, the steering headset and the pedals. The latest designs use new materials and new methods to tackle the two notorious weaknesses of bearings — their tendency to come loose and to wear out because dirt gets inside them and abrades the bearing surfaces.

▲ THE HEADSET:
THE STEERING BEARING

The headset lets the front wheel, fork, stem and handlebars all swivel together, independently from the rest of the bike. This component sits at the front end of the frame. The front tire spits mud straight into its face, and it's constantly being jarred by impacts from the front wheel.

So, while they're great at providing the steering movement, headsets tend to wear out prematurely, because of the dirt that makes its way inside, and to shake loose with vibration.

Since 1995, Aheadsets have become standard. They are 10%–20% lighter than the older style headsets and fix the vibration problem.

The Aheadset style is designed to be easy to adjust with a minimum of tools. As shown in the diagram, the steerer tube of the fork passes up through the headtube of the frame. The stem clamps onto the top of the steerer tube. The headset bearing is adjusted by loosening the stem clamp bolts, and tightening the top cap bolt. Since this screws into a nut wedged into the steerer tube, tightening the cap bolt pushes the stem down the steerer tube, tightening the headset bearings. They should be tightened until there is no play in the headset, while ensuring that the bars can turn freely. Then retighten the stem bolts firmly.

ADJUSTING HEIGHT

The older style headset had one advantage over the newer Aheadsets. With the old style, it was easy to change the height of the stem, and the handlebars, by loosening the bolt on the top of the stem, raising or lowering the stem, and retightening the bolt.

With Aheadsets, minor adjustments to the height can be made by swapping spacing washers so that they sit on top of or under the stem. More major adjustments to riding position can only be made by fitting a stem with a different angle, but if your stem is suitable, you can take it off and turn it over for a different riding position!

PROTECTION

So, how do you protect the bearing (i.e. the lower race) from daily off-road muck? Although grit doesn't appreciably increase the friction in the bearing, it does gradually scratch the ball and race surfaces so that they don't roll freely against each other and inside the casing.

The easiest way to stop that from happening is by sealing them inside a permanent cartridge which never needs to be stripped down for cleaning and regreasing. These are a little more expensive, but they do extend the part's life and are worth the extra expense.

HUBS

The hubs that the wheels spin on are not as maintenance-free as they seem. Their design hasn't changed much over the years so

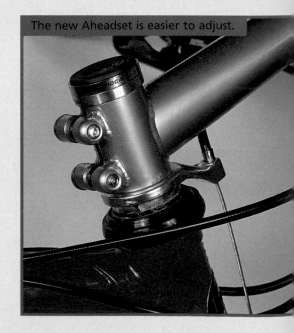
The new Aheadset is easier to adjust.

BEARING NECESSITIES
Ball bearing facts you didn't know you were missing!

■ **Ball bearings have a friction co-efficient of 0.011 — super-smooth! They have to be well-lubricated and clean to function this well.**

■ **Bigger bearings have less resistance.**

■ **The cup and cone design is effective enough to keep working, even if it's a little misaligned.**

■ **Bicycles were responsible for ball bearing design more than 100 years ago.**
(Source: Bicycling Science, MIT Press 1982)

upgrading is strictly a matter of improving aesthetics and saving weight and not at all about function, assuming that the bearings are kept dirt-free and stay well-adjusted, which is where bearings cause most trouble.

Non-cartridge, traditional hubs have adjustable cones that need slim cone wrenches for tightening or loosening bearing movement. Sealed hubs keep the bearings closed off. They are therefore are easier to maintain and there is a wide choice of them available in the stores.

SUSPENSION HUBS
Although all hubs are strong enough for the job, it is a good idea to opt for a rein-forced model on the front if you have sus-pension forks. They are called suspen-sion hubs and their axles are up to twice as thick at ⅝in (20mm) than the standard hub at ⅜in (10mm), to adjust to the unique forces of independently moving fork legs.

There are even hubs with four sealed bearings, rather than the standard two, for smooth turning all along the axle.

THE FREEHUB
The freehub body contains the bearings and pawls for freewheeling and backpedaling. These are designed so that the sprockets slide over the freehub body, but are held in place with a lockring. The design means that when the sprockets wear out, they can be replaced individually without replacing the freehub body.

The freehub body determines how many sprockets you can fit on your bike. 7-speed freehub bodies will only take 7-speed cassettes, but 8- and 9-speed freehub bodies are interchangable — either will take an 8- or 9-speed sprocket. Higher-end hubs have superior designs of the freehub mechanism, which makes freewheeling faster and pedaling more efficient.

BOTTOM BRACKET
The bottom bracket, the axle that the pedals revolve on, has the same troubles as the headset and hubs, but it also strains under all of the power from your legs. Almost all quality bottom brackets are of the cartridge

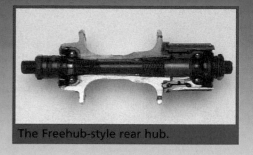
The Freehub-style rear hub.

type, to reduce the chance of dirt gettig into the bearings. A smooth running bottom bracket is essential to the efficiency of your bicycle, but it's easily neglected because you don't see it very often.

There are two main types of bottom brackets. The older type has a square section that tapers at the end of the axle, which fits into a square section hole in the chainset.

More expensive bottom brackets now have a splined end, and are fatter, for stiff-ness, and hollow, for lighter weight. A hollow titanium bottom bracket usually weighs only two-thirds of what a standard cromoly steel one does and has to be combined with a splined chainset.

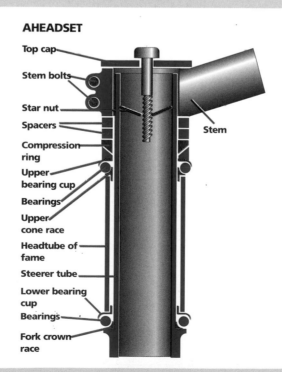

AHEADSET
- Top cap
- Stem bolts
- Star nut
- Spacers
- Compression ring
- Upper bearing cup
- Bearings
- Upper cone race
- Headtube of fame
- Steerer tube
- Lower bearing cup
- Bearings
- Fork crown race
- Stem

HEADSET
- Locknut
- Spacers
- Upper bearing cup
- Bearings
- Upper cone race
- Headtube of frame
- Steerer tube
- Lower bearing cup
- Bearings
- Fork crown race
- Stem
- Expander bolt
- Expander wedge

upgrading
pedals

CLIPLESS SPDs ▼

If your starter bike comes with platform pedals, the biggest improvement you can make in your entire equipment is to get a pair of SPD clipless pedals and matching shoes with an SPD cleat in the soles.

Clipless pedals are more accurately called "clip-in" pedals. It's true that they replaced toeclips and straps as the way of keeping the foot bound to the pedal, but the name is misrepresentative of the critical feature of the design, which is a mechanism in the pedal that grips the cleats in the soles of the shoes. It binds you to the bike and makes the most of your leg power.

Clipless pedals and shoes were first developed for road riding by Look and Time. They worked well in the saddle, but you couldn't, and still can't, walk in the shoes, because the cleat in the sole sticks out. If you haven't got a pair of cycling shoes with stiff soles and proper fastenings, then a set of clipless SPD pedals and shoes will be a good investment.

Shimano revolutionized the design by recessing the cleat inside the sole and created the first clipless system that worked in the dirt. Once you could walk, run and use double-sided platform pedals with clip-ins, there was no looking back.

The name SPD, which stands for Shimano Pedaling Dynamics, has become the generic name for the design, and SPDs are now made under licence by several manufacturers other than Shimano. Shimano and other licensed manufacturers make pedals and shoes that are all intercompatible. Less common types of spring bindings, like OnZa, for example, are not compatible with any other system.

Despite the cost and the adjustment period that comes with clipless pedals, they're an incredible invention. Acceleration is quicker, because none of your pedaling energy is wasted, and your handling of the bike over rough terrain is more accurate because you and your bike are locked together. You fall off a few times getting the hang of twisting in and out (so practice first!) but eventually it becomes second nature.

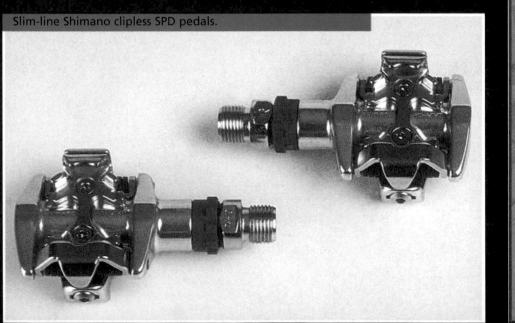

Slim-line Shimano clipless SPD pedals.

LIGHTER PEDALS

Pedals made of lighter materials are not as strong as regular ones. Lightweight trail freaks should go for pedals with lighter-weight spindles, shaved-down cages or pedals made from 100% titanium. But beware: pedals break, perhaps because they've been weakened by weight shaving. In the case of SPDs, the more likely scenario is that the bolt that holds the mechanism together came loose unnoticed and dropped out, or the pedal body came right away from the axle — usually from a crash or collision.

But their downside hasn't been fixed yet and the springs and cleat will clog up in muddy conditions so you can't clip in any more. Pedaling becomes really inefficient, and you find yourself craving for toeclips, which work no matter how bad things get. Be prepared to walk, or find a stick to clean them with.

Back at home, clean the springs and cleats thoroughly and squirt grease into the springs to help stop them from seizing up.

Having a degree of float is an advantage in SPDs. The side-to-side movement lets your feet pivot during your legs' imperfect rotation, while keeping them firmly attached. When you first get them, remember to set the angle of the cleats in the shoes to a comfortable position, otherwise you'll get sore knees.

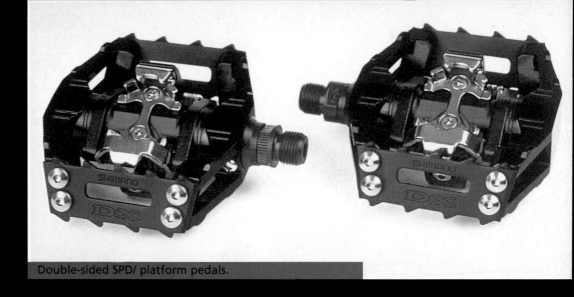
Double-sided SPD/ platform pedals.

SUPER PLATFORM PEDALS

As pedals for general trail riding get smaller, downhillers and trials riders are going for the largest, chunkiest pedals imaginable. It's not entirely clear why, because they rarely use them, their legs usually swivelling wildly in the air above people's heads.

Measuring up to 4in (100mm) across, vicious-looking platform pedals had all but died out before the full-suspension bike boom of the mid-1990s. Having your feet free for cornering on a downhill course and dabbing on a dual slalom course is vital. To make up for having no clip-in mechanism, the pedals have studs (sometimes replaceable) that bite into the rubbery soles of street and downhilling bike shoes. Downhillers virtually hook their feet around the pedals to carve and jump, and shin gouges are badges of honor.

Action platform pedals may be simple, but they're not cheap. The quality depends on the ratio of aluminum alloy in the cage to cheaper resin around the spindle.

SPD DOUBLE-SIDED PEDALS

The SPD double-sided pedal is popular with occasional cyclists for commuting to work as well as riding a local rail trial now and then. It has a clip-in mechanism on one side and plain platform on the other.

They're a great compromise between the demands of dirt riding and for reassuring cyclists who like to keep their feet free to hop off quickly. Off-road, they allow you to clip in for a full pedaling section, leaving you free to dab, pedal and dab again within seconds. In mud, the SPD mechanism clogs up, but then you have the option of using the platform side. In dry conditions, a platform pedal isn't as efficient as clipping in.

TOECLIPS AND STRAPS

Now old-fashioned, but always good to fall back on when SPDs have seized up, or when you are traveling in rougher, remote areas when you want maintenance-free pedaling, toe-clips-and-straps are rarely seen but always with us.

They never stop working, whatever the conditions, and can be adjusted to the width of your shoes (or even boots). You need to have good timing to get your feet into them when pushing off, though. Until you get used to it, there's a tendency to flick the pedal into a wild spin, then stand on the clip instead of slipping your foot inside it. Like most things, a little practice makes perfect.

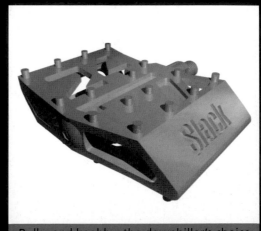
Bulky and knobby: the downhiller's choice.

upgrading saddles, cranks and stems

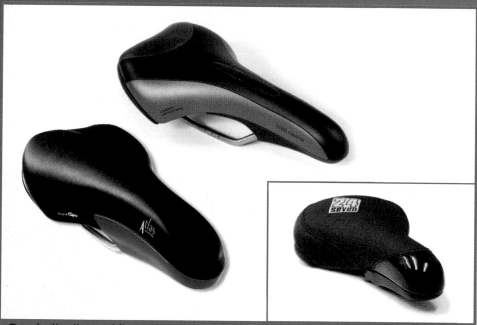

Tough slim-line saddles make good upgrades.

SADDLES

Saddles fall into three basic categories: softer and bigger for beginners and fair-weather riders, hard and light for tough-butted trail riders and cross-country speed lovers, and long and thin for style freaks. The majority of lower-end mountain bikes are fitted with comfortably-padded saddles that are just fine for an occasional ride, or for someone who just wants to try mountain biking out.

The important thing is to make sure that you're sitting on the bones of your pelvic girdle so that your genitals don't get squashed. Women's saddles are broader and men's are slimmer to match the differences in pelvic anatomy, but even then, a beginner of either shape should avoid the really wide saddles, which will chafe your inner thigh, push your knees out, and affect your pedaling.

A lot of recent research has been devoted to saddle designs that prevent genital numbness in both men and women. Various built-in features in saddles can take pressure off your genital areas in a number fo different ways, from a hole in the nose of the seat, to a lovingly-stitched-in soft patch. Gone are the days when it was macho to suffer in silence. Saddle soreness should only be temporary, and limited to the slightly bruised pelvic sitting bones.

No matter what, your first off-road ride will leave you with a few sore spots. Your body, which is remarkably adaptable, will toughen up in a few weeks, and the soreness will go away if you keep riding.

Once your butt gets calloused enough, you may want to put on a better saddle. It may have less bulk, with a slimmer nose and shallower sides, but will probably still be lightly padded. A gel pad can help, but they deform with age, (although less now than when they were introduced, when the gel tended to slip inexorably down the sides of the saddle).

By minimizing the shape and using titanium, magnesium or aluminum alloys for the saddle rails, the weight of a high-end racing saddle has been brought down as low as 5oz (150g). Lighter tends to mean more fragile, and off-road riding, with its run-of-the-mill crashes and scrapes, shortens the life of a saddle. The cheaper light-weight models don't last long.

Make sure you get a seat post, which attaches to your saddle, that allows you to adjust the angle of the saddle and slide it forward and backward for the most comfortable position. Women like to point the nose down slightly. Remember to keep the seat post greased or it'll seize to the inside of the frame and become impossible to adjust or replace.

CRANKS, CHAINRINGS AND CHAIN DEVICES

The crank is very simple; a bar of metal, usually solid, with a threaded hole at one

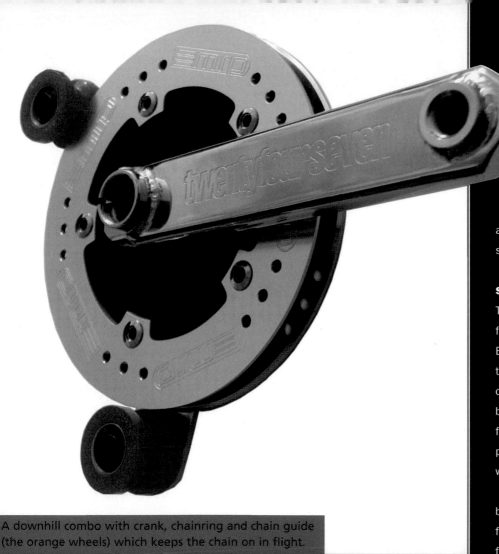

A downhill combo with crank, chainring and chain guide (the orange wheels) which keeps the chain on in flight.

around 700lb (318kg) per stroke, is the same as on a road bike.

STEMS

The stem connects the handlebars to the frame and doesn't seem to do all that more But don't be deceived. MTB designers can turn the simplest item into a complex key component. Mountain bike stems have to be strong, even though they're protected from the full force of the trail by front suspension; on a rigid bike the wheel and frame will fold before the stem will.

On cross-country bikes, stems need to be lightweight and simple. On downhill and freeride bikes, which have a way heavier front end and are subjected to more abuse from the rider, the stronger the better. All MTB stems need to be compatible with the type of headset in the frame. In mountain biking that means Aheadset-compatible where the stem clamps over the outside of the fork column (see p.71).

A chunky, hunky downhill stem.

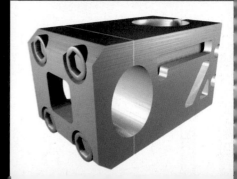

end that the pedal screws into, and a square hole at the other that fits onto the bottom bracket axle.

The design of cranks for cross-country mountain bikes peaked with lightweight configurations for the triple chainset (three rings on the front derailleur) that riders need for the range of speeds from very slow to very fast, and these haven't changed much in recent years.

In downhilling, design continues at an incredible pace. Nearly all downhillers, slalomists and street bikes use a single chainring. They don't need the lower gears, and they can fit guides onto the ring that stop the chain from flying off when the suspension destroys the chain tension. Single

chainsets need a slightly differently designed crank -- one that's usually stronger and more expensive. Shimano makes a downhill crank, and funkier designs surface constantly in the MTB world from companies such as Azonic, Gusset and 24Seven. They may have round-profile crankarms, tapered crankarms or straight fat arms — kind of like their riders really. Most are made from aluminum alloy, with a couple of carbon fiber versions making their way onto the scene.

One interesting mutation of crankarm designs is called the spider, where the right-hand crank fits into the chainrings, with either four or five arms.

It's also interesting to note that the stress placed on an MTB crank, up to

about suspension

Ask a silly question...

Why go suspended? Maybe you're looking for something that marks your identity as a rebel, maybe you've got too much money, or maybe you need something to talk about with your friends. All of these factors may come into play to some degree, but the main reason is because suspended bikes make riding easier, faster and more fun.

The idea of suspension systems is to separate the rider and/or bike from the direct effect of impacts between the tires and the terrain. This is done through shock absorbers on the front and back wheels, and also, occasionally, in the seat post.

With the shock of the trail partially absorbed you can go faster with more control. The wheels stay more closely in contact with the ground, because the shock absorption reduces ricochet. The rougher the terrain gets and the higher the speed, the wider the gap between the response of a suspended and a rigid bike. High-risk downhillers ride bikes with up to 7in (180mm) of shock travel at the front and as much as 10in (250mm) in the rear, to get as clean a line as possible and to handle high-pressure impacts and jumps.

Benefits

The benefits to beginners and cross-country riders are just as good. Suspension is forgiving, and if you handle your bike clumsily, it's not a big deal.

Although suspension was developed for downhilling, it's become standard on mid-range trail bikes, racers and freeriders, as the weight decreases with advances in design and materials. The net result — full suspension — is now possible even for cross-country riding because a fully suspended bike weighs just a couple of percent more than a rigid bike. High-quality full suspension bikes can weigh less than 25lb (11kg) or even less — which is pretty light by rigid bike standards.

That means that just about every cyclist can enjoy the higher speeds, the control and the lower physical stress that suspension provides.

Stress relief

Suspension is also a healthy addition where your other equipment is concerned. Back-country hackers who spend all day in the saddle, 5-minute downhill dashers and racing greyhounds will all have fewer flats and longer-lasting frames and components because of the reduced stress on the bike. A suspension bike frame can be built less sturdily to make it lighter, although the lateral reinforcement and extra parts it needs usually add that weight back on.

But remember, suspension shouldn't be seen as a cure-all for all off-road pains. A suspended bike is less sensitive on the trail, which is in itself one of the highs of mountain biking — and the injury rate in aspiring downhill pros is substantial. There's a fine line between skilled riding and losing control on a super-fast, super-springy bike!

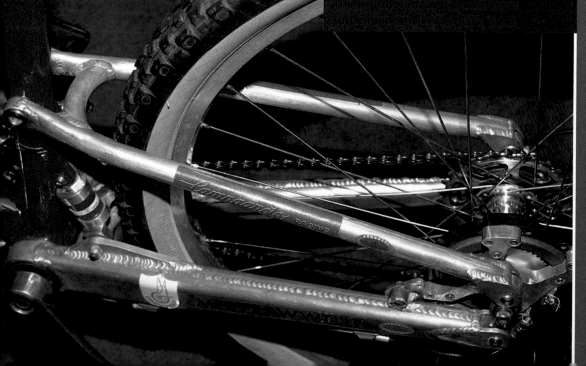

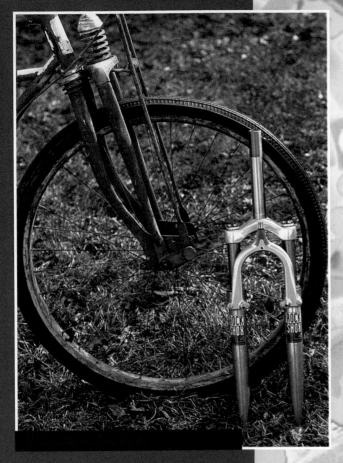

And another thing...

What about loss of speed when you're climbing? And the tendency for fully suspended bikes to pogo when the extra pressure on the pedals during a climb creates pedal feedback, an up-and-down oscillation in the rear suspension? Some professionals used to have suspension bikes for contractual reasons, not because they preferred them. Today, the big downhill bikes have rear triangles that eliminate bob (see the Santa Cruz V10) as much as they can, and the lighter-weight/less travel freeriders are bolted and reinforced laterally to stop side-to-side wobble when climbing out of the saddle, a small price to pay for the bonuses of suspension.

One day it may seem as exciting to ride a rigid bike again as it was when you first discovered suspension. No matter how imaginative designers are in experimenting

with the frame and parts of the bicycle, its performance always relies on the lungs and risk-taking of the rider. But, the sophistication and diversity of the suspension bikes they've developed supports their determination to push the capacity of the bike to some pretty high limits.

A brief history of suspension

The concept of shock absorption was taken from horse-drawn carriages and has been incorporated in some form on bicycles since they were invented in the second half of the 19th century. The roads were much rougher then than they are now, and any form of springing wasn't just efficient — it was essential just to keep the bike on the ground and in one piece. Now, suspension has become relevant again, as people have returned to the rough stuff voluntarily.

The low-pressure air-filled tire, patented by Dunlop in 1888, was a giant step forward from the solid tires of the very early years. Until then, sprung frames had been considered the answer, but they'd become loose quickly and stop working.

Sprung saddles help solve some discomfort, but they don't make the bike run any better and they do affect how extended your leg is while pedaling. UK designer Alex

Moulton is credited with first using metal spring and rubber on his 1960s bike, on which the small wheels and luggage-carrying capacity required some form of shock absorber.

The first major developments in successful MTB suspension were carved out by off-road bike pioneer Gary Fisher, and motorcycle engineer Paul Turner. Fisher teamed up with Harley Davidson factory rider Mert Lawwill and brought out an early swing-arm rear end on the 1990 RS-1 bike. It never made it commercially, but it did send a hundred new MTB inventors to the drawing board. Turner brought out the telescopic, oil-dampened RockShox fork in 1989. It was another influence brought over from the motorcycle and has revolutionized mountain biking. Its design remains fundamentally unchanged today.

Early full suspension bike developers were ProFlex, which used elastomer bumpers as shock absorbers in both a hinged stem — the FlexStem — and hinged rear wheel. The design of the rear end has continued to great success, but the idea of a flexible stem has been overtaken by suspension forks.

Cannondale took things further with more complex metal spring and oil dampening in a hinged rear triangle. And they followed that up by placing an internal shock unit in the head-tube, for a properly suspended front wheel, which still survives in their bikes today.

inside
suspension

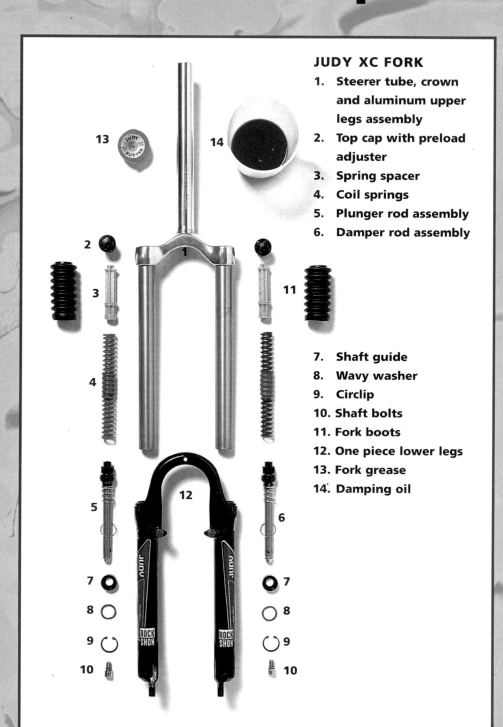

JUDY XC FORK

1. **Steerer tube, crown and aluminum upper legs assembly**
2. **Top cap with preload adjuster**
3. **Spring spacer**
4. **Coil springs**
5. **Plunger rod assembly**
6. **Damper rod assembly**

7. **Shaft guide**
8. **Wavy washer**
9. **Circlip**
10. **Shaft bolts**
11. **Fork boots**
12. **One piece lower legs**
13. **Fork grease**
14. **Damping oil**

Internal mechanics

Good suspension should absorb impact accurately and instantly, so that the bike can handle rough stuff and keep moving as fast as possible.

More than that, mountain bike suspension has become a specialized branch of technology, and has led to a culture where mechanically-minded bikers have an insatiable appetite for knowledge about how different materials and methods accomplish an ideal level of response.

Of course, you can enjoy the "boing" of suspension without having the slightest bit of interest about what's happening inside the greasy chambers of your fork and rear unit. But, ignorance isn't so blissful when it comes to the cost of maintaining a suspension bike. At least you can make on-the-trail repairs to suspension without knowing all of the ins and outs of it. If your suspension stops working while you're out on a ride, you'll simply clunk home, but you won't be stranded.

How does suspension work?

Shock absorption works by directing force in a controlled manner through compressible substances to isolate the subject from the force. The action divides into two stages and occurs no matter what the type of suspension.

First, there's the spring, which absorbs the impact, allowing, in this case, the moun-

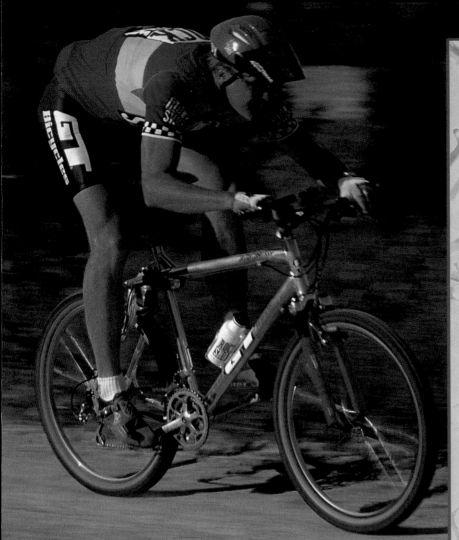

SHOCKS AT A GLANCE

METAL COIL

On cheap bikes, a spring on its own will mean uncontrolled bouncing. But it works well in combination with proper oil damping.

HYDRAULIC

Messy, because it involves oil, but highly tunable and cool. Partnered with a coil, considered best for big hits.

ELASTOMER BUMPERS

Mess-free, better at little bumps than oil, but with limited travel. Tunable by changing density of bumpers.

COMBINATION ELASTOMER/OIL

For a while, this system was considered to be the best of both worlds — the simplicity of bumpers with the big-hit hunger of oil — but the travel limits of bumpers quashed the design.

tain bike wheel to move relative to the ground instead of the rider and frame. The distance the spring travels depends on the amount of movement in the unit and the degree of stiffness.

Then comes the damping. The spring transfers the force to the damper, which is the dead end for the shock. It acts like the felt pad that stops a piano string from vibrating. The damper stops the impact from going into reverse and shooting back out through the spring with the same amount of force that it entered it with.

Different models of suspension fork/rear unit have their own pros and cons when it comes to functions like rate of absorption, travel and reliability.

HYDRAULICS

Hydraulic suspension uses oil-filled chambers to absorb the shock, and separates the spring and damping functions. The spring is either a chamber of air compressed by a piston, or an external metal coil.

The damper is a chamber of viscose oil compressed and extended by the spring. By opening and closing the aperture of the chamber's valves, you affect the rate of damping. And that in turn determines whether the suspension is tuned more for big or small hits.

ELASTOMER BUMPERS

In the 1990s elastomeric shock absorbers were big in suspension. On the front shocks, rubbers were arranged in lubricated stacks inside the fork legs. In the rear they appeared as fat, external units behind the seatpost. They worked simply, by compressing and releasing without separating the spring and damping, and tuning involved re-arranging colored bumpers of different density.

Most bumper development was done by ProFlex, the creators of the Flexstem. They produced a range of full suspension bikes that had a good reputation for a few years running.

In the mid-90s a more sensitive elastomer/oil shock appeared with separated damping, but a travel limit of 2in had been reached and bumpers were slowly phased out. Despite two advantages — no leakage and rare breakdown — rubber suspension has all but disappeared from the picture.

front
suspension

Almost all new mountain bikes now come with suspension forks. You have to work hard to find any model which isn't sold with a pair of shocks (or single internal shock in the case of Cannondales). Whereas riders once aimed to retro-fit front suspension on their hard-tail bikes, nowadays the upgrade entails fitting shocks that give more travel in the case of downhilling, weigh less in the case of cross-country, or have a little more travel and a bit less weight in the case of recreational full-suspension trailbikes (also allowing you to balance the bike between the front and rear).

Each year sees enhancements to the best models, and existing improvements getting cheaper and appearing on bikes from as little as $350. Rejoice that such a piece of engineering can enhance the riding of the regular joe. From the racer's experience, the ability to turn off the shock easily during pedaling is gaining ground, to the point where lockout could be the next chapter in the front shock story.

TRAVEL

Travel, the distance a shock absorber will compress, is the key factor in suspension. This governs how far the wheel will move independently from the bike in response to ground force, and the degree to which the rider is or is not ricocheted from the bike. Speedy cross-country bikes which require a bit of softening, better pedaling (so that on bumpy ground you stay in the saddle) and

speedy downhilling, get forks with around 3in (80mm) of travel. The fork is lighter, as the stanchions need not be so elongated to house the workings, and require less bracing and strengthening in the fork body.

Cannondale XC bikes, such as the 2002 Scalpel, offer 3in (70mm) of front suspension inside the head tube. A good quality lightweight XC fork is the RockShox SID, designed for serious sport or expert racers. Using air for the spring keeps the weight very low, at 2.8lb (1.26kg). Travel is midlength 2.5in or 3in (68mm or 80mm), designed for fast horizontal movement, not big jumps. Using a dial on top of the fork leg, you can lock it out at any time.

The new generation of in-betweenie full suspension playbikes are designed for riders to go all day and take the air at will. In this case, travel is around the 4–5in (100–120mm) mark, which also allows the suspension to be more or less equalized between the front and rear shocks. Typically, the Fox Vanilla fork achieves 5in (120mm) and the Marzocchi Bomber Z1 goes for 4.5in (110mm). The RockShox Psylo Race comes in a choice of 3in, 4in and 5in (80mm, 100mm, and 125mm) models.

It is the downhillers, who soar through the air highest and smack the ground hardest, who obviously need the longest suspension travel, and get it anywhere around 6.5in (160mm). At the opposite end of the spectrum from the lightweight XC fork, these beasts are super-strong, with longer

stanchions, extra leg thickness and a second cross-brace. Leading models are the Marzocchi Bomber Monster T (7in/175mm) and the RockShox Boxxer (7in/178mm).

LOCKOUT

The problem with suspension forks, as far as trail riders are concerned, is that they work. That's fine on rocky ground and descents at speed, but try climbing uneven tracks, or sprinting on even relatively flat ground, and you can see that fork giving way and wasting your power.

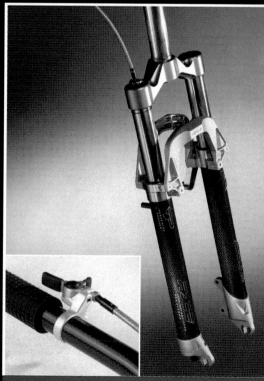

The lightweight air-sprung Pace RC38 Airforce fork has a handlebar lockout lever (inset).

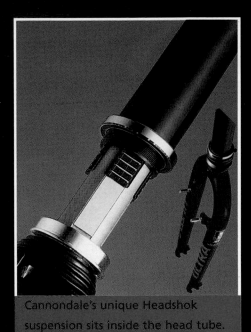

Cannondale's unique Headshok suspension sits inside the head tube.

To overcome this Achilles heel, researchers in the US and UK have come up with methods of letting you lock out the fork from the saddle, say at the beginning of a climb or heading into the finishing straight. Lockout may become standard on speed bike forks, since on the latest models the compression can be shut off using a lever on the handlebars. Experienced riders claim that flicking the lever acts like a psychological "go" button, as they use it subconsciously when they accelerate to power up slopes or attack rivals.

The bold US company Cannondale has been refining lockout for several years. Its biggest front shock design, the Headshok, is cleverly concealed within the head tube (for less weight and better stiffness) and has a lockout lever on top, where the stem fits on the head tube in the middle of the bars. This is within easy reach of either hand — but you still let go for a moment. Cannondale goes further with the lockout on the top-notch Jekyll 3000 bike. This uses an electronic button on top of the stanchion to turn off what is already a remarkable fork, the single-sided Lefty. This is again

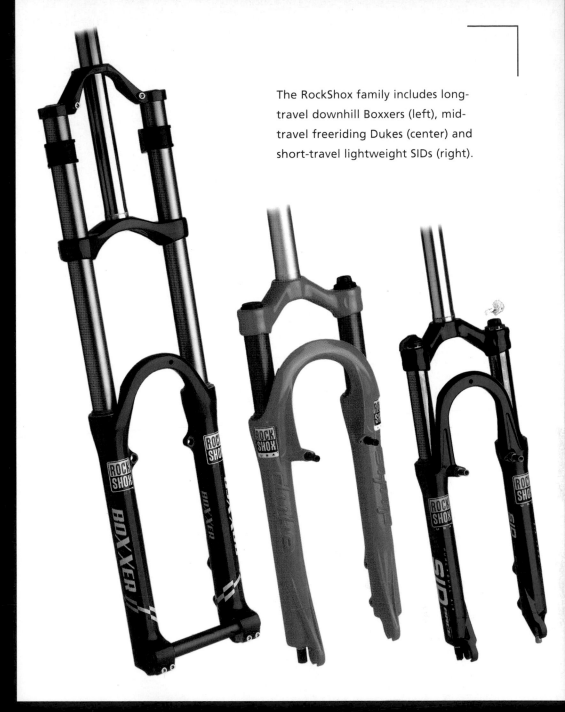

The RockShox family includes long-travel downhill Boxxers (left), mid-travel freeriding Dukes (center) and short-travel lightweight SIDs (right).

superquick on/off action, but you still take your hand off the bars.

The British developer Pace has made lockout-equipped front forks since 1998, starting with cross-country Airforce models with 2.5in (63mm) of travel, advancing to the longer-travel Pro Class, a mainstream fork for fun trail riding with 3.5–4in (80–100mm) of compression. The advantage of Pace forks is a customized lockout fixed right next to the gear levers — so there is no letting go when the sprint starts!

ADJUSTABILITY

Dials, knobs and valves on shock forks add up to hours of fun for riders who like to tinker with their equipment. Downhill competitors understand and fine-tune their forks precisely, but bike mechanics accuse amateurs of liking to muck about with controls without a clue how they work. Read the manufacturer's instruction leaflet to learn about pre-load (to set the shock to your weight) and spring & damper adjustments (for sensitivity to small and big bumps).

rear suspension

There's a line of thinking that says sooner or later we'll all be riding full-suspension bikes and that hardtails, still used by XC riders and regular trail-riders, will be a thing of the past. The reasoning is that, while rigid-rear bikes are fine for short, hard rides, if you spend a day in the saddle or race for over an hour, a fully-suspended bike will make you more comfortable and keep you going faster for longer.

Developments such as the Trek Fuel range show that full suspension can be fitted neatly and lightly onto a XC race bike just like you can bulk-up a downhill machine. The claim is that, for the weight of a hardtail, you get full suspension and a stiff back end.

Horses for courses

CROSS-COUNTRY BIKES

In most fully-suspended XC bikes the rear triangle remains intact and connected to the mainframe, usually through the pivot that serves the shock. Less travel means that you don't have to cut away the seat tube to make room for the wheel to dive in and out (like with some playbikes and downhill bikes). For cross-country riders, this keeps the back end stiffer like a hardtail. Cannondale's lightweight Scalpel bikes and Trek's similarly fine Fuels (pictured) both feature relatively discreet shocks with pivots bolted to the mainframe for rigidity.

The Foes FXC (see p. 26) does cut away the seat post as part of its aluminum box-work frame, for a confident fully-suspended look without the weight. Travel distances in XC rear shocks fall in the 2.5–3.5in (65–90mm) bracket, supplied usually by air-sprung units, such as the Fox Float shocks.

PLAYBIKES

Playbikes see a shift to bigger and some-what heavier coil-sprung suspension, with the powerful steel spring evident around the oil damping chamber. Now you're looking at travel distances of 3.5–7in (90–175mm), which give a range of choice to riders who jump as well as ride. This is the domain of, for example, the Fox Vanilla RC shock, where both compression and rebound damping are adjustable for sensitivity to both small and big bumps.

In some models (see the Rocky Mountain RM7FR, pictured), the rear wheel is now a swingarm fixed at the bottom bracket that uses the shock structurally as well as for compression. This dual job places a lot of stress on the shock, which is correspondingly strengthened so that it can keep the rear end together and rigid as well as compress.

DOWNHILL BIKES

In full-blown downhill bikes the seat tube is often cut away and the gap taken over by a

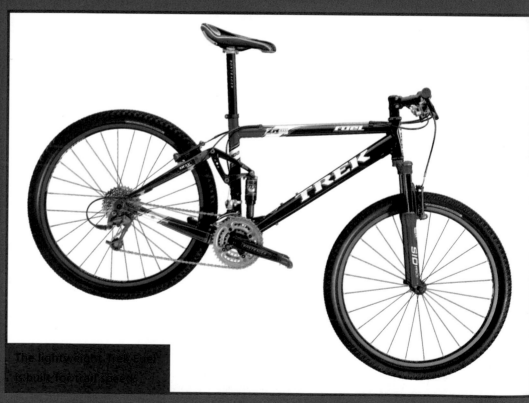

The lightweight Trek Fuel is built for trail speed

powerful shock with up to 10in (250mm) of travel (see the Santa Cruz V10 on p. 29). The shock operates a strong and chunky swingarm, which may be fixed on the downtube, or on an extra beam wherever space can be found.

Designers have found that downhill riders want rigidity as much as they want extra travel, so that's also become key.

Something new are the boxy aluminum Orange bikes, which attach the swingarm to the downtube with an axle right through the frame rather than individual bolts on either side. Orange also uses a standard front triangle, in bikes with big shocks but relatively simple design (pictured).

Different designs

■ Single pivot (see all bikes pictured): the simplest design, appearing in different forms on a lot of bikes from cheap to expensive, makes the rear wheel arc in a fixed line around one pivot. This style is easier to build and is less of a threat to the bike's rigidity, but doesn't track the trail so accurately. When the shock compresses, the rider drops in relation to the frame. Good examples of single-pivot models are, again, the Orange full-suspension bikes, where the rigid swingarm design remains the same whether the bike is for XC or DH. It's just the shock travel that gets longer. The regular diamond-shape of the Cannondale Scalpels and the Trek Fuels is deceptive. Their rear wheels also pivot in an arc, although only a small one.

■ Dual, floating or multi-pivot: this is the style that allows the rear wheel the most freedom. The wheel moves forward and backward and in rotation in relation to two or more pivots. This is supposed to improve the bike's tracking on rough ground, because it means that the bike doesn't always hit bumps head on. With the dual-pivot design, the rider tends to stay more level, too.

The Santa Cruz V10 (see p. 29) moves in an S-shape, due to what is called its "virtual" pivot point design.

■ Unified rear triangle: now outdated, the URT is still worth mentioning as a noble attempt on the path to improve MTB suspension. It grew from the problem that, when the rear shock compresses, the rear wheel moves more or less forward and the chain loses tension, which makes it jump the gears or drop off completely. To deal with that, the URT design dislocated the entire rear triangle including the bottom bracket (where the pedal axle is) from the main frame. This maintained the distance between the bottom bracket and the sprockets and the chain tension, but was over-complicated and created a bigger problem of how to keep the back end of the bike rigid. Chain tensioning devices developed at the same time and were an easier way of stopping your chain from falling off, and the URT faded from the mountain bike scene.

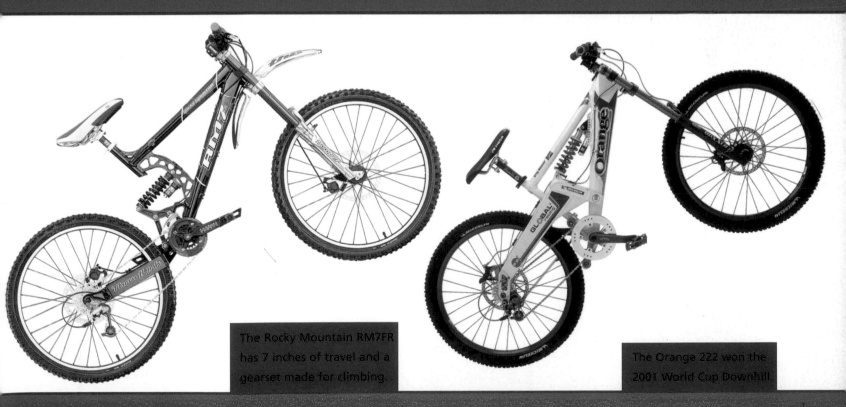

The Rocky Mountain RM7FR has 7 inches of travel and a gearset made for climbing.

The Orange 222 won the 2001 World Cup Downhill.

mud glorious mud

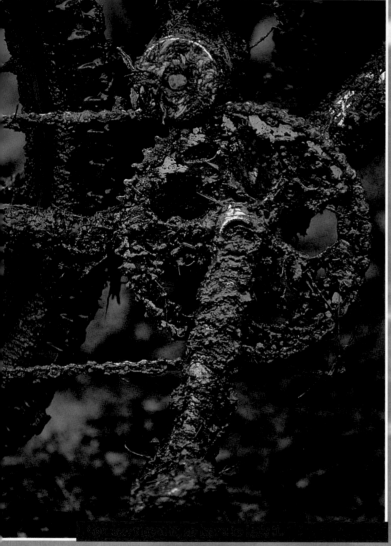

The ministry of mud defense

Tips to help you deal with the mountain bike and biker's favourite enemy — mud!

■ Go for the chunkiest tires your frame can accommodate (keeping ½in/10mm clearance). Wider knobs on the tread get rid of mud more quickly from the tire, depending on how sticky the mud is. Directional tires, like ones with a chevron pattern, are good, and there are also "semi-slicks", smoother tires which cut through surface slime to the firmer ground beneath it. Slimmer 1½in (40mm) tires are also better in mud.

■ Spraying your frame with lube in mildly muddy conditions will slow down mud build-up.

■ Thinner lubes like WD40 or GT85 are not intended for the chain. They're great for cleaning but will wash off quickly in mud and rain, leaving the links grating and scratching. Always use a thicker oil to lube your chain — the extra expense is worth it — and apply liberally if you're expecting hellish conditions.

■ Tire pressures should be low around 35–40psi, so that the tire can mould itself around objects for better grip.

■ Before starting out on a ride that'll be wet and gritty, either put new brake pads on, or pack a spare pair so you can change them mid-ride. Brake pads can wear down to the pegs or housing after a few long descents in wet and gritty conditions — the wetter it is, the more mud acts like sandpaper against the mud and rims. If the metal peg or housing is exposed it can split a rim and there's no fixing that out on the trail. Use the barrel adjusters on the brake levers every hour or so to adjust for any wear during your ride. And don't forget the 10mm wrench or Allen keys you'll need to adjust or replace the actual pads.

■ Wearing gaiters will protect your legs from getting wet and cold and will keep the mud away from your skin.

■ If you have any non-sealed bearings (bottom bracket, steering headset and wheel hubs) replace them with sealed cartridges. Until you do, you'll need to clean and regrease them frequently after muddy rides.

■ Hang your bike upside down to dry after a wet, muddy ride, to make sure water doesn't rust the tubes, especially around the bottom bracket (remember to remove the seat post before you do).

■ Install high-quality brake and gear cables, preferably PTFE or Gore-tex, for extra smooth shifting and braking when the mud gets serious.

■ Grease is a bike's protective layer. It protects it from the elements and helps give it a long life. Squirt the stuff into the little breathing holes in the chain stays, smear it around the headset races …

■ Check your bike for mud in hidden places: in the end of the handlebars, the end of the bar ends, underneath the fork crown going up into the fork column... The top of the fork legs, the gaps around shoe cleats, crank bolt caps, the spout of your water bottle, your ears, mouth and nose... (Only kidding!)

Muddy fixtures and fittings

■ Mud guards for the down-tube and front wheel — for maintaining a clean front.

■ A rear wheel mud guard — important for keeping the rear shock clean, as well as your butt.

■ A sprocket scraper — attaches at the rear hub during cleaning and combs away the crud from between the sprockets.

■ An anti-chainsuck plate — attaches beneath the chain stays at the chainrings and prevents a derailled chain being pulled up between the stays and the rings.

■ A chain retention device, because clogged rings easily derail the chain.

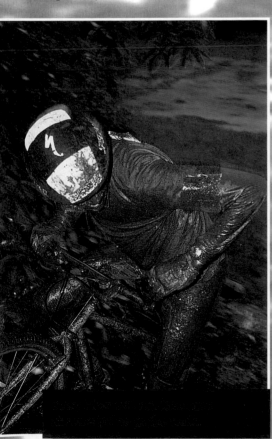

■ Make sure suspension fork legs are protected by gaiters. Lube the fork legs frequently. Service them to check that the seals are doing their job.

■ Clean out muddy allen bolts before undoing them, otherwise the allen key won't insert properly and the bolt will get rounded.

■ Spray the spring bindings of SPD-style pedals with lubricant — they're one of the first things to seize up. Or use SPD/platform combo pedals, or straight platforms, or just toe-clips-and-straps.

■ Don't remove the rubber covers on the brake lever pivots. Cover up the lower headset race with either a manu-factured neoprene and Velcro coat, or make your own from a piece of inner tube fixed with zip ties.

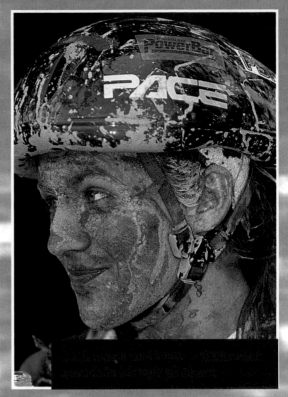

Mud and the mountain biker

■ Eye protection — wear it. It's not just mud that flies up into the eyes from Old MacDonald's farm — and it can cause infection.

■ Shiny rider — at home in the post-ride bath, don't forget to clean inside your ears! Get used to having lightly hennaed skin for a couple of days after biking in clay.

■ Gear grip — keep a grip on gripshift gears by getting covers with the sharpest profile you can find.

■ Clearance — make sure that the clear-ance between the chain stays and seat stays is big enough on the bike you want — before you buy it.

■ Seconds-serious racers can carry a sec-ond full water-bottle to flush the mud off the sprockets, and might want to consider on-the-move chain lubing devices. They could make the difference between a smooth win or finishing last with jumpy gears and recurring chainsuck.

■ In the car — buy or make water and mud resistant seat covers to keep the inside of your car clean. Keep some plastic bags in the trunk to stuff muddy equipment or clothing into. Carry around another couple of garbage bags for sitting on to calm pub owners, etc.

■ Sock sense — put aside a couple of pairs of socks just for muddy riding — you'll have to forget about their original color. Ditto, a few old and worn bath towels.

■ Recycle the mud you collect on your rides — wash the bike on a flowerbed.

■ Cleaning tips — thick mud is much more easily removed when wet and you'll also scratch your paintwork less. A thin layer of mud will come off more easily with a dry cloth when dry, but it can take the shine off new paint.

■ Stop-gap lubing — if you don't have time to clean and dry the bike properly after a ride, then at least spray some lube on the chain to stop it from going rusty overnight.

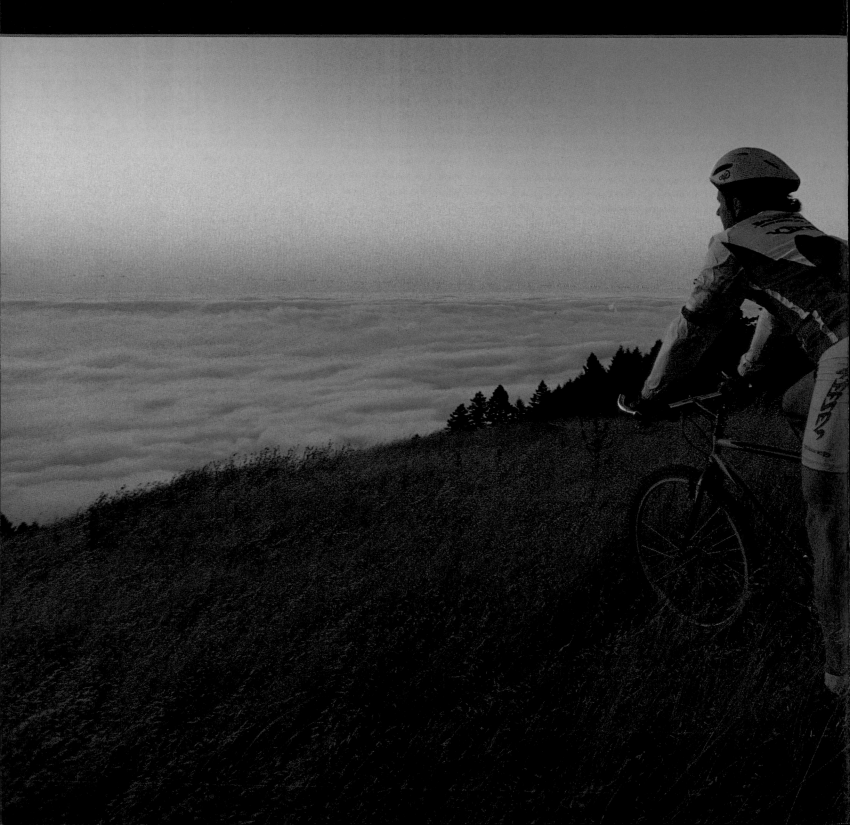

chapter two doing it

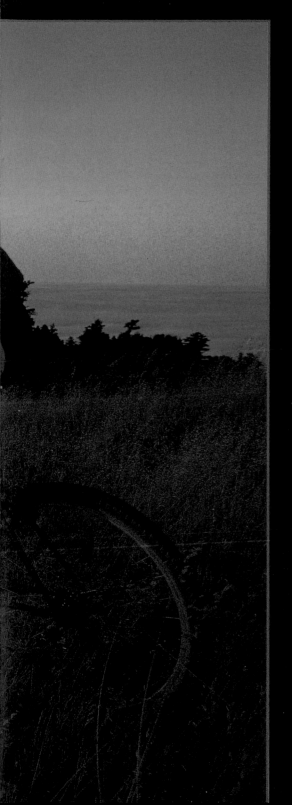

this chapter is concerned with building the mountain bike's engine — your body — and becoming familiar with how it operates so that you can get the most out of mountain biking. Don't be fooled into thinking that there's anything difficult about the sport. Anyone with a minimum amount of mobility is capable of riding and will improve with practice. It shouldn't be too difficult to find an easy-to-reach trail just a few miles from home — whether it's a state park, or an urban bike path.

The nutrition and stretching sections are here to remind you that mountain biking is an easy way to a healthy lifestyle and to show you, in easy steps, how you can get there. According to the British Medical Association, a regular cyclist has the body of someone 10 years younger. Regular exercise is also an excellent way to prevent heart disease. We explain how to train for a year from scratch, then how to keep training for racing. All the most important training issues are covered, from how to cross-train indoors and outdoors, to preventing colds and how to eat for energy.

Anyone who's looking for a way to fit MTBing into their busy lives, or who is unfamiliar with life beyond the city limits, will probably find their first try at it bruising — (mentally and physically) but keep at it! Try to think of every pedalstroke as a long-term investment that'll pay you back with better health, stronger legs and higher self-esteem.

Although riding a mountain bike can be as simple as swinging your leg over the saddle and keeping your balalnce, once you get the hang of it, you'll want to go faster, over more difficult terrain and over longer distances. That's the way to get the most from your bike and to get a feel for the landscape. Each time you're out on the trail you're intuitively using your balance in conjunction with the pedals and brakes to guide the bike forward or to resist the pull of gravity. The technique and terrain pages identify the handling skills you'll need to ride long and hard off-road. They also give detailed explanations of how to survive most of the surfaces and gradients you'll encounter.

Few mountain bikes are street virgins for long. You may use your bike between off-roading trips, to get around in the city, so survival in traffic is an important and crucial skill. Learn to recognize dangerous situations, and how to ensure your visibility in the dark. And remember, urban bike theft is big business.

When the call of the wild becomes irresistible, it's time to load your bike with panniers, get out the maps and get out there. In this chapter you'll discover the information and equipment you'll need to survive a long-distance trip.

William Morgan, a sports psychologist, claims that running is a wonder drug. Mountain biking is the same, but with better views and tales. What are you waiting for? Get out and ride!

getting in shape for mountain biking

Riding a bike is exhilarating and hard work — but don't panic. Inside everyone generally healthy is a conditioned body trying to get out, and what better to release it than a mountain bike?

A beginner's priority is to enjoy an afternoon's ride on their shiny new bike. But, even this needs a certain level of fitness, especially if you choose a hilly or muddy route. Athletic types, who regularly do aerobics, run or swim won't have any problems adapting to mountain biking, although the cycle-specific muscles in the calves and thighs take 6 to 12 months to develop. But, for the couch potato drawn to mountain biking by the call of the wild, the washboard stomach and trick componentry, that first afternoon will be a righteous challenge.

How fitness works

Whether you mountain bike regularly, or you consider walking to the burger joint an act of heroism, your natural body fitness is set at the following level:

Weekly demand + energy for emergencies = (un) fitness level

If you don't exercise much, your body will "relax". Exercise steadily and your body will feel as if it's resisting at first, but will eventually grow into a stronger core. Unfortunately, there are no shortcuts.

When will 1 be in shape?

Generally speaking, it takes a year for an adult's body to adapt from relative inactivity to a hard, hilly day on the bike. Younger women and men, teenagers and children have an abundance of energy and fewer bad habits, but their endurance may need some work.

In terms of individual training sessions, it takes 2–3 days to recover your energy after a session and a week or so for soreness to go away. It takes 3–6 weeks for your body to grow stronger in response to one of these sessions. It takes at least 3 years of committed training for endurance athletes, like cyclists, to reach their full potential.

Fitness tips

■ Avoid overdoing it — sometimes in their enthusiasm, people who are out of shape can overextend themselves, and will suffer a long-term loss of energy. Don't let your mind push your body faster than it can grow.

■ Quality not quantity — riding for a short time regularly is just as effective and more sustainable than once-monthly blowouts that will make you want to sell the bike.

■ Commute by bike — ride to school, college or work. These "invisible" miles benefit the environment and your heart and head.

■ Do hills get easier? Yes, but it doesn't feel like it. As you get into shape you'll find yourself wanting to climb bigger hills faster and more frequently instead of just sitting back and enjoying the smaller ones. It all means more mountain biking fun, rather than being able to laze on the bike.

How to ride into shape in a year

1 GOAL-SETTING
Set yourself realistic goals, reachable in the amount of time you have, otherwise you'll wind up quitting before you even got started.

For example:

■ In a month's time I want to be able to ride for 20–30 minutes, 3 times a week.

■ In 3 months time I want to be able to ride off-road for 1 hour without resting.

■ In 6 month's time, I want to be able to ride every day for short distances — commute to school, college or work, or do my first one-hour race.

■ At the end of a year I want to be able to ride all the way up "Grief Hill".

2 THE PLAN

The goal for your fitness program is to concentrate on steadily increasing the amount of time spent riding.

Months 1 to 3

Start with the three 30-minute sessions a week of exercise. Try riding, running, swimming or aerobics — any form of exercise that gets you out of breath.

Months 3 to 6

Increase one of the weekly sessions to a one-hour ride. By the end of this period you'll probably be able to spend a whole afternoon every weekend riding on rough terrain. Try to ride all the way up small hills, and practice better handling of the bike as your speed increases.

Months 6 to 12

Try your first fun, short (lasting less than an hour) race. Keep up the shorter sessions and make every other weekend ride an all-day one. Ride all the way up difficult hills, ones that require balance and strength. And how about marking the anniversary of buying your bike with a 2-day biking trip?

When the going gets tough

■ The first 20 to 30 minutes of riding feel awful. Rest assured that it's just a transitional phase when, as with any engine, your body's systems are adapting, trying to work more efficiently. After that, things get easier.

■ The burning pain in your legs when you're climbing a steep hill is lactic acid — a byproduct of the energy conversion process — which can't be expelled as fast as your body produces it. The burning stops when you rest, and the more training you do, the later and less you'll feel it.

■ If your enthusiasm dies in the face of pain or rain, it's not failure. Take a break from the bike for a couple of days. Change your plan and goals and review your equipment, but don't give up. Maybe your gear isn't up to the conditions you've been riding through? Treat yourself to an inspiring piece of equipment for the bike.

■ No matter how difficult or lonely the riding is, no matter how weak your body is feeling, the workout is doing your legs and heart a world of good. Be patient, and remember the goals you've set yourself, not the ones your friends set themselves.

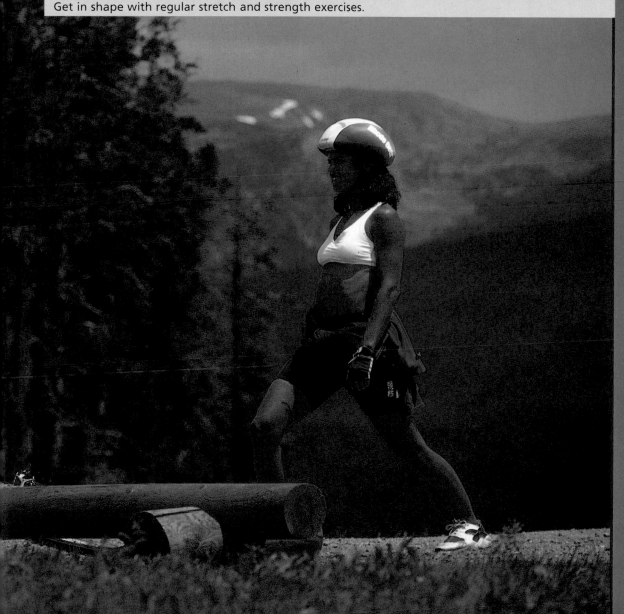
Get in shape with regular stretch and strength exercises.

strength & fitness

Once they've reached the point where they can comfortably ride off-road non-stop for 1 or 2 hours, a lot of bikers will choose to push their fitness level further. They're enjoying themselves and plan adventures in the neighborhood of 50 miles (80km) a day, spending their holiday in the mountains or even racing. Training doesn't always fit easily into a casual lifestyle. It needs performance goals, a seasonal training plan and usually some changes to the diet. Some of the old pastimes will have to go, but they're usually only things like watching TV.

The training plan

It's time to jack up the amount of time spent in the saddle by increasing the intensity of the workout. From now on, the quality of your workout matters as much as the quantity. The easier it is to make the effort, the longer you can ride. The harder the effort, the shorter the amount of time you'll be able to sustain it.

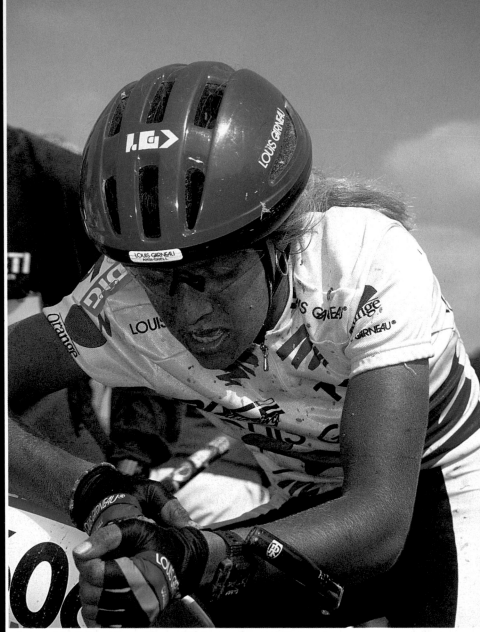

A good training plan will condition you for racing.

GUIDE TO TRAINING WITH A HEART RATE MONITOR

Effort level	% max effort	BPM	Produces	An/Aerobic	How it feels
LEVEL 1	below 50%	below 115	nothing	aerobic	gentle
LEVEL 2	50–60%	115–140	weight loss	aerobic	getting sweaty
LEVEL 3	60–80%	140–165	better fitness	aerobic	sustainably hard
LEVEL 4	80–100%	165–185	athletic fitness	anaerobic	unsustainable

The amount of effort you put into a ride gets divided into four percentage bands, all based on maximum effort and measured using a heart rate monitor.

The table, bottom opposite page, shows those four levels, all percentages based on a sample rider whose maximum heart rate is 185 beats per minute (everyone's maximum bpm is different).

In the off-season, racers do long low-intensity level rides to build endurance, like an all-day 70 mile (110km) ride with lots of stops. When the competitive summer season comes around again the rides are shortened and the intensity is increased to high level 3 and 4 efforts, to build strength and speed, like in a one-hour ride at level 3 or a set of one-minute repetitions (intervals) at maximum level 4.

Refinements, like rest days and weeks, are built into the plan to prevent over-training and to make sure the rider is at his or her peak for big events.

Motivation

When the novelty of training has worn off a lot of riders drop their training plans out of boredom or demotivation. Maybe you can't find the time to stick to an over-optimistic plan, or you're beaten in a race by someone you had no trouble pulverizing in the past. Also, mountain biking is one of those sports that's great fun in practice, but a lot of training work is done on the road, in the gym or on rollers.

Find ways to put fun into training. Build rewards into your diet, look for training partners to help you through. Don't abandon other fun parts of your life — entertainment, family and non-biking friends — but don't quit!

As with anything long-term, there will be highs and lows. Build as much as a 25% lost-time factor into your program to cover for sick days, relationships, family or loss of motivation.

ATHLETIC TIPS

■ Cross-country mountain bike racers train 75% on the road, 25% on the trail because pavement provides the predictable environment needed for controlled-intensity training sessions. Off-road work is crucial for developing faster handling. If you want to improve, you have to expose yourself and test your nerve and control on harder and harder obstacles and slopes.

■ Downhillers are purer trail devotees; in their split-second sport what counts is high-speed bike control as well as strength.

■ Train your weaknesses — whatever you work hard at you'll be good at. For example, if you ride for 100 miles (160km) steadily, that's the area you'll do best in, but your speed won't improve. If you suck at downhilling, sign up for a downhill race! If you can't mount the bike from the right-hand side, practice. If you fall behind on hills, write more climbing into your training plan.

■ Eat a balanced diet with approximately 55% carbohydrate, 30% fat and 15% protein. Eat fresh fruit or vegetables at every sitting, replace desserts with fruit,

and cream with yoghurt.

■ Keep a daily record of what cycling and exercise you have, or haven't, done. Don't waste time feeling guilty but try to understand why you haven't reached your goals.

■ Over-training will cause a long-term drop in performance. You've done too much too soon and your body, rather than adapting to the extra effort and becoming stronger, can't catch up and is defeated. An out of shape or semi-fit rider is just as much at risk from over-training as a professional, but the inexperienced rider is less likely to notice it happening.

■ Always rest properly between sessions, remembering that the harder the session, the longer the recovery period. Be patient — don't rush back into the saddle.

■ Trust your body. Don't expect to feel great for a few days or even a week after a big ride. It takes 3–6 weeks to feel the benefits from a training session. Without a full understanding of over-training, controlled rest is the only cure.

TRAINING AIDS

■ Good weather and exciting terrain.

■ A heart rate monitor.

■ Indoor trainers — indoor rollers or turbo trainers provide controlled cycling conditions and are highly effective if used to their full potential.

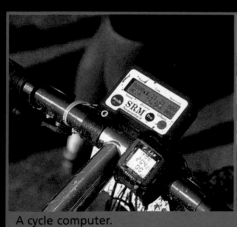
A cycle computer.

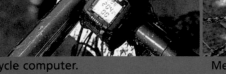
Measure your pedalstrokes.

eating and drinking
for mountain biking

Start with a
healthy diet

The average American eats double the amount of fat and half the amount of carbohydrate recommended for a healthy body. So the priority for active bikers is to get the daily balance right first, then tackle the finer points.

Experts recommend that the daily diet be made up of the following:

■ 55% complex carbohydrates — for energy. Carbohydrate is found in starchy staples such as bread, potatoes, pasta and polenta.
■ 10–15% protein — for growth. Protein is found in eggs, dairy products, beans, lentils, soya, fish, chicken and red meat.
■ 30% fat — an essential dietary aid. Good sources of fat are oily fish, dairy products, vegetable oils and margarine.
■ Eat fruit and vegetables at every meal and

you'll also be getting the other essential nutrients — fiber, vitamins and minerals.

What should I eat before a ride?

After 1–2 hours of solid exertion, glycogen, the body's fuel derived largely from complex carbohydrates and stored in the muscles, runs out. Suddenly, you start to shake and lose energy. This is called "hitting the wall", or "bonking". At best it's uncomfortable and if you're competing, it could mean that the race is over for you.

What happens is that your fuel system is switching over from short-term glycogen to long-term body-fat (your reserve tank). But for the hour or so it takes, you're not worth much as a rider. Eat, instead, for short-term energy. Munch carbohydrates in the form of sugary or mixed sugary starchy foods — for example, a banana or an energy bar — and you should be able to get back on your bike and pedal in about 30 minutes.

To avoid hitting the wall in the first place you need to carbo-load. Serious athletes carbo-load properly; they exhaust their glycogen supplies a week before the big event by working out really hard, then pack their plates with nothing but rice, potatoes, pasta or bread for the 3 or 4 days before the ride. That gives the body time to store maximum glycogen in the muscles. Carbo-loading for fun riders just means paying careful attention to your intake and eating more than your

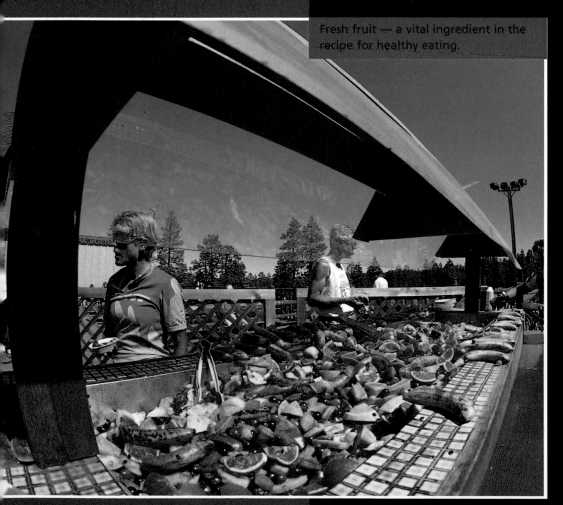

Fresh fruit — a vital ingredient in the recipe for healthy eating.

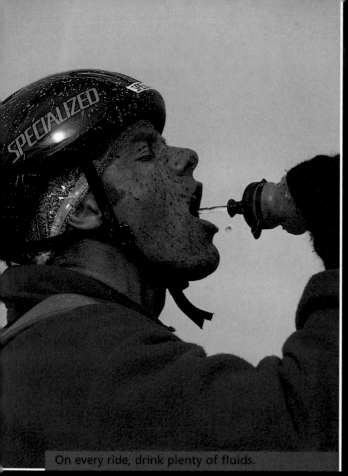

On every ride, drink plenty of fluids.

spirits need a boost, have an energy bar or a sports drink, but by preparing properly you should be able to avoid having to fall back on them.

AFTER

Eat carbohydrate-filled calories within 2 hours of stopping your ride, while your body is still efficiently converting that energy. Studies have shown that eating then will help your body bounce back faster.

Liquid-fuelled

Three and a half pints (2 litres) of water is the recommended daily quantity that all adults should drink. Cyclists can hardly get too much of the stuff, using and losing it at an incredible rate. Always drink a glass of water before you start a ride — whether you feel like it or not.

Your freshly filled water bottle is an essential piece of equipment on any ride, so use it. Start sipping from your water bottle 15 minutes after you've started your ride. Try to remember to drink a little water every 5–10 minutes for the rest of the ride, and at least another full glass as soon as you finish.

The human body can process about 2 pints (1 litre) of water an hour, so it's easy to leave it too late to catch up with the amount you've sweated out.

Post-race headaches are caused by dehydration, just like hangovers. If you get a headache, even if you don't feel thirsty, try steadily drinking a pint (half a litre) of water, and another, if you feel like it. Some racers in hot climates hydrate themselves before an event, to the point where their urine starts to run clear.

ENERGY BARS

The advantage of commercial energy bars and drinks is their portability, and how easily the high-energy ingredients can be digested. If you're riding in a remote area those bars can be survival aids, and they make great comfort foods when the going gets tough!

A typical bar will contain a solid mix of complex and simple carbohydrates for instant and long-term energy, plus minerals. But you really don't need or use them unless you've hit rock bottom. Remember that a big banana, a home-made oatmeal and raisin cookie, or water with added fruit juice may be just as effective at restoring your energy.

Whatever you choose, eat it slowly and chew it well, and pause before you ride off.

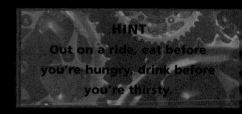

HINT
Out on a ride, eat before you're hungry, drink before you're thirsty.

Cool water feels great on a hot, tired mountain biker's body!

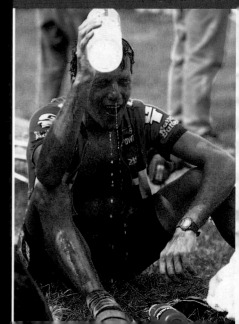

usual amount of carbohydrate-based food in the days running up to a big ride.

When and what should I eat?

For any ride over about an hour, eat a hearty breakfast of cereals, toast or muesli, but nothing heavy, like bacon and eggs, which take time to digest. Allow 2 to 3 hours between your last meal and the ride, because when you start riding the blood is drawn away from your digestive organs to the muscles, and anything undigested will stay that way until you stop. Worse, there's a risk of getting stomach cramps.

DURING

Don't bring a big meal along on the ride. Snack here and there instead, before you get hungry. Pack your backpack with ready-made moist starchy sugary foods that you can eat while riding. Try dried fruit, sultanas or raisins, energy bars, bananas, chewy cookies. If your legs and

stretching
for cyclists

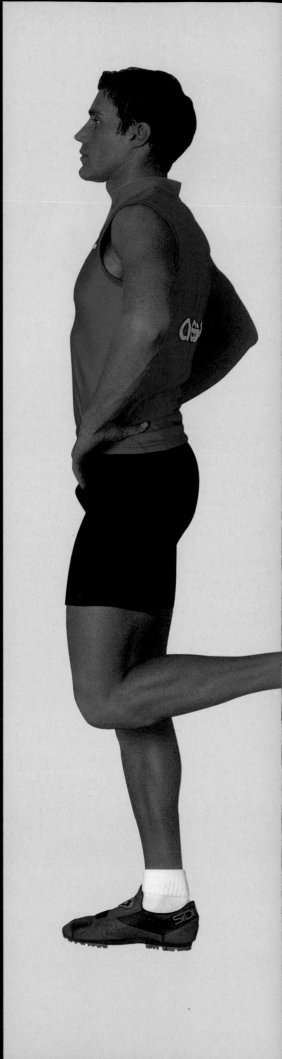

Why bother?

Stretching is excellent for cyclists because it helps prevent injury and soreness of muscles and increases flexibility. Stretching always feels good, but as with any exercise program you should consult a doctor before trying anything new.

Stretching is not enough to get you in shape, but what other form of exercise can be so easy and such fun to do? Whether you work a single throbbing muscle for a few seconds while you're waiting for lunch, or do a half-hour head-to-toe routine, stretching can feel great. It has a few things in common with yoga and other relaxation techniques, and has the ability to stimulate deep concentration and a sense of well-being. When training feels like all work and no play treat yourself to an extra dose!

For racers stretching is not a luxury. It's important for the maintenance of muscles stressed by riding hard or training. When a muscle activates it contracts. After working hard, muscles shorten and become tight. Stretching opens out the muscles, tendons and ligaments again, by pulling them gently in the opposite direction of the contraction.

The movement also flushes whatever part is being stretched with oxygen- and nutrient-full blood, which is necessary for basic function and healing after exercise. It also feels nice. The pulling and flushing protects the rider from the side effects of heavy exercise on muscles and joints as they're being strengthened.

Soothing, preventative, stretching

A stressed muscle shortens while it recovers. It feels like something between stiffness and soreness, and is, in fact, the body's warning not to use the area. The muscle loses its normal flexibility and can be damaged by day-to-day movements, which you wouldn't normally notice, let alone expect to cause damage.

While the muscle is healing, sudden exertions, like bending over to pick something up off the floor or racing to a meeting, could actually tear a muscle, ligament or tendon. This would entail long-term rest. Stretching prepares the body for day-to-day movement until the muscles have finished recovering and/or growing and return to their normal flexibility.

> Gentle stretches performed on a regular basis are always good, whether you cycle or not. They'll stimulate the blood flow and increase your flexibility.

THE KNEECAP AND ANKLE

A shortened muscle can pull and harm the joints next to it. If a joint becomes sore after training, think about what muscles are attached to it. The muscles around the joint may feel fine, but by stretching them gently you may find that the soreness in the joint starts to feel better right away.

The ankle joint is connected to the calf muscles by the Achilles tendon, which runs from the heel bone to halfway up the calf. If the calf muscles shorten they pull on the Achilles tendon. This may limit the movement in the ankle, to the point where it affects how you walk. In this state a short sprint may be enough to tear the tendon, a serious injury that takes a lot of time to heal and can happen again and again. It's important before any exercise to stretch your calves to loosen the ankle.

Stretching the quadriceps (the extensor muscle in the front of the thigh) can help avoid misalignment in the cyclist's most crucial and exposed joint, the knee. Just like

CAUTION!

■ Stretch gently — don't bounce. It's risky, ineffective and hard work.
■ Over-enthusiastic stretching done too quickly or taken too far does damage. Don't hold a stretch beyond the point where the muscles or joints aren't able to relax into it. Ease off the moment you feel pain, or if you start to shake.
■ Stop if you're in doubt about whether a stretch has turned into a pull. Take care not to overdo it.

1 Achilles tendon (lower calf)
Straddle the bike with one foot on the floor, the other on the pedal set at the bottom of the stroke. Straighten the pedal leg, so that the ankle swivels below the pedal. Repeat on the other leg.

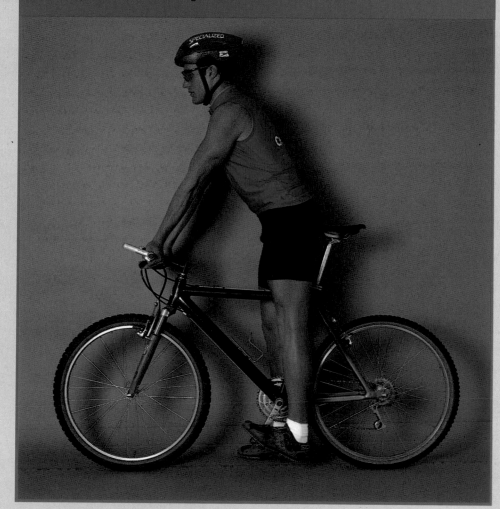

a warped wheel, the patella (kneecap) can be pulled out of true as the thigh muscle group adapts to training. Hardcore cyclists may ride enough so that the proportion of their muscles are changed.

The quadriceps are a powerful four-muscle group that provides most of the force in pedaling. But, if you're not careful they can change the alignment of the kneecap. Three muscles in the group attach to the outer edge of the kneecap. The inner edge of the kneecap is held only by the single vastus medialis muscle. When the thigh grows stronger, the outer muscles begin to pull more than the single inner muscle. This can mean a painful misalignment, as the kneecap gets pulled out of the groove that it travels smoothly along with each flex and release of the thigh.

DIAGNOSIS

Try stretching to cure minor aches, but consult a doctor if the pain lasts more than 3 days. Be careful not to work a joint or muscle that you suspect is damaged, not just strained. With experience, you'll be able to tell whether an ache requires a visit to the doctor.

2 Quadriceps (thighs)
With your back to a wall, place the lower leg flat against the wall, the knee on the floor touching the wall. Place the other foot flat on the ground, in a comfortable position away from the wall, with your hands on either side of the front foot for balance. Get comfortable, without stressing the knee. This stretches both thighs simultaneously, but after a minimum of 10 seconds it should be repeated on the other side.

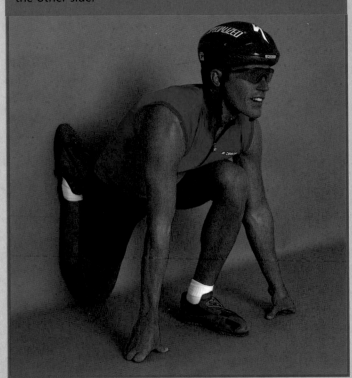

3 Head
Tilt your head to the left, then to the right and forward. You can also tilt it back as long as you do it gently. Turn it to the left and right, but don't rotate.

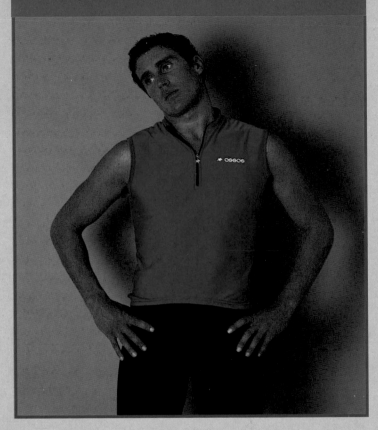

Warm-up and cool-down stretching

Stretching before you get on the bike can improve a warm-up routine, but it shouldn't be used in place of a controlled 20–30-minute build-up on the bike!

Warm-up stretches prepare the muscle responses. Concentrate on the legs and back. Do a few gentle knee-bends of no further than a 90° flex, and calf and quadriceps stretches, as shown here (or use variations). Rotate your ankles and swing your hips. Lean your head from side-to-side.

After a good workout, muscles will be relaxed and their stiffness and soreness can be lessened with more gentle leg and back stretching. This will also help flush stinging lactic acid (a by-product of energy production) from the muscles. But, stretching shouldn't replace a low-key 10-minute cooling-down ride. That ride will let your body temperature and heart rate fall slowly back to normal, and will also help get rid of lactic acid.

The developmental, "big" stretch

Deep stretching makes you extra flexible, and is good for everyone, not just athletes. Men, being less flexible than women, should definitely follow some sort of developmental stretching regime at all ages, from puberty to retirement. For mountain bikers, who squat to fix flats, jump on and off the bike, crash, recover and carry 30lb (14kg) of rubber and metal about on their shoulders, added flexibility from stretching can only be a good thing. Watch the pros — every one of them will be able to bend over and squat easily, as well as nail twisting, heavy motions, like pulling the bike out of ditches, without a problem.

Developmental stretching is easy. You need to be patient, though, to hold the positions for longer than the recommended minimum of 10 seconds and to take the stretch further after you've practiced it

4 Hamstrings, upper calf, lower back and shoulders
Face the bike. Place one hand on the handlebar, lift the same leg and place it on the top tube, placing all of your weight on the standing leg. Keeping the raised leg slightly bent, put your other palm on the raised knee and lean over gently. Repeat on the other side.

5 Upper back
Straddle the bike, both feet flat on the floor. Grab a hold of the top tube behind you with both hands. Lean gently back — not far — and hold for a few seconds.

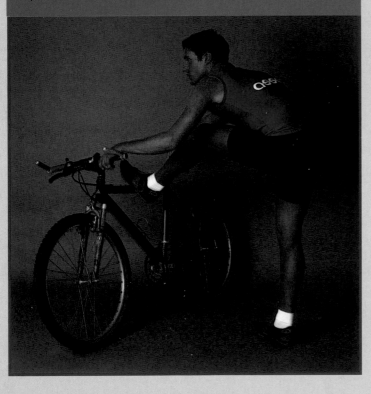

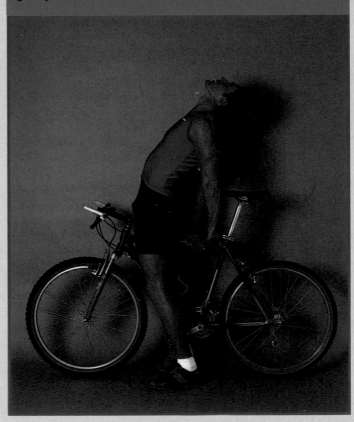

regularly. It's during these sessions that the pride and joy of having gotten into shape can be overwhelming.

Stretch technique

■ Warm the muscle up for the stretch by flexing it gently and relaxing it once. This gets the blood moving.
■ Stretch to a point of solid resistance then relax back. Settle at two-thirds full stretch.
■ Feel and hold the stretch, for between 10 seconds and as long as you like. Relax into it. Think of opening up, rather than pushing or forcing. The move is an extension, not a contraction and it shouldn't speed up your heart rate. Think about the specific muscles and joints you want to work, and shift the pressure around to make the stretch as full as possible.
■ Remember to breathe! An even slow breathing rate will help you relax into the stretch.
■ The muscle will gradually relax into the stretch. Be patient and enjoy it.
■ At the end of that stretch, either return to a normal position, or gently go further to two-thirds of the next degree of complete resistance and repeat until your time or patience runs out.
■ Shake out gently after the stretch.

When to stretch

Regular riders and racers should stretch daily, and do developmental stretching once or twice a week to increase their flexibility; they should also do warm-up and cool-down stretches before and after riding. New riders should stretch before riding, (but rarely do) and after riding, for recovery, plus regularly for general mobility. And everyone should stretch just a little when they get out of bed; with knee-bends — no further than a 90° flex — neck and back.

Illustrated stretches

This is a sample of five stretches out of about two dozen or so geared for cyclists. Most of these can be performed in different positions. Three use the bike as an anchor, but any convenient floor or wall will do. Hold each stretch for a minimum of 10 seconds.

Cross-training

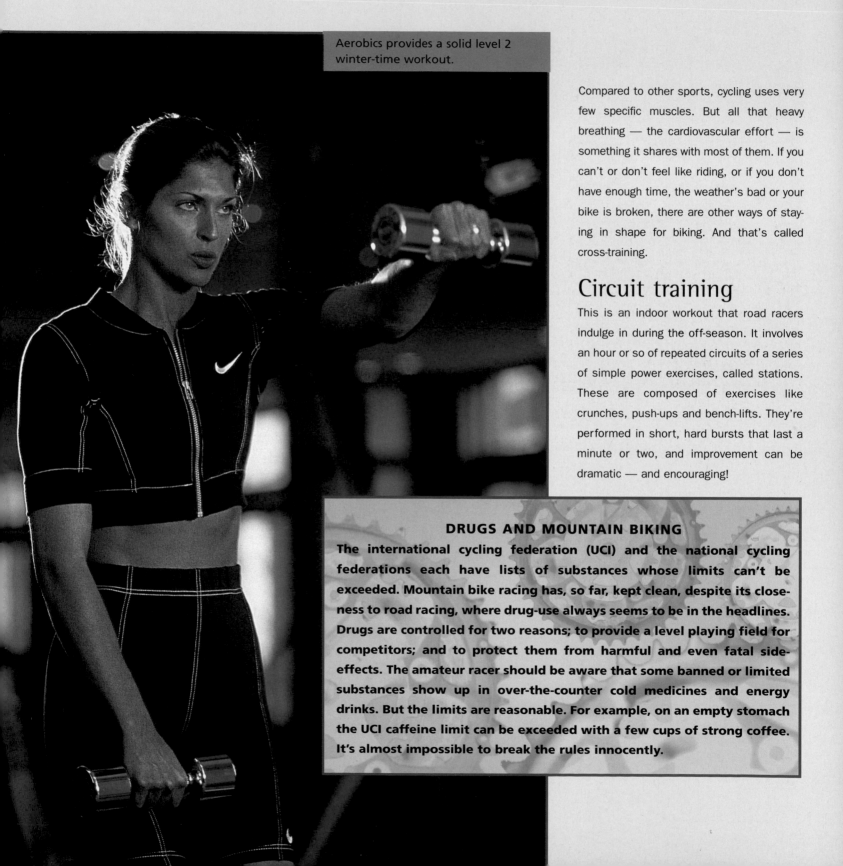

Aerobics provides a solid level 2 winter-time workout.

Compared to other sports, cycling uses very few specific muscles. But all that heavy breathing — the cardiovascular effort — is something it shares with most of them. If you can't or don't feel like riding, or if you don't have enough time, the weather's bad or your bike is broken, there are other ways of staying in shape for biking. And that's called cross-training.

Circuit training

This is an indoor workout that road racers indulge in during the off-season. It involves an hour or so of repeated circuits of a series of simple power exercises, called stations. These are composed of exercises like crunches, push-ups and bench-lifts. They're performed in short, hard bursts that last a minute or two, and improvement can be dramatic — and encouraging!

DRUGS AND MOUNTAIN BIKING

The international cycling federation (UCI) and the national cycling federations each have lists of substances whose limits can't be exceeded. Mountain bike racing has, so far, kept clean, despite its closeness to road racing, where drug-use always seems to be in the headlines. Drugs are controlled for two reasons; to provide a level playing field for competitors; and to protect them from harmful and even fatal side-effects. The amateur racer should be aware that some banned or limited substances show up in over-the-counter cold medicines and energy drinks. But the limits are reasonable. For example, on an empty stomach the UCI caffeine limit can be exceeded with a few cups of strong coffee. It's almost impossible to break the rules innocently.

Aerobics

An hour of upper level-2 workout is tougher than it looks. The instructor warms up the group, then takes it up to a heart-thumping non-stop level-2 all-round workout. Sometimes a step is used to increase resistance — good for cyclists' calves and thighs — and some instructors will also use hand and wrist weights. An aerobics session shouldn't be under-estimated.

Snow sports and skating

Cross-country Nordic skiing is both low-impact and leg-based, just like mountain biking. Snowboarding is good training for speed and quick response, and snow-shoeing is a great high-resistance workout. Rollerblading also helps with mountain biking, because you need to have good balance and coordination.

Running and swimming

Running and swimming are good cross-training activities that can be done at whatever level you want. Running is high-impact, but can jar a cyclist's highly-tuned legs, and swimming gives the arms and lungs an excellent workout. It's also much less likely to pull a muscle or tendon in swimming.

Weight loss by cycling

Mountain biking is famous for transforming tubby guys and gals into lean machines without a change in diet. Losing weight by getting in shape instead of dieting has a lot of advantages. First, it's fun, which makes it easier. Second, you burn calories not only when you ride, but when you're recovering — including while you sleep — as your body gets ready for the next ride. Third, you don't need to cut down much on the quantity of food you eat, but keep your intake balanced and below the amount you burn up on rides. One afternoon's hard ride could burn up more than a whole day's worth of food. Six months of more riding and a balanced diet could mean substantial weight loss. Keep at it for a year or two, and it can transform an overweight person's life and outlook.

A healthy, balanced diet by its very nature usually means less calories, because it reduces fat to the recommended level of 30%. Cut portions of dairy products, processed food and red meat by a third. Cut out and replace chips, cakes and cookies with bulky or low-fat carbohydrates (pasta, potatoes, bread) and fruit. Eat fruit and vegetables at every meal.

A healthy level of body-fat is about 25% for women, 15% for men. An athletic level of body-fat is around 15% and 10% respec-

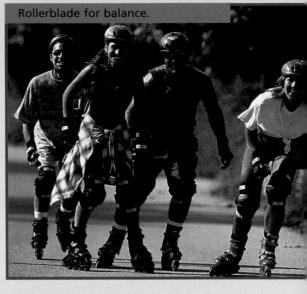

Rollerblade for balance.

tively. Endurance rides burn fat instead of glycogen (carbohydrate), but for most people, just getting out on the bike regularly will do the job.

A healthy daily caloric intake, which keeps the body functioning and supplies energy for effort, for adult women is about 1,800 calories, and around 2,500 for men. Eat regularly (and not just when you're really hungry) to avoid sugar highs and lows (i.e. bonking).

There is no harm in counting calories and it may help you but don't let it become an obsession and never embark on a fad or crash diet. They rarely produce long-term slimness and can damage your health.

One hour's steady riding burns about 350 calories, but during a race, you may burn as much as 600 calories. With these figures, losing weight becomes as easy as falling off a bike.

If you stick to the recommended calorie amount, ride twice during the week for an hour, and do a day ride or race on the weekend, you'll be slimmer in a few months. Equipping your bike with lighter componentry is one way to lose a pound or two, but slimming your body means time spent having fun on the trails and in the kitchen.

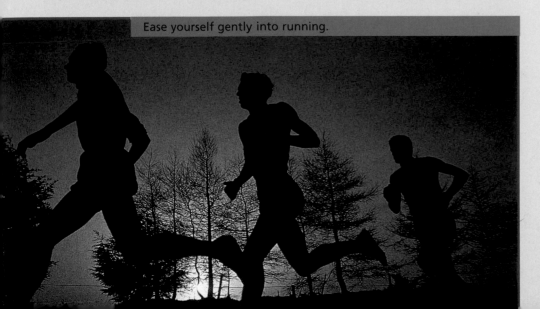

Ease yourself gently into running.

young and old

Mountain biking is a new sport that has only been improved by participation from women and those ready to retire. It can be practiced at any level from a gentle afternoon ride to racing. As long as you're in good health — a check-up at the doctor will determine whether you have a condition that may prevent you — and have a bike you can ride on, off-road cycling can be celebrated by people from six to sixty. An active lifestyle is the greatest natural defence against bad health.

Health tips for men

Men are naturally less flexible than women, and should stretch a few times a week (see pp. 94–97). Also, beware those evenings in the pub with your friends!

Health tips for women

■ Osteoporosis is a devastating and common condition in post-menopausal women that involves crumbling bones caused by calcium deficiency. It can be avoided by lots of physical activity throughout one's younger years. There's a general shortage of women involved in mountain biking, and that's reason enough to get teenage girls and young women out on rides.

■ If you want to lose weight, concentrate on riding on a balanced diet, not a skimpy one.

■ Women may need to take iron supplements to protect themselves from mineral loss during menstruation.

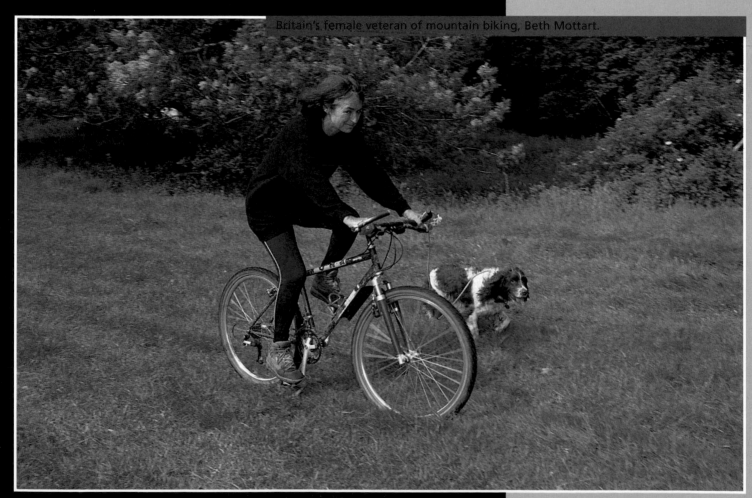
Britain's female veteran of mountain biking, Beth Mottart.

Mature riders

The older you are, the more difficulty you may have in learning how to handle the trail, and the longer it may take to recover from a long ride or a crash. But, as long as your health is generally good — have a check-up — there's no reason why you should miss out on the fun. People who have been riding all their lives have a hard time slowing down. It's got something to do with the cardiovascular and endurance systems — road racing men and women in their fifties are infamous for showing up-and-comers how it's done. Mountain biking's in its third decade, and the veteran, master and supermaster race categories are growing in leaps and bounds, proving that an enthusiasm for biking fades at a much slower rate than performance.

Younger bikers

■ Kids love to ride bikes, and mountain biking is definitely the coolest way of doing it. Traffic-free trails can plant a respect for the land and a healthy awareness of self-sufficiency. Generally, kids of age 10 and older are fine on their own bike, but make sure that it's not too big for them and has gears. It goes without saying that they must wear a helmet. Try putting a younger child on a trailerbike, a one-wheeled trailer with a saddle and pedals that attaches easily to a regular bike. That way, they get to ride, but you decide where, and you don't have to do all the work!

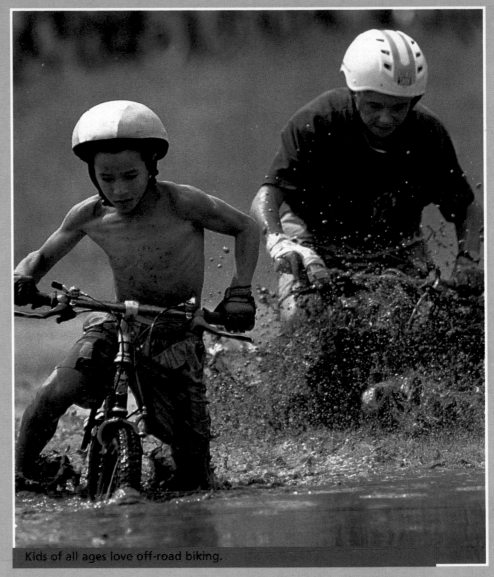

Kids of all ages love off-road biking.

■ A lot of parks have graded mountain bike trails made for children and family groups. If yours doesn't, how about organizing and building one?

Leading mixed rides

■ Successful group rides go at the pace of the slowest rider. Send faster riders ahead, asking them to wait at junctions, and don't drop anybody.

■ Most women tend to tackle harder terrain with strict self-control, where men are more likely to take risks and assume they can ride something dicey, even if they can't. Be aware of both styles and carry encouraging words and a first aid kit.

■ Be prepared for breakdowns and a wide range of mechanical knowledge in any cycling group, but let riders learn to do the repairs themselves.

■ Childrens' energy can exceed their stamina, so make sure that a ride isn't too long for them. Their bike can weigh more than they do! It's a good idea to carry a variety of small snacks for them, as children also need regular refuelling.

■ Novices tend to race ahead, or to the top of a climb without warming up properly, and burn out fast. Pace the ride, and don't destroy their enthusiasm.

injury free

Cold Free

Most cyclists can expect at least a few scratches.

premature return to riding comes at a great personal or even national loss. Protecting your health is an important part of a racer's lifestyle. Casual riders are also at risk, usually because of inexperience.

A lot of cyclists swear by taking high doses of vitamin C while they have a cold, but a balanced diet will provide the recommended daily amount. Any excess will just be flushed out of the body.

Hypothermia

Hypothermia, a condition where the core body temperature drops to a dangerously low level, can kill unless the patient is warmed up quickly and safely. A loss of three or four degrees is enough to stop some organs from functioning. Impaired judgement is often a key symptom — a patient may deny that there is anything wrong with them. Warm the person up with blankets, bodies and warm (not hot) drinks. Try to carry an emergency blanket on any long rides.

A lot of mountain biking is done in exposed areas and in low temperatures. Before heading out in below-freezing temperatures, especially if it's wet or slushy, make sure that everyone is wearing enough warm, windproof clothing. Always make sure you know the weather forecast and plan rides with alternatives or contingency plans so that you can get people home in case the ride is too much for them or the weather deteriorates quickly.

Sticks and stones break collarbones

The most common fracture in mountain biking is the collarbone, usually caused by pitching over the handlebars at a high speed and landing upside down on the shoulder, or on an outstretched arm. It is not a serious break, because the collarbone acts as a static strut, but it is painful and needs binding. Riders are usually back in the saddle after 3 weeks, a little longer if it's a multiple fracture, although full movement returns after another month or so. What's usually more debilitating is the loss of confidence in your riding, which will need re-building.

Nurse your knees

Unfortunately, knees can't be replaced if you wreck them (yet). It's hard to care about a kneecap when you're out enjoying a ride with friends, but keeping your knees healthy is a hidden skill of cycling. Take advantage of the fact that mountain biking is a low

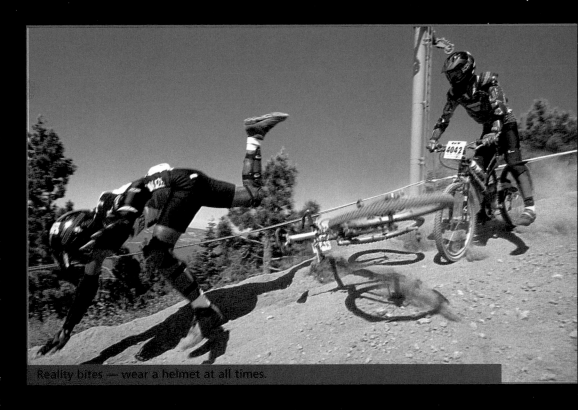

Reality bites — wear a helmet at all times.

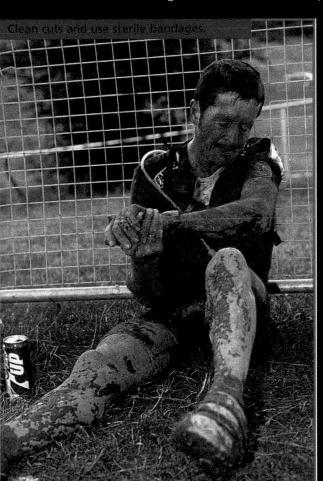

Clean cuts and use sterile bandages.

impact sport. High impact sports, like running, pound the body, and knees can take a real beating.

Take every ache, soreness or pain in the knees seriously. Is it caused by riding too hard or too long? If you're not sure, stop riding and see a doctor. The damage may be temporary and you may only need time and rest. If rest is recommended, make sure that you carry it out properly. But the damage may be permanent if the patella has been dislodged by an uneven pull from developed thigh muscles.

TIPS FOR HEALTHY KNEES

■ Equipment — get your saddle height right (see pp. 22–23). Your knee should almost straighten with every stroke. The angle in the bent knee should be comfortable. Make sure that SPD (clip-in) shoes are set at the right angle for your foot, and that you're pedaling with the ball of your foot. Wear over-the-knee shorts during chilly weather, to keep your knees warm.

■ Pedaling — warm up your knees with a few gentle bends and quadriceps stretches before heading out. Start and stay pedaling slowly until the stiffness has disappeared. Don't rush. If you're in any doubt, stop riding.

■ Home treatment — stretch your thighs, so that it's not temporary contraction in recovering quadriceps muscles that's affecting your patella. Stay off the bike for a while. If the pain recurs or makes it impossible to ride, go and see a doctor.

Staying healthy is a hidden skill of mountain biking.

handling the bike

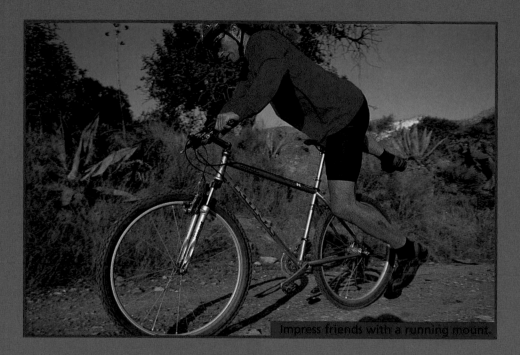
Impress friends with a running mount.

Good technique begins before you even get on your bike. The ability to "handle" your bike, (i.e. to manage it when you're not actually pedaling), is necessary on any ride. The techniques included here require practice, perseverance and patience.

TURNING IT UPSIDE DOWN

Stand with your legs apart beside and facing the bike, lean over it and place your hands as far down the seat tube and fork as possible. Turn it over, pulling the saddle toward you. The further down your hands are, the easier it'll be to do.

LIFTING A BIKE

Stand with your legs apart, facing the bike and bending your knees (not your back),

place your hands as far down the fork and seat tube as possible so that most of the bike's weight is above your hands. Then lift. If you're hanging the bike up, warm up your arms first so you don't strain them.

Getting on your bike

MOUNTING FOR ABSOLUTE BEGINNERS

Put the bike into an easy gear and straddle it. Use your toe to position the right pedal at 2 o'clock (10 o'clock if it's the left pedal). Put your foot on the pedal and give it enough of a push to allow yourself enough rolling time to hoist yourself into the saddle and to get the other foot on the pedal and moving.

STATIONARY MOUNT

Put the bike in an easy gear. Stand beside it, lift your right (left) leg over the saddle, put it on the right (left) pedal and push down. Slide on to the saddle and start pedaling.

MOVING MOUNT

This takes a little practice, so make sure the bike's in an easy gear. Lift your right (left) leg over the saddle. Push off with the leg that is still on the ground and slide onto the saddle. For a brief moment both feet will be in the air before they find the pedals but the bike should still have some momentum to carry you through.

RUNNING MOUNT

This is really just a faster version of the moving mount. You need predictable ground, but once you have it mastered, it can save several seconds in a race. When done properly, the running mount is impressive, but if you do it wrong you could injure yourself. Work up to it with the moving mount.

Put the bike in an easy gear and with your hands in position on the handlebars, run along beside the bike, pushing it. Using the same motion (but faster) as the moving mount, push off with the left (right) leg, with the right (left) leg lifted to clear the seat. You

FOR THE LEFT-LEGGED
Instructions for cyclists who favor their left legs are in brackets.

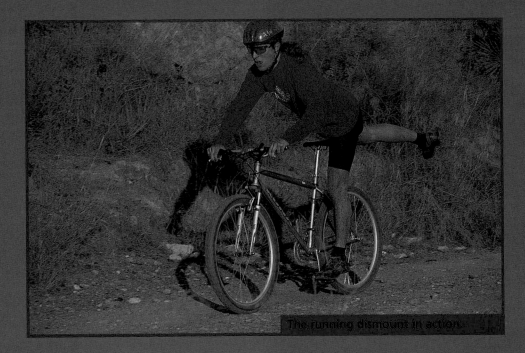
The running dismount in action

Stand beside the bike, keeping it steady by putting your left (right) hand on the handlebar. Bend your knees and crouch to put your right (left) arm through the frame. Now stand up, with the top tube resting on your right (left) shoulder. Keep the bike steady by holding either the stem, or the right or the left handlebar with your right (left) arm. Use the other arm as a counterweight to balance while you're walking or running. Racers don't use shoulder padding, but beginners may want to use one to prevent bruising.

USING THE MOUNTAIN BIKE AS A PROP

When you're crossing streams, gullies, or bogs, you can use the bike as a crutch to jump from rock to rock or safe point to safe point. You may even be able to climb up on to high walls, and down the other side using the saddle as your ladder.

THE SHORT, QUICK LIFT

If you're running alongside the bike, the fastest way to get it over a small obstacle, is to take the weight off the front end, using the handlebars, and the back end using the down tube or seat.

should land on the seat in your normal riding position.

UPHILL MOUNTING

Put the bike in a very easy gear. Place the right (left) pedal in the 2 (10) o'clock position. Hold the bike steady with the brakes on. Swing your right (left) leg over the saddle and slip on to it. For maximum momentum, get the right (left) pedaling foot properly inserted into the toeclip or SPD pedal before you push off with the left (right) leg, and let go of the brakes.

Getting off your bike

STATIONARY DISMOUNT

Unclip your left (right) foot from the pedal and slow down, straightening your leg. Stop the bike, transfer your weight to place your left (right) foot on the ground, and swing the other leg over the saddle

RUNNING DISMOUNT

While you're riding, unclip the right (left) leg, and stand up on the leg that's still clipped in. Swing the right (left) leg over the back of the saddle, pass it between the left (right) leg and the bike, and step ahead on to the

ground. Unclip the left (right) leg quickly and hit the ground at a run.

Push or carry?

Tackling unrideable terrain on foot with a firmly shouldered bike can be easier than pushing it through. You don't have to find a line for the wheels *and* your feet, or push the bike over obstacles. But you will be carrying around 30lb (14kg) — especially if it's muddy, which will add to your load. And lifting the bike onto your shoulder can be awkward.

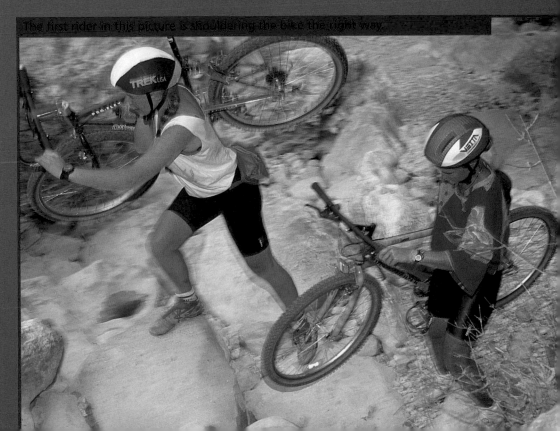
The first rider in this picture is shouldering the bike the right way

mastering pedaling and gearing

Good pedaling

Although pushing the pedals in a circle — spinning — rather than pumping them up and down like pistons is preferred, the style of pedaling you use most of the time — assuming you're even thinking about it — depends on the kind of terrain you're riding on. The method that feels natural to you is probably right.

Spinning is an efficient road riding technique that works at medium to high speeds off-road. On predictable, but not necessarily straight track, you can pedal in smooth circles at a high cadence, between 80–100rpm (revolutions per minute).

This is a great way of picking up speed quickly after a corner, but you need to be in shape to keep it going. Keep your upper body motionless — no swaying — and all your weight on your butt, not your legs. It may help if you go into a bit of a crouch. If you're clipped in pull on your feet as well as pushing them down. Once you're at full speed, spinning takes on a momentum of its own — feel that wind!

GET YOUR SADDLE HEIGHT RIGHT

Efficient pedaling is difficult if your saddle isn't at the right height. See pages 22–3 for information.

When you're climbing, and each stroke feels like your last, pumping the pedals is unavoidable. Visualize pushing down on each stroke. Pull on your arms, rock as much as you like and pray you make it!

Changing gear

Terrain can change so quickly in mountain biking that the ability to time a perfect gear shift is crucial to your riding. It makes the difference between a smooth ride and hard work. Like all mountain biking techniques you need to practice and expose yourself to different tracks and speeds. Gear components now have pre-set gears and ramps built into the sprockets and rings to help the chain slip easily from one to the other. All you have to do is shift the right lever the right way at the right time!

HOW GEARS WORK

■ Mechanically speaking, gearing adjusts the pedaling load so that you can adapt to fluctuations in terrain. Your speed changes accordingly.

■ A gear is described by the number of teeth on the rings you're using. A 36–18T gear means the chain is on the 36-tooth chainring and the 18-tooth sprocket. A gear can also be described in inches, telling you how far the rear wheel travels for one pedal stroke. To see how your gear is measured in inches, use this equation:

front ring teeth ÷ rear sprocket teeth x wheel diameter.

Typical MTB gears are 22–109in. The easiest gear is 24–28T, the hardest gear is 46–11T, a range that means you can pedal at any speed from a walking pace, approximately 1.8mph (3km/h), to the speed of a cruising car — around 30mph (50km/h). A typical road gearing has a range of 41in to 117in — or 42–28T to 52–12T.

If speed is what you want, change up to a 100in-plus gear, described as big, hard or high. For slow work or singletrack, where you persistently recover lost momentum, change down to a small, low or easy gear, below 40in.

GEAR RATIO

A gear ratio is the relationship between the front chainring and rear sprocket in use.

If the chainring and the sprocket have the same number of teeth, (e.g. 32), the rear wheel turns once for every pedal stroke, and the gear ratio is 1:1. If the chainring has 34 teeth and the rear sprocket has 17 teeth (a commonly used gear) the rear wheel revolves twice for every pedal-stroke, making the gear ratio 2:1.

On slow ground, when the sprocket has more teeth than the smallest chainring, the wheel turns more slowly than the pedal stroke, with a negative ratio; for example, 24T:18T would have a ratio of 1:0.75.

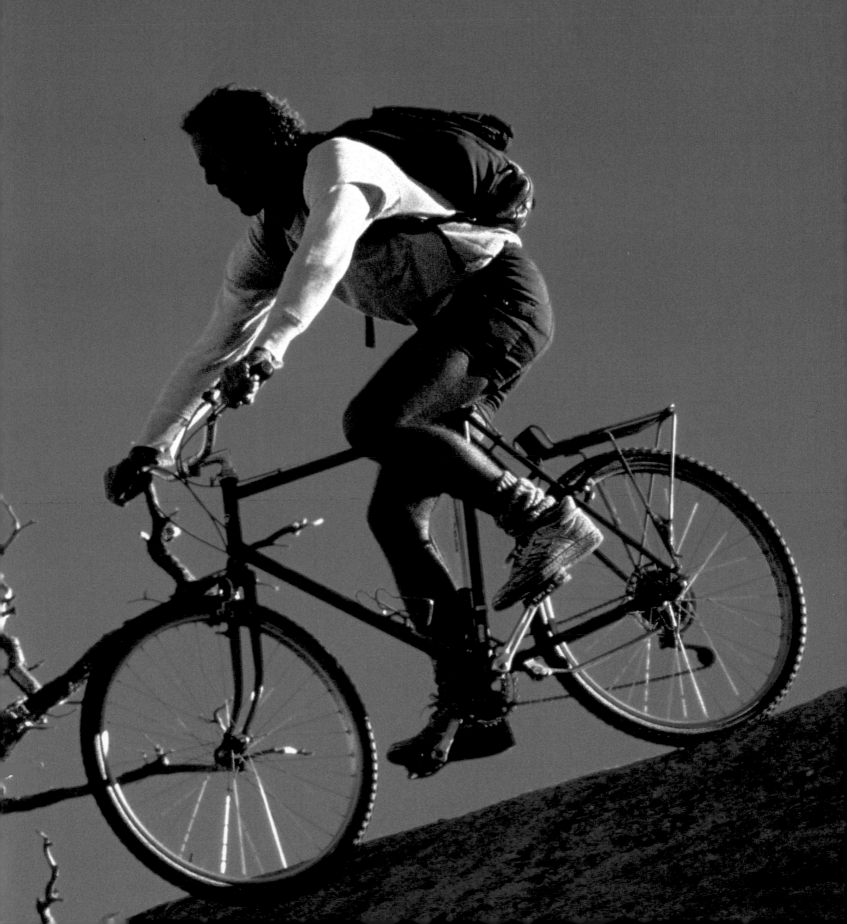

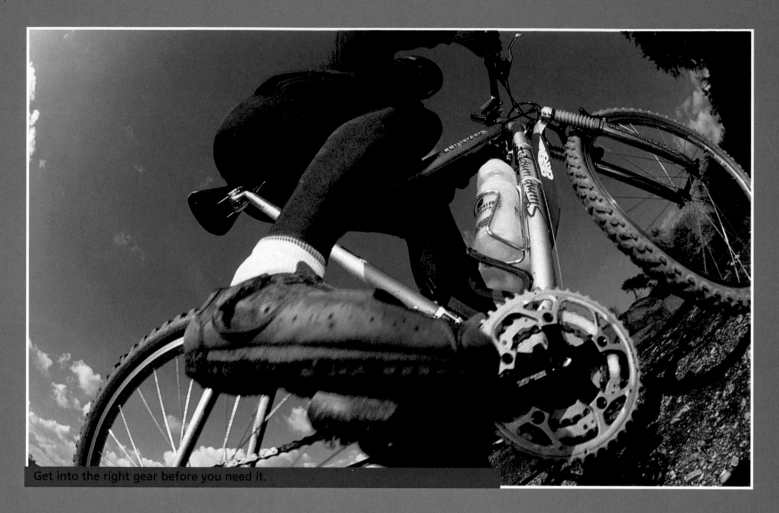

Get into the right gear before you need it.

UNDERSTANDING RATIOS

The bigger the chainring and the smaller the sprocket, the bigger the gear ratio. The bigger the gear ratio, the larger the pedaling load and the higher the speed. The idea behind gear ratios is that different combinations of chainring and sprocket provide the same amount of resistance. For example, the 48:12 gear is the same as the 52:13 (a road bike ratio) — a ratio of 4:1. Understanding gear ratios is the key to realizing that having more gear combinations does not mean higher and lower speed limits, but a finer distinction between gears and a larger choice of combinations.

KEEPING A STRAIGHT CHAIN-LINE

The chainring and sprocket combinations you can use are limited to those that keep the chain in a relatively straight line. You can't use the big-to-big (i.e. big on front, big on back) or small-to-small combinations for two reasons. With those combinations, the chain runs diagonally, which damages the chain plates; also, the ideal chain length is not long enough to go all the way around the big chainring and the big sprocket. If you get your chain into that combination, you may find that it won't come off again!

If the chain becomes too slack, as it would if you used the smallest chainring and smallest sprocket, there's a risk of it bouncing off. But you can find the same ratio in the middle chainring with a mid-range sprocket.

Try to use the largest chainring with the smaller sprockets, and smallest chainring with the bigger sprockets. Gear toward the bike for easy pedaling and away from the bike for harder pedaling. The middle chainring is the most used, and you can safely combine it with both the biggest and the smallest sprocket.

INDEXING AND OVERCHANGING

All MTB gears are indexed, which means that they're pre-set, and will click into place. Changing into a bigger ring or sprocket is a push because the movement is against the spring tension in the derailleur. Push the lever a little further than the resting position before releasing it so that the chain can make it up onto the bigger chainring.

On under-bar or top-bar mounted levers you need to do this with your thumb, because it's stronger. With gripshift gear changers, you have to turn the barrel towards or away from you.

Changing to a smaller ring or sprocket is an easier motion, because the lever is releasing the spring tension, letting the derailleur fall naturally into position. On under-bar or top-bar mounted levers this is done with the index finger. But with gripshift gear changers, you rotate the barrel one way or the other.

You can change more than one gear at the same time, either with one movement or several quick clicks, depending on your gear levers. If the chain falls right off the chainrings or sprocket cassette, the derailleur needs adjusting (see pp. 52–53).

Beginners tips for good gearing

■ You can't change gear without turning the pedals. To change gear when you're not on the bike, stand on the bike's left-hand side. Pick up the rear of the bike with your right hand and keep holding it up. Change the gears while turning the left pedal with your other hand.

■ Sprockets are used for small changes in speed, such as when you're climbing a long, steady hill. To make small changes with the right-hand gear lever, start with the chain on the middle chainring (front) and the middle sprocket (back). Try riding and clicking the right-hand lever until you can make the pedaling harder or easier without even thinking about it.

■ Chainrings are for bigger changes in speed, such as going over the summit of a hill into a descent. Using the left-hand gear lever, start with the chain in a middle sprocket, ride and click the lever up and down to change the chainrings. See how

much more of a difference there is in resistance between each chainring than between the sprockets.

■ The ideal gear to begin cycling in is usually somewhere in the middle of the sprockets and the middle chainring.

■ Beginners tend to focus so hard on steering and pedaling that they forget that the gears are there to help them — remember to change gear.

Gear changing hints

CHANGING DOWN AHEAD OF TIME

Get into the right gear before you need it. Trails are composed of tricky obstacles and rises waiting to try and steal your energy and speed. Keep up that speed by dropping your gear way before the trail slows your pedaling power. You will find that reading the trail ahead becomes second nature.

MISCALCULATING THE GEARS

There's nothing more frustrating than climbing up a hill, holding the line by a hair, knowing you have got a gear left, and then finding out that you've run out of them. Keep tabs on which gear you are in, either by reading the indicators on the gear levers, or by looking down at the rings and sprockets. Getting the hang of this will take some practice, but it pays off. It'll help you avoid miscalculating and accidentally jamming or dropping the chain.

TRICKY GEAR CHANGING

If you need to dramatically drop your gear and speed, a smooth gear change will stop the chain from jamming or being thrown off.

Again, this needs practice and the best place to practice high speed large-ratio gear changes is on a stretch of rollercoaster-like track where you can roll fast down one side and then crawl back up the other. As you approach the bottom of the dip, which will probably be at a high speed, decide well in advance the gear that you need to be in for the upcoming climb. Pick as smooth a line as possible through the dip so that you're able to focus on braking and changing gear, instead of having to keep the front wheel under control.

When you actually hit the bottom, change down to the lowest gear — smallest chainring — at the front, and down to the third or fourth sprocket at the back — that'll save a couple of sprockets for the hardest part of the climb. Shift both gears simultaneously. Then wait for a second to give the chain, which will have lost all its tension, a chance to catch the new teeth and for the derailleur to take up the slack, so that it doesn't get thrown off.

Be prepared to spin the pedals like crazy while the bike slows down to its new speed, from a ratio of 4:1 say, to 1:0.75. For a few seconds, before the bike gets into gear, you'll probably find yourself spinning without resistance.

On bumpy, fast tracks and downhills keep the chain in a large sprocket and middle or large chainring to prevent it from bouncing off.

SINGLE-SPEED MOUNTAIN BIKES

Single-speed bikes have only one gear. That means that the bike has only one chainring, one sprocket and no gear levers. The simplicity of the design is attractive in a mountain bike world that seems to be always increasing in complexity.

good climbing technique

Climbing is the great challenge of cycling. And the mountain bike is designed specifically for taking on the challenge. The broad, grippy tires, the position of the rider over the back wheel and the 2mph (3km/h) gearing give the MTB a caterpillar-like ability in tackling tricky ascents.

Mountain bikers have a love-hate relationship with climbing. It is hard work, but it makes life clearer. Day-to-day issues like money, friendship and the future can be complicated. But in mountain biking, the goal — reaching the top — is simple. Whether you're a beginner or an expert, there's nothing like the feeling of accomplishment that greets you at the top of a climb. And the descent is always sweet.

Technique summarized

In the hands of a good rider, a mountain bike can handle inclines of close to 45° on badly broken ground. The key factors are two things that can be learned by everyone; balance and power. Balance is gained through awareness and practice. Power is gained through repetition, an investment in muscular and cardiovascular strength.

CLIMBING AIDS

1 **Centre of gravity.**
2 **Use wide, knobby tires to provide grip.**
3 **Bar ends offer a variety of hand-holds to open out the chest slightly and provide a distraction when the going gets tough.**
4 **A frame with short chain stays, under 16.5in (420mm), will keep the rider's weight at the back of the bike for balance, power and grip. Radical frame designs that tuck the rear wheel further under the saddle may have elevated stays or kinked seat-tubes.**
5 **Suspension has its pros and cons in climbing. It wastes rider energy but increases grip, so set adjustable shock absorption harder for the best of both worlds. It's also important that suspended bikes, which have extra joints and pivots, are laterally strong.**
6 **Adjusting the saddle so that its nose points slightly downward will relieve pressure on genital areas if you have to crouch-climb.**
7 **SPD-style spring binding pedals and shoes make climbing easier — once you're used to them!**

Lower total weight of bike+rider = less work

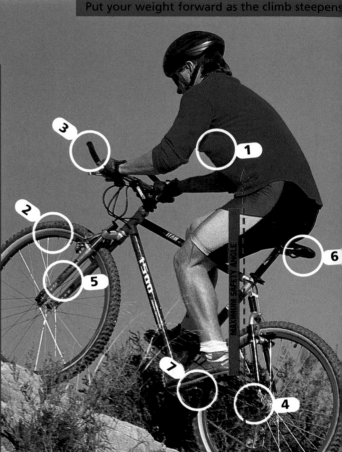

Put your weight forward as the climb steepens

CENTRE OF GRAVITY

The centre of gravity of a bike and rider is the abdomen. To hold the line and to avoid falling off backward while climbing, draw an imaginary line from where the rear wheel touches the ground to your abdomen. It should never be greater than 90° from a horizontal. Pull your body weight further forward as the climb gets steeper, otherwise the front wheel won't have enough weight on it and it'll lose grip or lift up, and you'll lose your line or fall off.

On the other hand, if your abdomen is too far forward, the rear wheel won't have enough weight on it. It'll spin and your momentum will be lost, so much so that you won't be able to stay in the saddle. It's a question of constantly and minutely adjusting your position for the optimum performance.

STANDING UP
In a middle gear the most effective and — until you're strong enough — painful way to climb is to stand on the pedals. It adds your body weight to the muscular force of your legs pushing on the pedals, but because of that it also takes more strength. Rocking the bike from side-to-side maximizes the weight on each pedal, but you may be using more energy than you are gaining.

SITTING IN THE SADDLE
When things get really steep, keep your weight as far forward as possible without losing grip on the back tire. Slide forward on the saddle and get into a crouch by bending your arms, and dropping your wrists and back — concentrate on your position.

This sitting position is only used in mountain biking, and takes practice and strength-building. The back and abdominal muscles have to resist the invisible force of gravity, instead of the pedal or handlebar.

GEARING
The grade of the terrain will tell you what gear to be in. Getting it right comes with practice.
■ Get into the right gear a fraction of a second before you need to be in it.
■ On a long haul try changing up for a few seconds into a harder gear, so you can stand up and pump the pedals for temporary muscle relief.
■ Try to keep one last gear, for emergencies.

PICKING A LINE
Grip is the number one priority when you decide where to steer. You'll improve the more you practice on different kinds of terrain.
■ Look ahead.
■ Follow other tire tracks.
■ Choose a line that's clear of loose stuff; leaves, gravel or dust.

Beginners' tips
■ Every time you push down on your pedals you become a stronger cyclist, which is one of the keys to better climbing. The more you ride, the better you'll get at climbing hills.
■ Don't get down. There are no shortcuts to good climbing, so every time you expose

Pearl Pass (12,705ft/3,874m) between Crested Butte and Aspen in Colorado was first conquered by a team of mountain bikers in 1976. The ride is now a focal point of the Annual Crested Butte Fat Tire Festival.

yourself to a brutal new ascent, or get something wrong, you're learning!
■ Don't compare yourself to other riders; measure yourself against yourself. Try to ride further up a difficult hill every time you head out.
■ Climbing gets more rewarding, but not necessarily easier!

Advanced training
■ On or off-road hill repetitions are the most effective — and painful — way to improve your climbing. Ride up a hill a bunch of times as hard as you can in a half- to one-hour period, with a brief rest of just spinning the pedals easily in between.
■ Rest sore legs for a couple of days after a training session, or just ride gently. If you do it regularly, you'll start to enjoy hard riding, but don't overdo it.

PSYCHOLOGY NOTES AND TIPS
■ Don't think about falling off. If you do, you will. Let the bike lose its grip before you do.
■ Feeling sick on a climb just means you're trying hard. It happens because the blood is moved quickly away from your organs, including your stomach, so it can supply the muscles with oxygen.
■ Racers approach a hill thinking about going over it instead of up it.
■ Climbing is a test of patience. When you begin to wonder if you can stand the pain, distract yourself. Think about the rewards; the descent, the cold beer at the pub at the end of the ride, what you're going to eat tonight. Say the alphabet backwards, sing a song in your head, or go through all your friends' birthdays, dates of battles, Shimano part numbers, the states and their capitals, recite your favorite scene verbatim from *Pulp Fiction*.
n Break up the climb into sections mentally, and tackle them one at a time.

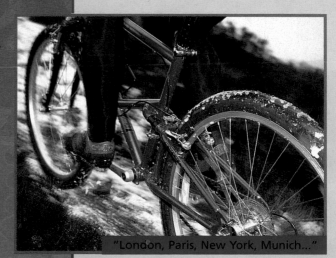
"London, Paris, New York, Munich..."

descending
techniques

Descending is the fun part of mountain biking; anyone can enjoy it, regardless of strength or skill. But, the faster you go, the more in control you have to be. Here are techniques that improve your speed, as well as your chances of survival.

Descending principles

The centre of gravity of a bike and rider is the abdomen. To stay on the bike down a steep descent an imaginary line drawn from where the front wheel touches the ground to the abdomen cannot be greater than 90° from the horizontal behind you — the opposite of when you're climbing.

If your centre of gravity falls ahead of the line on a descent, you'll go over the handlebars, or at least have to dismount before you do. Keep the centre of gravity behind that vertical line, and the angle of slope that an experienced rider can descend can be steeper than 45°.

CONFIDENCE TIPS
The mountain bike can stay upright on incredibly angular slopes, so trust the bike and let it give up before you do, just as you would when climbing. A skid can make you feel like you're out of control, but if you practice, you'll learn that you're not.

KNOW YOUR LIMITS

Descending is a combination of balance, will and applying the brakes at the right time. You need to have nerves of steel to be a competitive downhiller, as well as an explosive strength to power yourself out of corners.

There's not much mystery behind downhilling, but every cyclist does it differently. In all mountain bike techniques, becoming competent and safe is a matter of practice, but with downhilling, each rider has a personal speed limit that's hard — and usually painful — to exceed. Don't ever let yourself be pressured into riding beyond your ability. Crashing does more damage than having to buy a round of beer because you were the last one home!

Beginners' descending

1 Sitting down on a descent only works on gentle, smooth slopes. As soon as the ride gets bumpy, you need to stand up to let your legs absorb some shock. This frees the bike up from your weight and lets you shift around. A descent technique popular with beginners is to grip the saddle with the inside of the thighs.

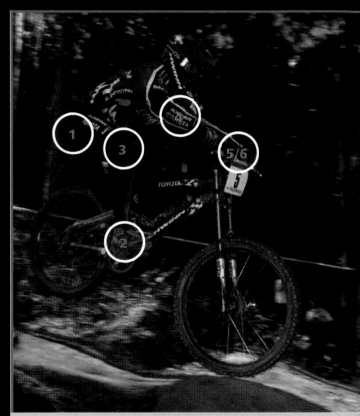

The steeper a hill the further back your weight should be.

2 Make sure that the pedals are horizontal — a common MTB technique that's used when riding over obstacles and uneven terrain.

3 Keep your legs slightly bent, and use them as shock absorbers.

4 Straighten your arms and bend your legs the steeper the hill gets, to keep your weight as far back as possible. On extreme slopes, you can apply stability and traction by slipping your butt over the back of the saddle.

5 When you're going downhill, it's better to use the front brake, not the rear. Use it to

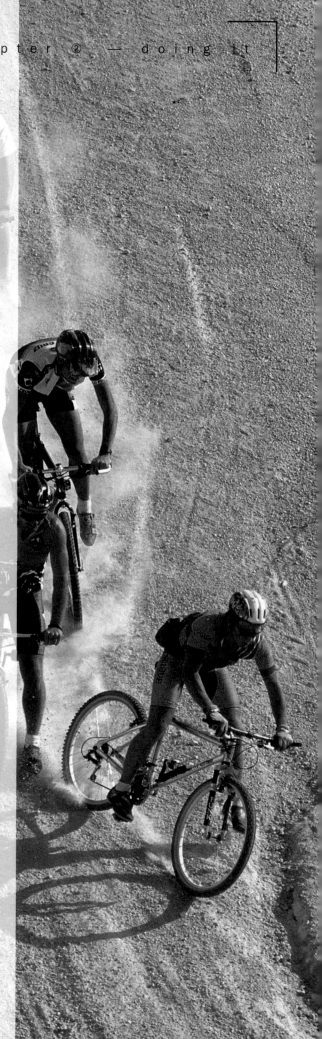

control your speed and steering. Be careful though — the front brake reacts much faster than the rear one. Slam it on too fast and the moving weight of the bike and your body will get pushed over the front wheel. The rear brake takes longer to react, and is better used in combination with the front brake, for controlled skidding and emergencies.

TIPS AND SPECIALIST EQUIPMENT

■ **Always wear a helmet, preferably a full-face one. Body armour is a good idea for playing around and is required in competitions.**

■ **Keep your brakes serviced and done up. Julie Furtado, one of the world's most successful racers and the only ever winner of both the downhill and cross-country world titles, was the favorite to win the 1992 world championship cross-country, but had to drop out when her front brake cable pulled through at the brake pad and forced her off the trail.**

■ **Suspension bikes are made for downhilling. The shock absorbers go to the limit to keep you in line and in control.**

■ **Flat pedals are great for specialist downhillers, who use their extended legs as stabilizers on the corners. The rest of us find SPD clipless pedals the best way to stop our feet from being shaken off the bike. A good compromise is double-sided pedals, giving you an SPD on one side and a plain platform on the other.**

6 Over very fast, bumpy ground, lock your thumb and forefinger around the handlebars (to stop yourself from going over them), keeping the middle and fourth fingers free for braking.

7 Look at where you want to steer, a few metres ahead of the bike.

8 The best way to improve is to repeatedly practice a steep downhill or drop-off that you find uncomfortable. Once you've conquered it, try the next most difficult descent. Racing is good for downhill technique, because you repeat descents on each lap.

Speed descending

■ Descending is all about letting gravity do the work, while you concentrate on braking and distributing your weight. Think ahead on rough terrain and corners, and slow down enough to flow over or around them. Try not to brake so much that you lose momentum.

■ Speed itself can help you stay on the bike. A fast spinning wheel is a rigid structure that will carry you over rough sections that might give you trouble at a slower speed.

■ Take the shortest line, cutting corners closely, and going for the smoothest piece of track you can see.

■ Keep your wheels on the ground. Low jumps, taken in a crouch with bent arms and legs, help keep a clean line, and the wheels level. Traveling through the air more than a couple of inches will slow you down.

Safe descents

Be aware of other trail users — just because you're the fastest thing on the trail doesn't mean you have the right of way. Hikers and horses using the trail have priority over your screaming downhill. Slow down for people and stop completely for horses. Know your terrain — never let loose if you don't know what's around the corner.

cornering

For successful cornering watch out for:
- Balance
- Braking
- Progressive position of the bike around the corner.

Like all mountain biking techniques, improving your cornering comes with exposure and practice — which basically means that you learn by riding! On any ride you'll turn dozens of corners, over grass, on loose gravel and in ruts, steeply downhill or sharply up. On some pieces of track you won't travel in a straight line at all. That's one of the big differences between off-road and speedier on-the-road biking, which generally runs along straighter lines. It also helps explain why mountain bike design is more concerned with strength and maneuvrability than aerodynamics.

Watch the champions

You can learn a lot from watching a professional downhill or cross-country race and having a first-hand look at the lines the riders take. It's on the corners, the most common part of the trail, that a race can be won or lost.

Centrifugal force at work!

When you corner the centrifugal force tries to push you outward off the trail. Centrifugal force involves three factors — the sharpness of the bend, your speed and the combined mass of you and your bike — and you can manipulate each of them with good technique.

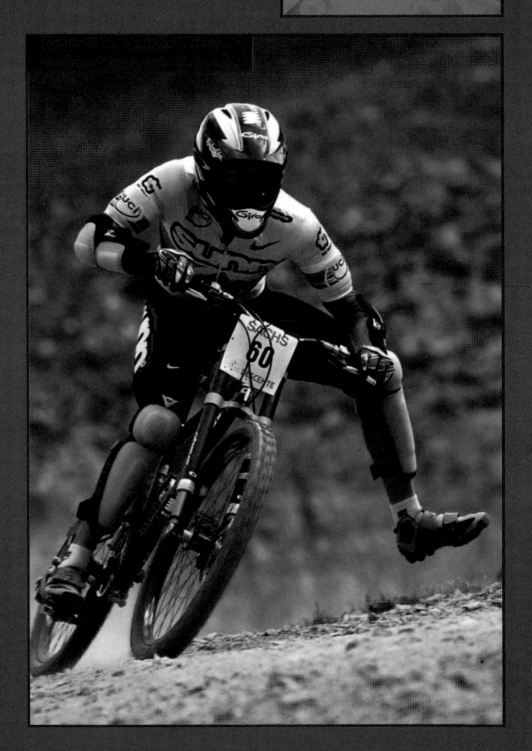

The theory of cornering

1 SOFTEN THE ANGLE

The tighter the corner, the more powerful the centrifugal force, so the goal is to soften the angle of the curve, keep the speed higher and make a quick exit. You can do that by completing most of the turn in the first half of the corner. As you approach the curve, swing away from its sharpest point, then turn inward and aim for it. By the time you're at the sharpest point, you should be facing more or less the right way.

Use the full width of the track if you need to. Sweeping around a corner that way saves speed and feels great.

2 CONTROL YOUR SPEED

Centrifugal force increases exponentially as speed increases, so you need is to enter a corner slowly and exit quickly. If you keep your speed at maximum, as if you're still going in a straight line, you'll be shot right off the trail.

To take a corner any faster than at a low-key cruising pace, use the brakes on the way into the bend and the pedals on the way out again. Get into the right gear for the exit and brake before you hit the bend, to allow for that outward swing.

Keep your fingers over the brake levers as you go around, applying them equally. Don't panic and jam on the front brake, which could suddenly stop, probably shoot you over the handlebars, and may twist the front wheel.

Start pedaling when you've handled the corner, which may even be before you hit the sharpest point. Assuming you got the gear right, stand on the pedals if you can to sprint away.

3 USE YOUR BODY TO BALANCE

Lean your weight to the inside to minimize the centrifugal force; the sharper the corner, the sharper your lean. Bending the inside elbow helps pull your weight forward and inward. Standing up is tricky, but useful, when you are experienced, for bumpy corners, because it lets you use your legs as shock absorbers and determine where you're going to throw your centre of gravity.

Sitting down is good for smooth, fast corners. It lets you to bend your inside knee and press down on the straight outside leg, to push against the force. Resist the temptation to lean backward; the front wheel will become less weighted, and you'll have less control over the grip and steering.

BEGINNERS TECHNIQUE

Slow cornering off-road is simpler than it sounds because MTBs are so well-designed. If you want to take a sharp bend easily, the wide, knobby tires will help you all the way around — just as long as you keep up the momentum.

If you are just getting the hang of how the bike feels there isn't even a need to swing it out before the corner, or stick out your knee. Those techniques come into play at higher speeds. Just ride around at your own pace, and think about the next obstacle. Most people find left-hand turns easier than right-hand ones, so practice the right-handed ones!

ADVANCED CORNERING

The more familiar you are with off-road biking the more you use your body's weight instead of your brakes to get around corners without losing momentum. Put your body to one side, then the other, off the saddle, stand up and sit down, hammer for the best position around a corner.

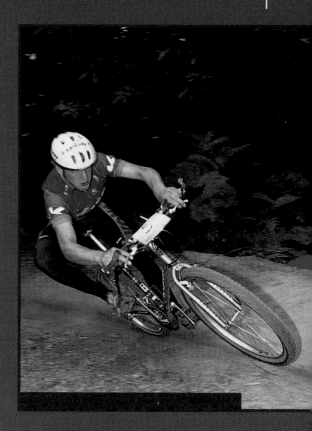

What you're riding over is critical. Try to plan the move so that you get as clean a surface as possible. Ruts are dangerous so keep clear and avoid wet roots at all costs! Sand is like a sponge, gravel is risky. Mud is a better bet than most of these, believe it or not, and a puddle usually has even better grip, but be aware of the powerful braking effect that water can have. If it's more than a couple of inches deep, it can send you flying over the handlebars.

SKIDDING

Experienced riders use skids to get around corners quickly. They brake hard with the back brake once they are well into the curve and lock up the rear wheel so that they skim across the ground's surface with rapid deceleration. A well-executed skid is thrilling to watch, and a useful skill to master, but they're more tricky to control than rolling wheels, and an unpredictable off-road surface means more chance of a painful fall.

airborne techniques

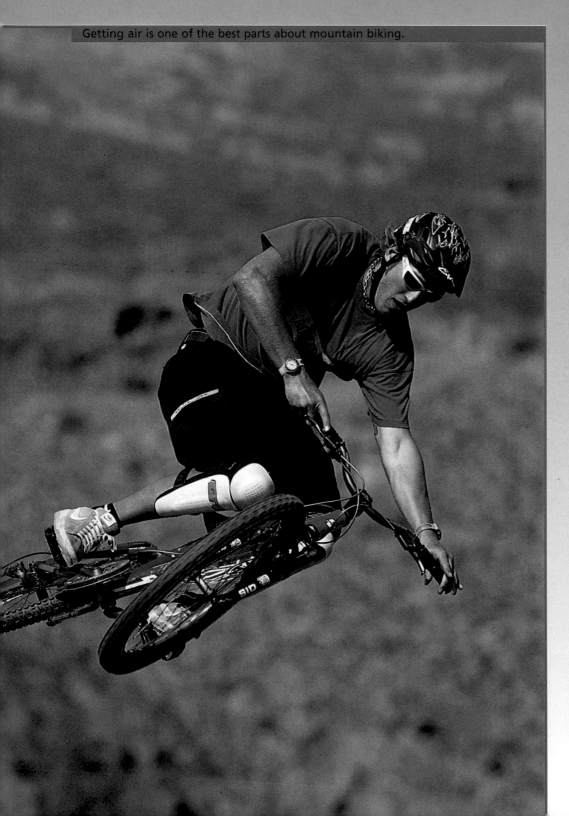

Getting air is one of the best parts about mountain biking.

Getting the bike off the ground

Unexpected obstacles litter the route of the off-road rider, just waiting to bring you down. So the most useful handling skill to have is the art of getting air, that is, to be able to lift the wheels off the ground, either one or both at a time. This technique can be applied to anything between a simple log-roll to a full-blown jump, with bunny hops somewhere in between. Once you've mastered it, you'll ride faster and more confidently — and impress your friends.

Log hops for beginners

To hop or roll over a log, lift the front wheel in a controlled wheelie, and then pull up the back wheel, but don't completely leave the ground.

Find a 6in (150mm) log or make your own log-like substitute on flattish ground with enough room to approach and get away from it.

Pick up enough speed, to get yourself over the log — you may need an extra push on the pedals. When you're a yard in front of the log, stop pedaling, place the pedals in a horizontal position (so they don't hit the log), and, still sitting down, shift your weight backward to get you weight off the front wheel. Just before you hit the log, push the pedals another half-turn (finishing with the

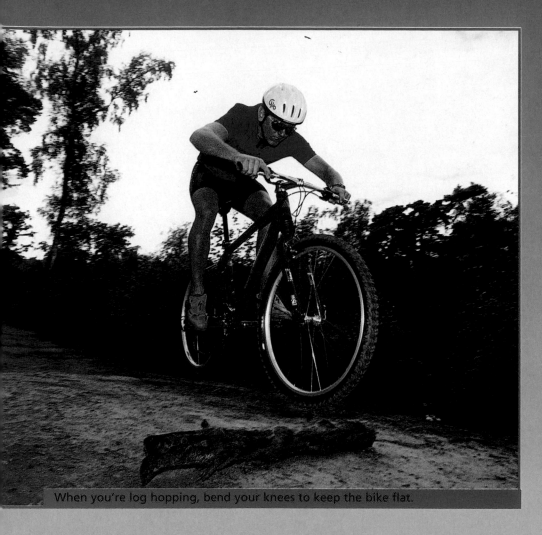

When you're log hopping, bend your knees to keep the bike flat.

logs, or even just painted lines on the ground, which aren't so frightening!

Approach the obstacle at a medium speed. A yard or so in front of it, stand up, crouch and bend your elbows and knees and shift your weight forward to take the weight off the back wheel. Jump up, bending your knees and pulling up on the pedals to bring the bike with you, and keeping the bike as flat as possible. Your arms do a lot of the work. Beginners tend to pull up too much in the front while the back wheel stays planted on the ground.

pedals horizontal again), and pull up on the front wheel — all your weight should be at the back of the bike so that you're not just pulling up against yourself. The wheel should pop up into a wheelie and glide over the top of the obstacle.

The second the front wheel hits the ground again, stand up in the pedals, push your weight forward and bend your knees to pull up the back wheel. This will minimize the impact and let the back wheel bump over the log.

If the chainring teeth catch on the log, give the pedals a push to keep the bike rolling — it's not very cool to get stuck see-sawing like this.

Bunny hops

A bunny hop is, as the name implies, where the bike lifts completely off the ground with both wheels at the same time. It is a useful

trick for getting out of all kinds of trouble such as unexpected potholes on the road. You'll probably enjoy the feeling of clearing heights of 2in (50mm), but practice enough, and you'll see how easy it is to break bunny hop records.

The most difficult part of a bunny hop is lifting the back wheel up. SPD pedals and shoes are a huge help and don't solve the mystery of how stunt riders do such big jumps using just plain pedals and shoes.

For the less talented, a bunny hop can be done just by getting the approach speed right. If you're traveling fast then it's easier to get the bike airborne. But, a true bunny hop moves more vertically than horizontally, and you should practice doing them with no momentum. To do that, you need to time the moment when you jump with your body to bring the bike up and along with it you, in a smooth motion. Practice going over smaller

Jumps with launch pads and lips

Using ramps and edges it's easy to make air, but you need to know how to land safely. Even a medium speed is enough to fling a bike and rider way above the ground, and the last thing you want is a front-wheel touchdown. The bike will rise through the air, level out and then flip downward, hitting the ground vertically. You end up either going over the handlebars or having the front wheel twist out of control and falling to the side.

To stop that from happening, as soon as you've taken air, get the bike ready for a horizontal landing, both wheels touching down at the same time. Put yourself in a crouched position, straighten your arms and bend your legs and push the whole bike forward underneath you.

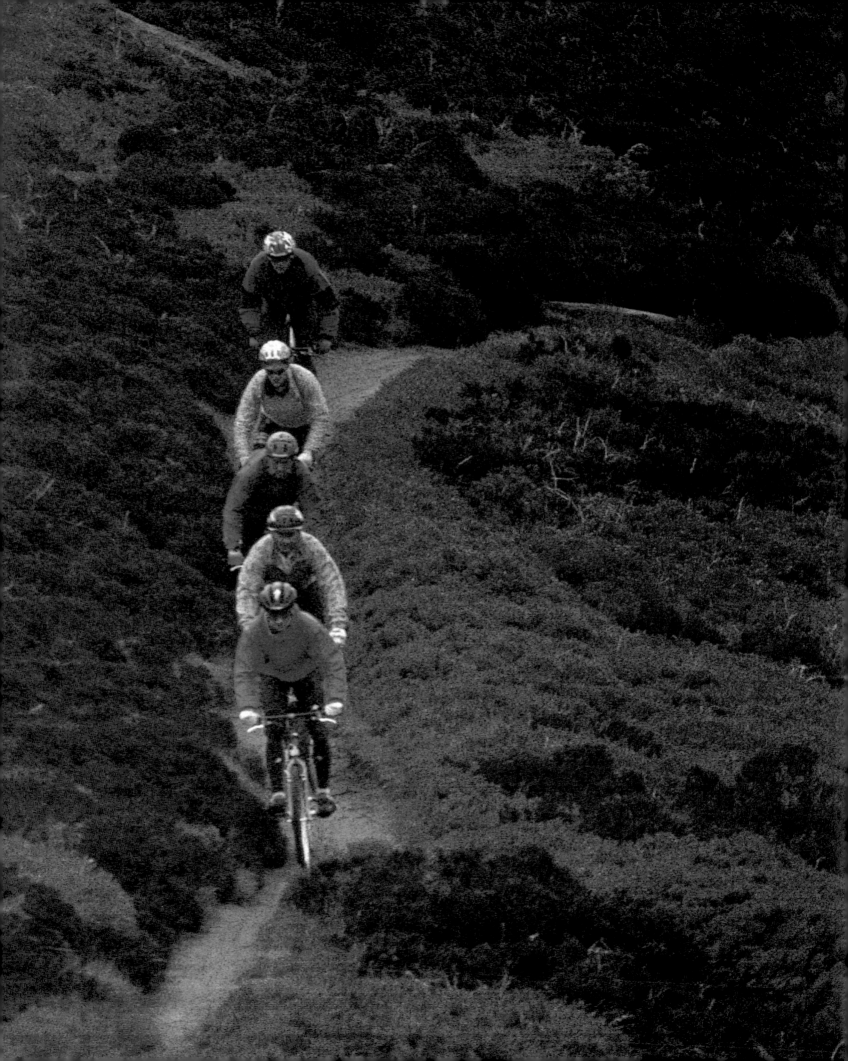

riding
single-track

Single-track riding can be all things to all people. Most mountain bikers rate single-track as second only to a good downhill. It can be fast, but not stressful and your quick reactions can turn it into an ego ride. Single-track is the cream of the crop of all varieties of trail, because no two sections in the world are the same.

Shifting your bodyweight from one side of the bike to the other and timing acceleration means a more intellectually stimulating kind of riding. In a single-track's twist and turns, a bike and its rider become one unit.

Or, you can cruise along comfortably, taking time out to enjoy the view and looking out for wildlife.

So what is single-track?

Single-track is exactly that. It's different from wide double-track, which is named after the tire marks cars and trucks leave off-road. A single-track trail is inaccessible to vehicles. It is rough, narow and no wider than a bike. It's definitely too narrow for horses but will sometimes be used by walkers, who don't know what fun they're missing. A bike's footprint is only 2in (50mm) wide, so an inch or two more each side to clear shoulders and hips, and the mountain bike can slip through anything 2ft (0.6m) wide. At full speed, it's invigorating fun. Just watch out for foot traffic; you usually can't see much farther than the next tree.

Techniques of single-track riding

Riding single-track is simple and can even be appreciated by a novice. It is as close as you will get to a crash course in mountain bike control, because pure single-track is 100% balance, steering, braking and pedaling. You can tackle it at whatever speed you want, since there is no painful grade to pedal or to brake up or down.

Try to maintain as high an even speed as possible for the whole length of the track. Practice will increase your speed and your timing, which will need to be tighter and tighter. The key to doing it as fast as you can is all in your concentration. Anticipation and cornering, and knowing when to put in a blast of power, are things to master. You'll improve more with exposure to trails than you will with being in shape. Eventually you'll reach a stage where a little feathering of your brakes and a few pushes on your pedals will create a momentum that floats and feels really good.

The best single-track is in naturally forested areas — as opposed to grid-like tree farms — where the track twists and turns around tree trunks over fallen logs, slimy roots, and through puddles. But variety is the spice of the trail and more open sections can be equally rewarding, where you can catch a quick glimpse of a stunning view over the mountains in between concentrating on guiding the bike.

SINGLE-TRACK TIPS

■ Cut the corners tightly, because your speed isn't going to be high enough to throw you off a banked curve, and start pedaling again as soon as you are pointing the right way.

■ Bringing your handlebar as close as possible to tree trunks is a thrill of single-track, and a way to gain a nano-second of speed over riders who are less brave. The consequences are nasty if you mis-time it.

■ Learn to pedal from any position so you can cruise through rough sections, roots or bumps and to pull and push the bike.

■ Some single-track can narrow right down to a tire's width — and this is where you get in trouble with overhanging branches whipping the arms and face. Expect to steer one-handed if thorny bushes close in on one side. Wear gloves and a helmet.

■ Brake and change down gear ahead of sharp corners or bumpy sections.

■ Dry conditions are best. In wet conditions be ready to bunny-hop damp roots, which can take out the back wheel.

■ Crested Butte in Colorado, USA, is renowned for its narrow, fast woodland single-track trails.

Surviving
the street

Beware inexplicable gaps in the traffic

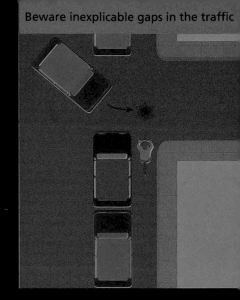

Opening doors

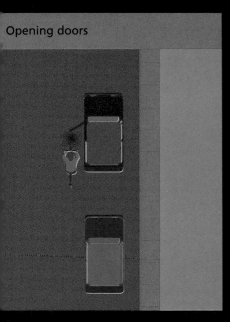

Sudden turns without time to react

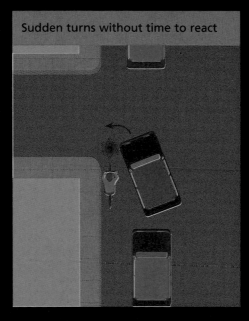

Drafting

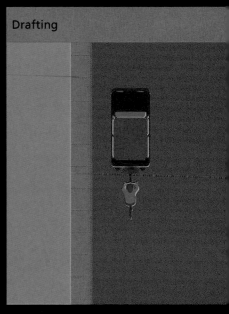

Watch out for turning trucks

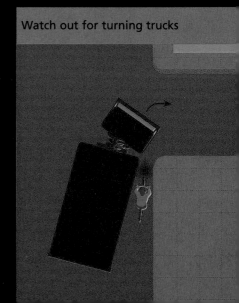

No mountain bike is ridden just on trails, so a mountain biker has to adapt to riding on roads, and learn to avoid cars as well as trees. On the street, a driver's vision is more restricted than a cyclist's. A cyclist can hear and feel the effects of speed, but a car driver is in a vehicle that blocks out noise.

Safe practice

■ A little visual dialogue goes a long way. Don't be too shy or too cool to use hand signals in traffic. Make eye contact and let drivers know when they're being helpful.

■ Know everything that is going on around you. If you don't understand the traffic's movements then approach cautiously with your hands over the brakes.

■ Going with the traffic flow disrupts drivers less, and makes it easier for them to accom-

modate you. But you do need to be in shape to keep up with the cars.

■ Use bike lanes where they are provided. Try to convince your local politician to cut back on vehicle dependency and to improve the bicycle network.

Danger spots

■ Opening doors — give parked vehicles at least 3ft (1 metre) of clearance, a door's-width, to avoid being hit if a driver swings one into you.

■ Car escape routes — when riding beside a line of waiting cars, be aware of for the side streets and be prepared for drivers to turn onto them suddenly to escape traffic.

■ Watch out for inexplicable gaps between vehicles ahead. Sometimes cars will leave space open for an oncoming vehicle to access a side street.

- Beware of trucks at all times — their drivers can't see you beside them and may not hear you shouting to let them know you're there. Try not to get on the inside of a turning truck, because what starts out as a huge gap is reduced to nothing. A large number of cycling fatalities are due to cyclists being crushed either against railings or by the wheels of turning trucks. It's not worth the risk for a few seconds gained.
- When you're changing lanes, use your hand signals. Cars joining traffic from a yield lane may look behind you for oncoming traffic and not see you at all.
- Riding fast — vehicles and pedestrians underestimate how fast you can move on a bike. So they'll turn or step out in front of you because they assume you're moving much more slowly than you are.
- Drafting or slipstreaming behind vehicles is fast and fun, but it's also dangerous. Vehicles brake and slow down faster than bikes, especially in wet conditions.

Bicycle thieves

Beware of the bicycle thief. A shiny bike has the bonus of also being a getaway vehicle that is easily converted into cash and difficult for the police to track down. You can never be sure that your bike won't be stolen, but you can try to prevent that by using a good lock, and ease the pain with a good insurance policy.

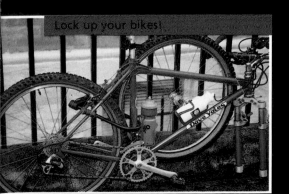
Lock up your bikes!

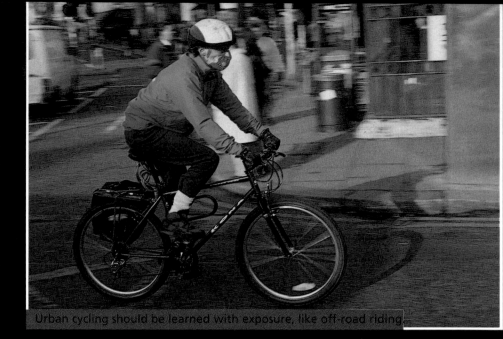
Urban cycling should be learned with exposure, like off-road riding.

Insurance

Your annual cycling budget should include about 10 per cent of the original cost of the bike for insurance. If your bike gets stolen, the insurance repays itself in a second so it's worth having. Ask your cycling friends about their own policies, or go to your local cycling club for advice. Your bike should at least be covered on your household policy. You may also have to pay a supplement, and make sure you read the fine print.

The right lock

A steel U-lock is the king of bike protection, but it is still not 100 per cent theft-proof. The flexible, covered heavy-duty motorcycle cable or chain is also popular, but also is not completely theft-proof.

Locking up

- Find an unmovable object.
- Remove the front wheel. Place it between the rear wheel and the object. Put the lock through the rear wheel, frame and front wheel, placing the actual lock in a position that makes it awkward for anyone with a lock-breaking tool to get at.
- Remove everything loose — lights, pump, wedge pack and front wheel — even the front wheel quick-release if you are in a high-crime area.

Where's the risk?

- Your bike's also easily stolen from a garage, so lock it to something or even bring it inside. And it's probably not a good idea to leave it in the hallway of an apartment building.
- On the car. Either U-lock the bikes to a rack which can be locked to the car roof, or never let them out of your sight.
- Parked outside a shop — the "I only left it for a second" scenario. The opportunistic theft is the most common one — don't risk it.
- At your work. If you ride to work every day, it's easy to get lulled into a false sense of security about your employer's bike racks, but they probably don't pose much of a challenge for a thief.

Precautions

- Cut down on the time your bike is parked and exposed to theft. Use a less attractive bike for commuting or booting around a city.
- Write down the number of the key for the lock, so you can get another one cut in case the bike is locked up when you lose it.
- Write down the frame number (on the bottom of the frame), keep a description of the bike and take a picture of it. Register the bike with the police.

unmissable — night-time visibility

Don't be put off by a false sense of modesty from making yourself as visible as possible on the road. The colors of specialty biking clothes may not be pretty but they may save your life.

During the daytime, make your presence known with bright colors. When it's dark, use reflective strips and bands and powerful lights both to light up the road or trail and to signal your presence to other road-users.

High-visibility clothing

Most cyclists identify with environmental issues, and then they clothe themselves in a fluorescent yellow that's too ugly to occur in nature. A bit of Day-Glo never does any harm, and anything that reduces a sense of vulnerability, which puts so many people off cycling on the roads, is a good thing.

A neon-yellow or reflective, strip-coated breathable waterproof jacket is essential on wet days when drivers can't see as well as they normally can. On drier, warmer days, neon jerseys are easy to see, and a thin Pertex shell will keep the wind out.

Reflectives

REflective clothing can be as effective as lights and will score you points with drivers. For daytime riding, grey Scotchlite-type

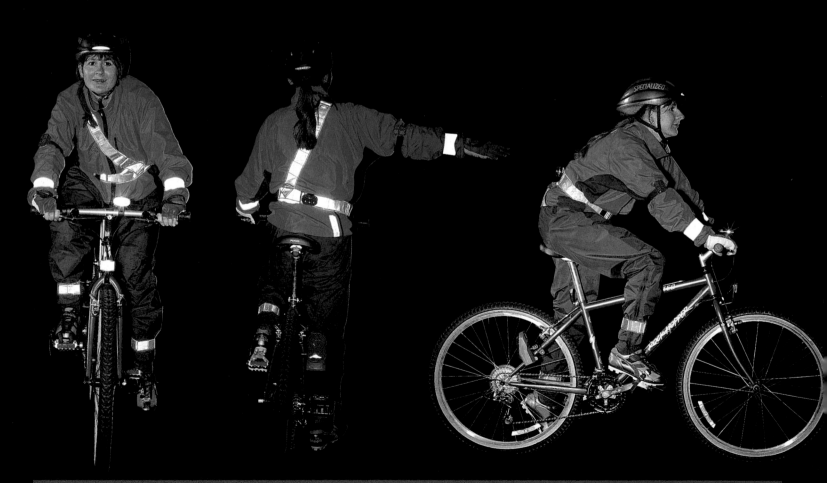

Light up the night with Day-Glo strips and clothing.

coatings are easier on the eye. At night they are turned into a reflective silver by headlights.

For extra visibility try wearing fluorescent velcro ankle straps. They're especially noticeable because they move (and flash) up and down with your legs. Wrist straps are great for making turning signals in the dark and putting fluorescent tape on your helmet helps too.

A little silver piping can go a long way. When a backpack covers the reflective strips on your jacket, put patches of reflective material on the backpack. They can be bought pre-cut or by the yard. Stick them over everything that's visible from the rear; the seat stays and fender, the back of the helmet, and even your shoes and overboots.

Reflective tires with a bead of Scotchlite tape around the side wall are compulsory in the Netherlands, and very effective. They're recommended for commuters and anyone else riding after sunset.

But, no mountain biker would be caught dead with reflectors on their front and back wheels. It's too bad, because the front reflector not only lets cars see if you've forgotten or lost light from your front light, but catches a snapped front brake cable before it snags the front wheel and throws you over the handlebars.

Lights

A light's primary job is to let traffic know you're there. There is a wide variety of lights on the market — most of them good and easily removable. They usually use "AA" batteries. Rechargeable batteries save money and are more environmentally friendly, but they're slightly dimmer and fade faster and faster the older they get. Do not forget to charge them after each ride.

When it comes to the bulb, halogens use up the batteries quicker, but it hurts even to look at them. LED (light emitting

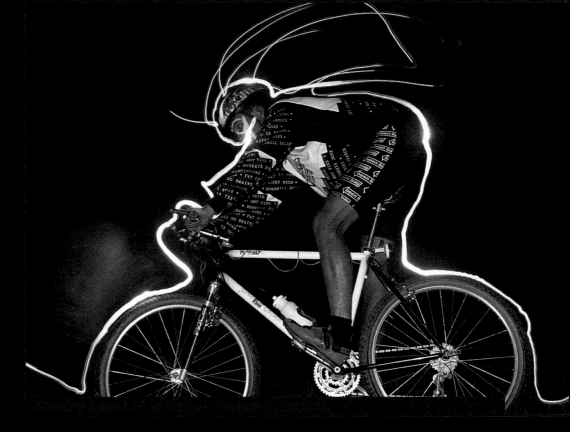

diode) lights are light, cheap and last longer, especially if you set them on flash, but are only supposed to be used with standard bulb lights.

There's a theory that the flash setting is a distraction to drivers. But anything that attracts a driver's attention can only increase the cyclist's safety; and any driver who genuinely mistakes them for a car's blinker signal shouldn't be on the road.

The best place to mount lights is on the bike frame, but you can also attach some to your body and on your accessories; on the helmet, attached to a belt, on your arms or wrists and even to pannier pockets. Most lights come with special clips so you can do that. Lights like those should only be used on their own in emergencies.

Seeing your way on the road

There are also brighter lighting "systems" so you can see, and be seen, like car head-

lamps. Their bulbs range from regular 6 watt (W), strong 10W and a dazzling 50W. They are excellent for urban visibility, unlit back roads and nocturnal off-road rides, when they can be used with a helmet-mounted light.

Most super-systems are front light only, some with two lamps for an option of dipped/full, narrow or wide beam and more or less wattage to conserve the battery. Powerful remote battery packs can be mounted on the bike, either in the bottle cage or underneath the top tube, and provide the extra power needed to light up the night. They weigh a lot, though, and are bulky; not the easiet thing to take off and carry around when you park and leave the bike.

If you're on a longer off-road trip and camping, your bike lights are going to be invaluable, both on the trail — remember that the country is very much darker than an urban nightscape — and round the camp. You'll probably need extra batteries.

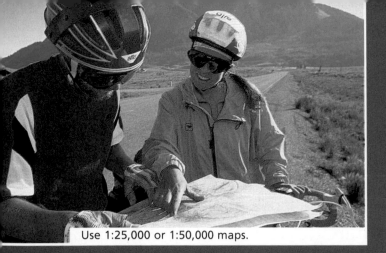
Use 1:25,000 or 1:50,000 maps.

planning
your ride

Day tripping

The essence of mountain biking is the afternoon, day or weekend ride, done by most bikers for the exercise, the sense of discovery and as an easy way to make and spend time with friends. All you need is a map and a banana and you have the keys to a new world at the end of the road.

The pleasure principle

■ Build in meal or drink breaks where muddy bikers are welcome.

■ Try to include viewpoints or historical areas. Use your imagination. Sometimes you can follow a professional road race by taking off-road short-cuts.

■ Flat routes along the bottom of valleys or alongside rivers, lakes or canals are great for beginners, children and older riders.

■ The ideal air temperature for a ride is around 60°F (15.5°C) with a gentle breeze. Not too hot, not too cold.

■ Check out the undiscovered land that lies between the back roads close to your home.

■ Head out for enjoyable, thrilling descents and challenging, satisfying climbs.

The challenge

■ Try to break your own records for distance, altitude climbed and time.

■ Enjoy the mountain air by riding on steeper trails. Even in bad weather, it can be fun and exciting.

■ If life in the city gets boring, get back to nature for an afternoon.

Where to ride

There's a thrill in exploring a new area without having a clue where you are or where you're going — but make sure that you don't wander too far, and that you have good weather. It doesn't take more than a couple of rides for off-road innocence to fade and for the biker to crave bigger riding opportunities and a closer connection with nature.

For those who want longer distances ridden at high speed, you'll need a map.

To plan a route, read bike and outdoor magazines and ask other cyclists for their recommendations. Get the right map in the right scale (see pp. 126–7) from an outdoor store or map shop. Using a fluorescent highlighter pen, mark the route you want to take or all the legal trails in the area.

You can buy a device that runs over a map and adds up the miles for you. Or, use a piece of thread to follow the twists and turns of your proposed route and then add them up on the scale at the side of the map.

How far to go

Decide how long to make your ride, according to the daylight hours available, how

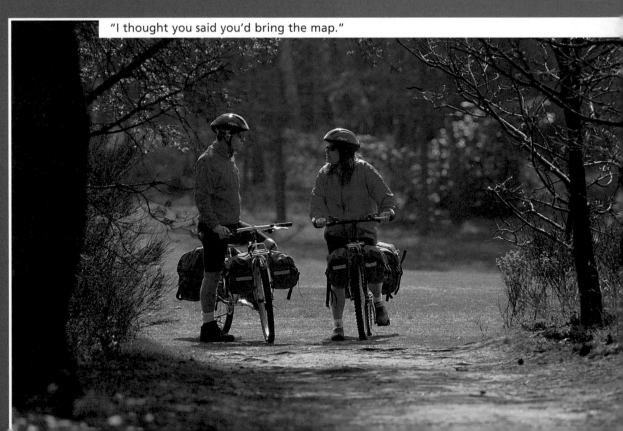
"I thought you said you'd bring the map."

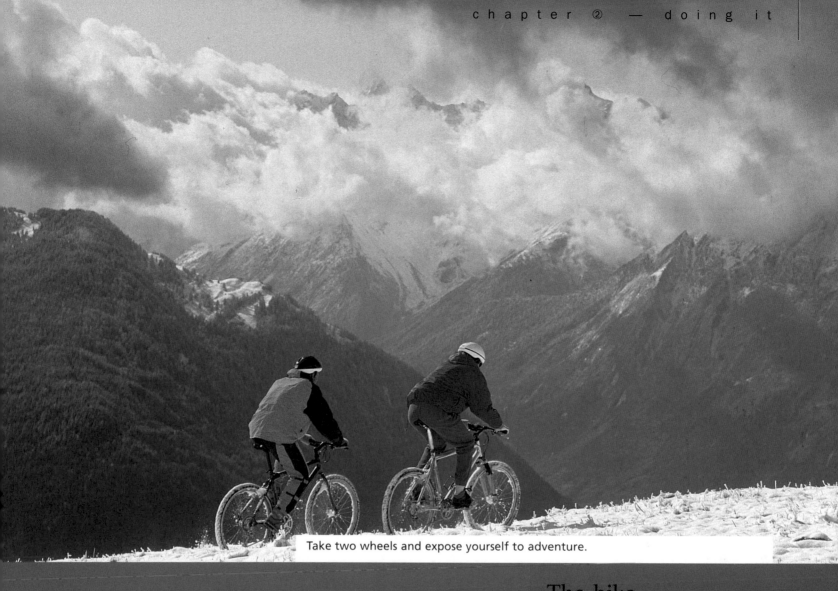

Take two wheels and expose yourself to adventure.

many rest stops you think you'll need and cal-culate the distance relative to your average off-road speed. Most racers travel at about 10mph (16km/h), so bear that in mind. Excuses for getting home late include:

■ "I had to buy a round of beer at the end because I was last."

■ "I'm fat and out of shape."

■ "I got a flat and the bike broke."

■ "I got lost."

■ "I crashed."

■ "The group went slowly."

■ "We had to keep stopping to read the map."

Or bad conditions:

■ A sudden strong headwind, rain or snow.

■ Darkness.

■ Too much climbing.

■ Rough under-tire conditions, including rocks and mud.

■ Having to carry the bike.

Be realistic

A realistic distance to cover in an afternoon ride is 10–15 miles (16–24km), but it may be a lot less, depending on terrain and the age and strength of the riders. A day's ride with a few stops for lunch and snacks can range from 20–25 miles (32–40km).

Strong riders in dry conditions without any chance of getting lost can tackle 50 miles (80km) of off-road in a day. But it's not done without pacing yourself and taking lots of rests.

The bike

Having a properly working bike is more of a priority than having an expensive, high-quality performance mountain bike. For day rides a basic, well-maintained mountain bike is just fine, although the more challenging the grades and terrain the more a perfor-mance bike will be useful, if only for its light-ness and handling.

Every cyclist knows that their bike needs to be trailworthy. But, when faced with sun-shine and friends, it's a rare person who won't head out, putting their faith in the spirits of the trail and ignoring the awful noises coming from their bike. Putting off repairs can only lead to a disappointing ride so remember the pre-ride check (pp. 36–7).

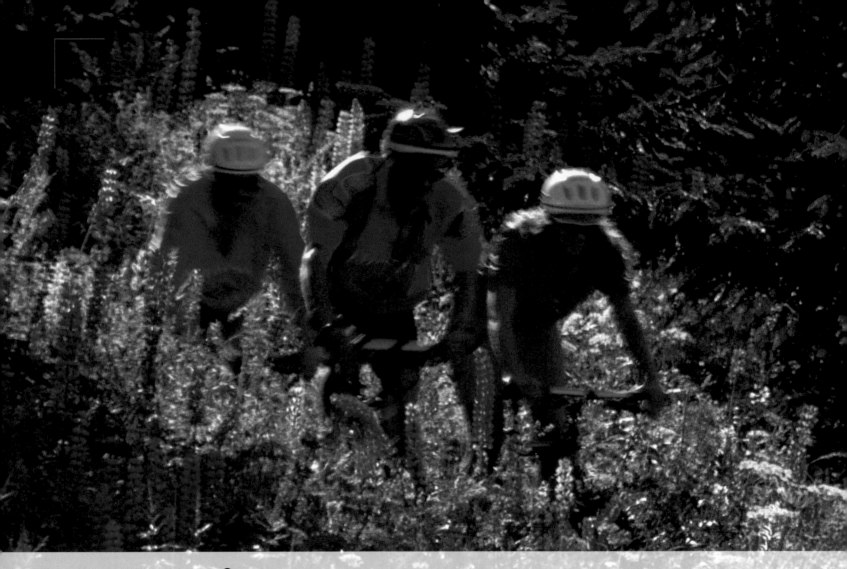

equipment
for the trail

Bicycling bags

Traveling without baggage is something that takes practice and is usually learned the hard way; by making miscalculations that leave you cold, starving or with a long walk back. It's a rite of passage that'll only make you tougher.

Traveling lightly can be done using the back-pockets of cycling jerseys and jackets and stuffing saddle pouches with the bare minimum of tools, a spare inner tube and levers. Mount the pump and water bottle on the frame. Most windproof shells scrunch down to a manageable size and can be squeezed into in a backpocket.

WAISTPACKS

A waistpack is great for carrying all the essentials for a simple day ride, and it leaves your shoulders and back free and dry. The best models are waterproof and padded on the body-side, with a strong snap-clip. Unless you're riding in weather that's so hot that two water bottles on the bike aren't enough, don't use a waistpack with bottle containers. They are intended for runners and the disadvantage is that they tend to crumple maps. Also, when the large models are overloaded, they turn into a wagging spare tire around your middle. In this case, the only way is up, to...

LUMBAR PACKS

In between a waistpack and a backpack is a hybrid called a lumbar pack. It's a high-framed waistbag with the capacity of a small backback that climbs halfway up your spine. It was first developed for runners and has minimal bounce straps, so that it stays glued to your back no matter how bumpy a descent is — and is big enough to stop maps from getting chewed up.

BACKPACKS

The biggest thing you should ever carry on your back while riding is a regular daypack that hikers and climbers would use. Anything bigger or heavier will throw you off balance, and you should use panniers, instead of a bigger backpack. Your shoulders may get tired and a bit sore with a backpack, but as long as it has a waist-strap, you can cram enough for a month-long (non-camping) trip inside one. It can hold the usual snacks, tools and light clothing, and its extra depth means room for rain gear if you're expecting bad weather. You can also squeeze in a full-length pump if it won't mount on the bike. A waterproof external map pocket is a good idea, because it can be frustrating to keep stopping and taking off your pack to get the map out.

Some specially-designed cycling backpacks are available, with good padded frames for protection from things like big tools. They also have compression straps, mesh pockets, key and pump clips. Hikers' backpacks are designed to be waterproof, and are the most waterproof of all the packs. If you're going to wear one, choose on with a wide waist-strap to minimize bounce and to distribute the weight over the hips. Some packs have a chest-strap too to keep it in place when it's packed full, and when you're hacking down a brutal trail.

Day trip gear list

■ Pack the right tools. Wrap and pad them so that they don't bounce around or dig into your back. Use lightweight multi-tools. (See emergency repairs, pp. 38–43.)

■ Think about rain gear. Remember that the temperature drops approximately 2°F (1°C) for every 300ft (100m) climbed, and never, ever forget that the wind can really reduce a temperature. The temperature difference between the trailhead parking area and the top of your climb could be as much as 36°F (20°C). Ask yourself if the weather could get worse. Are you going to be climbing high? Is it windy? Are you going to be back late? Do you have a change of clean clothes for the end of the ride? A plastic bag is great to have for muddy clothes or to protect upholstered seats or chairs.

■ Make sure that everyone in your group has a helmet and is fully equipped.

■ Remember to take a map.

■ Money — either pack bills in a ziploc bag or take coins.

■ Trail snacks. Energy bars can save you on a long day ride, with their convenient packaging and concentrated starch/sugar and nutrients. Natural options include bananas and dried fruit, or cookies and cake from the local café. You need to pack these more carefully, though. An uneaten banana at the end of a bumpy ride can be a pretty messy thing. Take extra food for emergencies, in case you get lost and wind up being out longer than you thought.

■ First aid — an afternoon ride can turn nasty if someone in your group has a bad crash. Antiseptic cream and bandages will provide temporary relief to cuts, although they'll have to be scrubbed out and cleaned later. An emergency blanket could save a life. Take bug repellant if you think you'll need it and anti-histamine tablets in case someone in your group reacts to a bug bite.

Don't forget the sunscreen. Remember that you won't feel the full heat of the sun if you're riding with a breeze in your face and you can get burned without realising it.

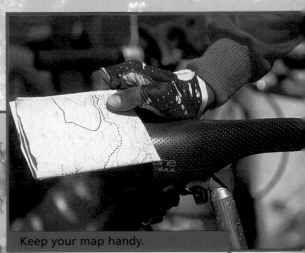
Keep your map handy.

MAPS

What scale map for mountain biking? The larger the second number the smaller the area and greater the detail. The best scales are 1:25,000 — 12 x 6 miles (20km x 10km) per oblong sheet, showing boundaries, naming properties and tree types, or 1:50,000 — 25 x 25 miles (40km x 40km). Standard hiking maps usually show enough ridable trails for several all-day looprides.

■ **Read contour lines, which are probably set at 150 or 300ft (50m or 100m) vertical intervals, to know how much you'll be climbing and descending. The closer they are, the steeper the grade — a solid block means a sheer cliff. Use the maps to help you plan your ride more effectively.**

■ **Weatherproofing. A wet ride can be enough to turn that crucial green line on your map into soggy, illegible pulp, which winds up being expensive and could turn your trip into an adventure you weren't expecting. You can buy laminated maps, which don't fold all that well, or laminate them yourself.**

trail protocol

THE OFF-ROAD CYCLING CODE

1 Stay on the trail
Only ride on marked bike trails. Avoid footpaths. Plan your route in advance, using maps.

2 Horses and hikers have the right of way
Make sure they hear you approach. Slow down when you pass them.

3 A large group riding abreast is annoying
Ride in twos or threes to let others pass.

4 Respect birds, animals and plants
And keep an eye on your dog.

5 Prevent erosion
Skidding is bad trail etiquette.

6 Close gates behind you
Don't trespass on private property.

7 Stay mobile
Wearing a helmet will reduce the risk of a head injury.
Take a first aid kit.
Carry enough food and water.
Pack rain gear and warm clothes.

8 Take pride in your bike
Repair it before you leave.
Take essential spares and tools.

9 Be tidy.
Take your garbage home.
Guard against fire.

10 Keep smiling

Never ride alone. You could crash and break a limb, and there would be no one there to help — it's better not to ride solo in exposed areas, especially in bad weather. Two is ideal and three is fine. A group should ride at the pace of the slowest rider, but usually what happens is the faster riders will ride ahead and wait for the slower ones to catch up at junctions or on the tops of climbs.

Like the off-road code says, mountain bikers in bunches are annoying to hikers and horseback riders, so try to keep it to under ten people — resist the power of the mob mentality.

Holy slopes

While mountain biking is pretty well established as a wilderness sport, authorities still do have the power to take cycling rights away from riders. Bikers need to respect the land, and to be friendly and accommodating to hikers and horseback-riders. With horses you should come to a complete stop well ahead of them, because they're easily spooked by bikes. You'll need to give up on the idea of downhilling if there are hikers anywhere on the trail — no one likes a close call, especially at 25mph (40km/h).

"The Mountain Bike Terror"

"Mountain bike craze sparks ban call". That's the sort of publicity that needs to be avoided and it's the responsibility of every rider to make sure it never happens. Ride on land that you won't permanently destroy, or reduce the bike's impact by sticking to the middle of the trails, so that they don't

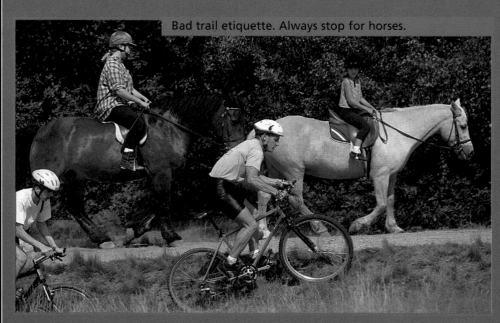
Bad trail etiquette. Always stop for horses.

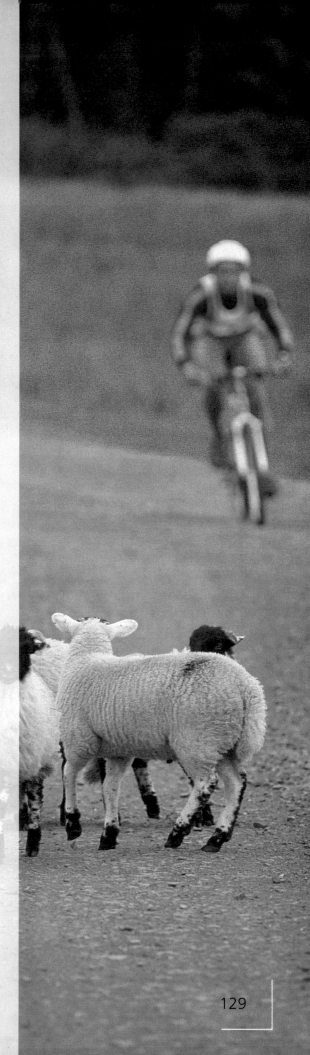

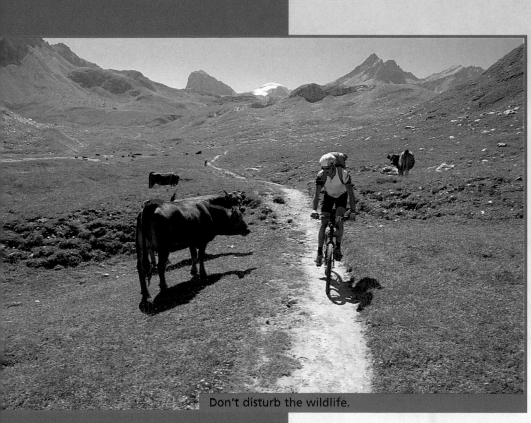

Don't disturb the wildlife.

erode. Tires themselves don't cause erosion; it's caused by water washing away soil and stones that have been dislodged, which is common in alpine areas.

In fragile areas, such as the desert of Moab (see pp. 162–3) or on tundra like that found in Iceland or Canada, vegetation can take more than 50 years to grow back, so if you're in doubt, don't ride over it.

On legal bike trails, erosion is a reality that designated land can handle. The mountain bike lobby wants governing bodies to understand that it's reasonable and containable, without distinguishing between boots, hooves or tires.

Tire marks tend to cause more of an uproar than the other two sports, but studies have shown that the area and depth of tire imprints on a trail are no worse. Mountain bikers will have to continue to prove themselves worthy of their trails.

The law

Where you can and cannot ride varies from area to area, but there is now a worldwide network of hundreds of thousands of miles of trails.

In the UK there are two main types of trail; footpaths, which are out of bounds to cyclists, and bridleways (horseback-riding trails) which are bikeable, but most other countries aren't as strictly regulated. Generally, the less populated an area, the less restrictions.

Popular destinations, such as the National and State Parks, the European Alps and Pyrenees, each have their own legislation, which is usually printed on maps and trail signs. As a rule of thumb, you should be satisfied with staying on marked trails.

In the less developed world, designated highways can be challenging dirt tracks and "off-road" can take on a new meaning.

equipment for long-distance trips

For any long-distance biking the best mountain bike to take is a rigid one with brazons for pannier racks. The one you don't want is the old, reliable and much-loved bike. The fact that your faithful pre-suspension bike hasn't given you any problems for 3 years is a warning — it's about time something major came loose or broke, such as the bottom bracket, a crank, a pedal, the headset or a wheel.

The best bet is a new-ish ridden-in bike, or one that's been well-maintained, with good parts, and where you're familiar with the wear and tear on each of the components. A major breakdown in a remote area could mean the end of your trip.

Componentry

■ Keep the componentry simple. If you're using SPD clipless pedals, keep them well-lubricated, or go for old-fashioned toeclip/straps. Use parts that need only minimal tools for maintenance. Performance lightweight componentry will not survive a round-the-world trip.

■ Suspension is great for comfort, but needs maintenance and difficult-to-find parts, like special oil. Stick to just suspension forks, or even a rigid bike.

■ Know your saddle. Wear it in, so that you know you can survive sitting on it for hours and days (although some soreness will be unavoidable at first).

■ The cables should have stretched, but always carry backups.

■ Take chainlinks, or a complete chain, and make sure it's the right kind for your bike.

■ Your wheels should be young. Rims get worn thin by the brake blocks and if they

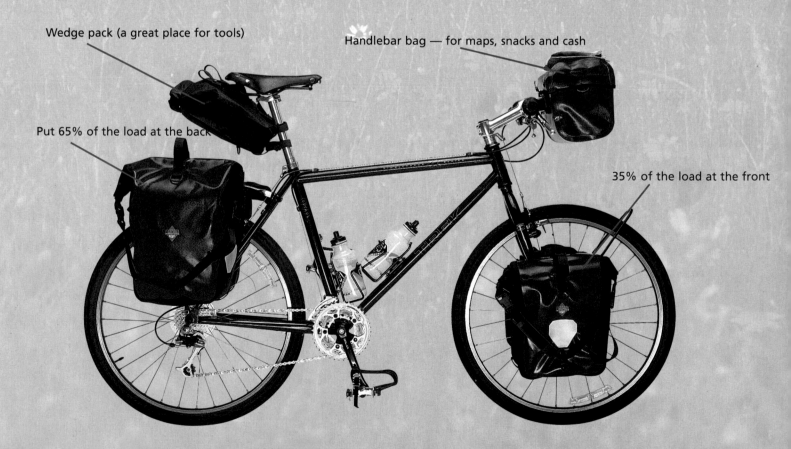

Wedge pack (a great place for tools)

Handlebar bag — for maps, snacks and cash

Put 65% of the load at the back

35% of the load at the front

TOOLS
For a trailside toolkit
see pages 38–39.

split you could have a collapsed wheel within a few minutes.

■ Fenders keep you dry in wet conditions, but they bend easily and may not survive a major trip.

■ The headset should be worn-in and problem-free. The now-standard Aheadset almost never comes loose.

■ The bottom bracket should also be worn-in and never come undone. This is normal.

■ Start with new, high-quality tires. They have a life-span of about 620–1,240 miles (1,000–2,000km), so take spares for longer trips in remote areas. Slicks and knobbies can be switched around according to the terrain to minimize wear and weight.

Traveling equipment

PANNIERS

Good panniers should have a reasonable capacity, secure rack clips (which have in the past been problematic), easy to access pockets and should be waterproof.

Some travelers prefer front-loaders, which don't affect steering, but most use back-loaders with a handlebar bag that holds frequently needed items, such as the map and valuables. It should be kept light for climbing out of the saddle. For a full load use both front (35% load) and rear (65% load) panniers, keeping the overall weight as low as you can.

Leave the luxuries at home and give yourself enough space for things you may buy along the way.

THE PANNIER RACK

Break a pannier rack and your trip could be

over. It's crucial that you buy a high-quality rack, such as one from Blackburn, or one recommended by the pannier manufacturer. Cheap steel versions bend and snap. Check the bolts frequently to make sure they don't shake loose. Try glue if they do.

FIRST AID, POTIONS AND LOTIONS

Carry a complete, waterproof outdoor athlete's first aid kit. Adventure Medical Kits make a variety of them, large and small. The one you choose should have all the equipment and instructions you need to deal with accidents and emergencies, and it should all come in a waterproof pack. Travelers in remote places should ask their doctors about what they should carry.

Use the strongest bug repellant you can find if you're traveling through wet areas during biting season. For sunny climates, sunscreen is essential to avoid burning, which can cause peeling and blistering on the trip and skin cancer up to 25 years later. Use lip balm, with a high Sun Protection Factor (SPF), especially in sunny or snowy conditions.

SLEEPING BAG

Lightness, compactability and the right degree of warmth are what you want in a bike traveler's sleeping bag. Pick a two-, three- or four-season grade to match the night-time temperatures you'll be dealing with. The better the bag, the smaller it will be in a compression sack. If you feel you need a

sleeping pad, use something like a portable, inflatable Therm-a-rest.

TENT

Low weight and simple tents are easy to find nowadays, but you'll want something small — so be prepared to be cramped (but dry).

COOKING

Stability, easy fuel supply, low weight and compactness are what you want in a camping stove. There are lots of stoves out there with all those qualities.

Survival aids for every trip

On any trip, knowing how to navigate with a map and compass will help you enjoy the back country. With a compass you can decide on the right trail, re-find yourself after getting lost and figure out an escape route in bad weather or if you have an accident. Landmarks disappear in cloud or fog.

Another essential is water- and windproof clothing. It keeps your body temperature and your morale at the right levels. It's particularly important to recognize the value of seam-sealed, windproof jackets and pants, so that even if you're wet on the outside, you'll be relatively warm on the inside.

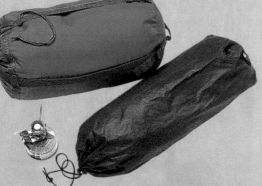

FIT TO TRAVEL?
Are you healthy and strong enough to enjoy your trip? If you don't cycle regularly, then start at least three months before you leave. Have a medical and dental check-up to avoid becoming the victim of an emergency tooth extraction in a remote area.

winter
biking

The mountain bike comes into its own in ice and snow, both as a plaything and as a work-horse. In cities, when public transportation grinds to a halt in a snowstorm, when people can't walk to the corner without slipping and falling and cars are trapped behind snow-banks, the mountain bike finds a unique urban niche.

The bike always gets through — as long as the rider can stand the conditions — and the fat-tire townie can silence the smart-ass who's constantly pointing out the rest of the time that there aren't any mountains in Toronto, Boston, Berlin, Paris or even Manchester.

Leaving city slush behind, there's plenty of snow in the country or mountains that the bike is happy to cope with, and it's great for beginners. In the silence that envelops a wintry landscape sometimes the only noise is the soft, continual "crump" of snow crunching under the knobby-tires, as steam rises from the backs of riders after a big climb.

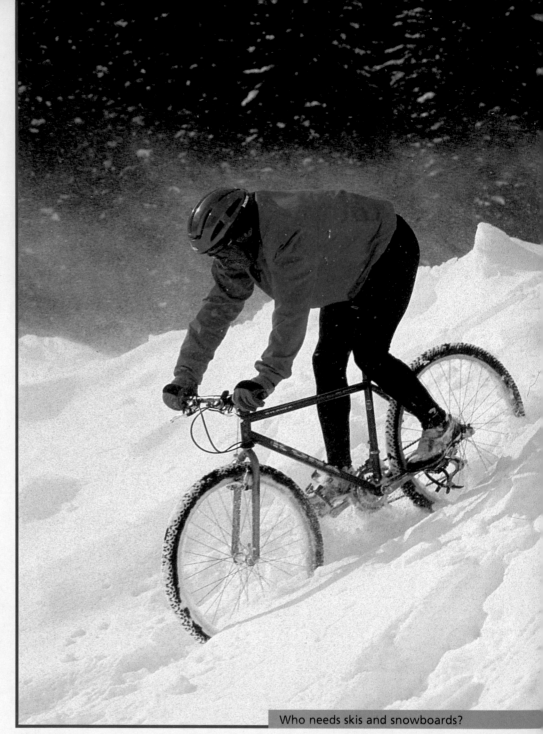

Who needs skis and snowboards?

In the right conditions (a little below freezing) you may even be able to relax your handling a little. The grip of the tires reacts to the forgivingness of a few inches of pow-der. You can mess around in the snow with-out much consequence. When you fall, you fall on to a soft wet mattress. There's noth-ing like marking your presence on a piece of white virgin trail. If you're not the first there, try to guess the kind of tire that has beaten you to it.

Watch for ice build-up on the tires, and clear it off before tricky descents, which will be less snowy if they occur in the forest. On exposed slopes, be prepared to lose the front wheel in a drift or depression. Watch out for hidden boulders on rocky single-track where the snow can fill up the spaces in between.

The trickiest sub-freezing surface to predict is an icy patch. Where streams cross paths or stone slabs, an ice rink a few inches thick can form. If you take your chances and pedal onto the slippery slab, just try to stay upright — the tires will have absolutely no lateral grip. Lean to the side at all and you'll go down — hard. Rough ice is sharp, and tough as concrete, so wear a thick, strong shell if you can, to stop your clothes from getting ripped.

A word of warning — don't venture far in winter if a blizzard's expected. Swirling snow and cloud can obscure even a well-known landscape almost immediately. After riding on slushy, salted highways, rinse off your bike. The salt can do more corrosive damage than a winter's worth of muddy rides.

Snowy events

The best-known off-season extreme event is the Iditibike race in Alaska, which takes 2 days to complete. The route follows sled-trails and frozen rivers and the race is performed by a small, experienced group. Alpine countries usually just turn to skiing in the winter, but biking events are sometimes held too, like coursing down the Olympic Cresta Run at St Moritz in Switzerland or doing time trials around high Alpine frozen lakes in France.

Winter equipment

STUDDED TIRES

Just like hikers use crampons on their walking boots when it's icy, ordinary MTB tires can be augmented with screws and a little patience. Take four hundred ordinary ⅜in (10mm) screws, and screw them through the tire lining from the inside, so that they protrude a fraction above the tread. Space them regularly on the sides and on top so that about four are in contact with the ground at any given time.

EFFECTIVE GLOVES

When venturing out on snowy rides, your gloves need to be warm and waterproof. If the temperature hovers around freezing, then the wind-chill on soaking wet fingertips can be the first step to painful frostbite. The macho-est of men have been reduced to whimpering fools by the agony of thawing fingertips.

Lobster mitts are a great idea. These mitts have the body of the glove split into two pincers so that fingers can keep each other warm while still being able to feel and work the gear and brake levers. Ski gloves or mountaineering gloves tend to be a little bulky but are extremely warm.

OVERBOOTS

They may look stupid, but like good gloves, overboots can mean the difference between a great day playing polar explorer, and a day spent in misery.

When you go to the store, buy your pair a little on the large size; most of them are made for road shoes, and may be tight, and maybe even restrictive.

If you are expecting to spend the whole of the day in deep snow, wear a pair of solid hiking or mountain bike boots with gaiters. You may have to change your SPD pedals to platforms, or even to wide open toeclips/straps, but it's not a bad idea in cold conditions anyway, when the spring in SPDs freezes up, and the cold seeps through the cleat.

SHADES

Bright snowy days are made for wearing cool, dark shades to block the glare from snowfields. Choose glasses that wrap tightly around your face, to cut out reflections on the inside of the lenses.

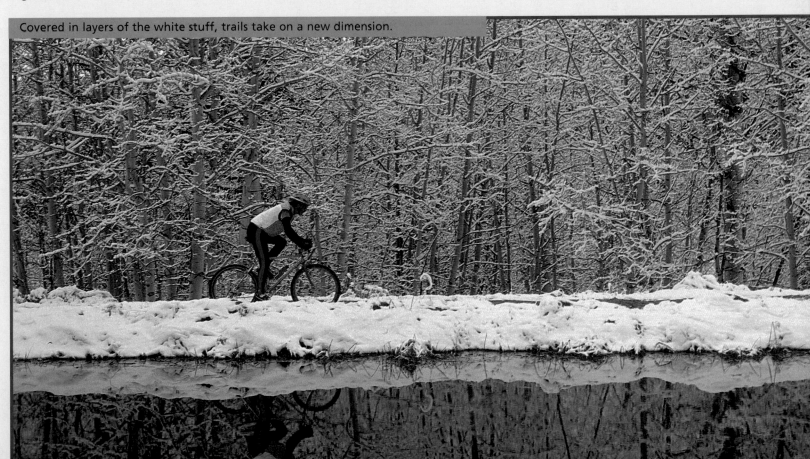

Covered in layers of the white stuff, trails take on a new dimension.

coping with rock, sand and grass

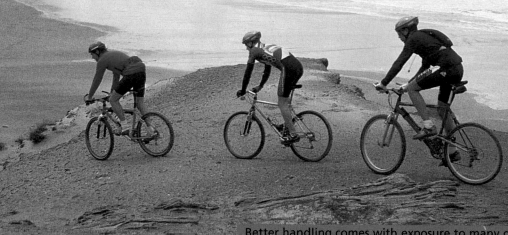

Better handling comes with exposure to many different surfaces.

Sand

It's safe to say that the majority of riders will never tackle sand on a Saharan scale, but you will encounter it sometime, and it's tricky enough to be worth mentioning.

A dusting of it here and there is harmless but, as soon as fine sand is more than a couple of inches deep, riding in it becomes like riding in molasses. Even when it's dry, it can somehow be slippery. There's nothing more frustrating than slipping around like a novice on a previously muddy, but ridable trail that's has been sanded to provide "grip".

Sand patches make you wipe out. If you're going around a sandy corner, enter it a little more slowly and in a lower gear than normal in case you lose traction. The front wheel can tweak out at an angle and bring you to a stop. If the back wheel spins out, that's less of a problem — as long as you're

in that low gear. Just stay sitting to keep the wheel weighted and pedal as hard as you can. As long as you have about 50 per cent grip you should haul yourself through and back on to a pure surface.

Beware of hitting sand patches at high speed; this can feel like someone else is slamming on your brakes without telling you and this could then throw you over the handlebars.

Equipment-wise, sand and water wear down brake pads rapidly. Anyone living in a sandy, wet area should keep their bearings tight — a grain of sand in the races won't turn into a pearl, it'll ruin them.

On beaches, you can ride below the tide mark where sand is firm enough to hold you, but remember that the salty air and water will corrode the bike and it should be rinsed off as soon as possible.

The sand dunes that are situated above

beaches are usually fragile, protected areas and as a result you should treat them as out of bounds.

Rocks and stones

Rocks and bikers are a challenging mix. Boulders are the props of trials races, inspiring the more experienced to mount, pirouette and jump. They're the thrill in single-track downhills and the curse of the paramedics.

There are three explosive-free ways of beating a big mid-trail rock. One extreme is to get off and carry your bike, the other is to jump the rock and the third is to ride it. Even though textbook tips follow, better rock riding only comes with exposure. The more differently shaped rocks you tackle, the better you get at dealing with them.

Learn to wheelie — get all of the weight off the front wheel and pull up on the handlebars, balancing on the rear — to lift the wheel onto the obstacle. That keeps up the bike's momentum and minimizes the risk of slamming into it and sending the rider flying forward onto the stem.

Balance, not strength, is the key to rock riding. Stand up in the pedals on your approach, and keep your weight back, especially if you're riding downhill. If you have enough speed, the back end of the bike will follow the front end over the top. Try not to bail out prematurely. Trust the bike to finish the maneuver without sending you forward or backward.

It may help to visualize yourself cruising over the obstacle, and let the bike give up before you do.

Dry rocks present no surface problems, but moss and rain change their nature completely, making them harder to control. Gravel and stones present all sorts of difficulties. They destroy traction on corners and lie around looking innocent until the front wheel hits one at the wrong angle and

speed and sends the rider into a perfect trajectory ... off the bike. Don't get lazy on the trail. It's full of tricks and surprises — which is why we go mountain biking.

Grass

The most abundant plant on earth's surface, grass moves in mysterious ways. It usually isn't a problem but when it's long and tough, or tussocky, riding across it becomes really hard work.

One of the hardest surfaces to ride in the mountain bike world is a meadow without a marked trail.

Be careful on banked grass trails, especially if they're wet — you could lose traction and slip. If you feel like you're about to go into a slide or a spin (whatever the surface you're riding on) stand up in the pedals for quick weight distribution and slow your speed. In muddy conditions grass won't matter, but it can sling mud on the bike, and make clogging worse.

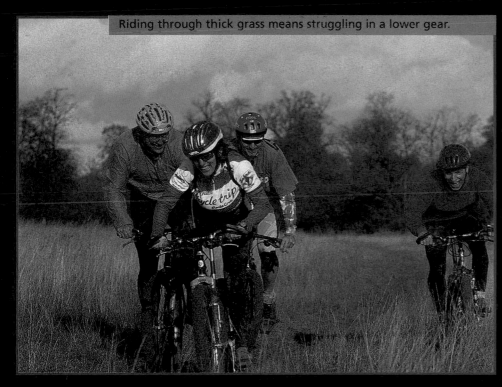
Riding through thick grass means struggling in a lower gear.

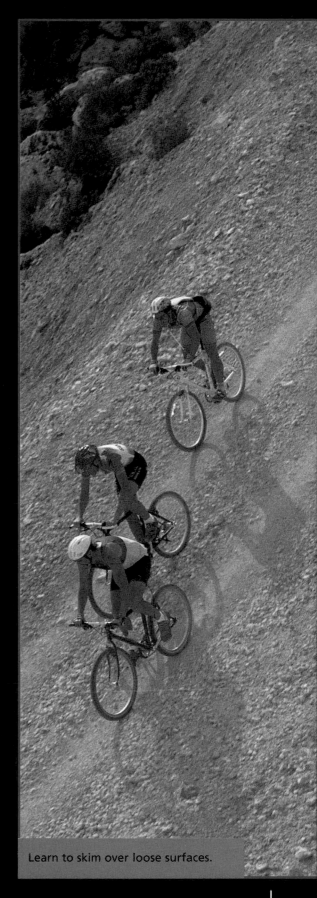
Learn to skim over loose surfaces.

the water factor
mud, puddles, rivers and streams

Mud

Mud, a variable-strength solution of water and planet, makes itself familiar to most mountain bikers some of the time, but there aren't many ways to solve the mess of what it throws up. Like most obstacles in mountain biking, you have to learn to play mud by ear.

The more you ride, the more you'll become used to the way terrain changes beyond recognition according to the season and amount of rainfall. What may be tortoiseshell during the dry season turns into swamp during the wet one. Your handling adjusts as a response. One of the marks of a true mountain biker is an ability to keep a steady pace whatever the terrain.

Usually, the more dilute a surface is, the better grip it has. Rain doesn't make trails unridable — the sunshine after the rain does, so don't cancel a ride in the middle of a rainstorm, thinking that mud will prevent you from continuing.

Apart from being slippery, mud will slow you down — climbing, descending and on the flats. Soaked ground on trails can be more of a problem, because the bike sinks with every pedal-stroke. It's best to avoid equestrian trails during or after a rainstorm; they can turn a fun ride into a really boring, frustrating one.

Traction is usually less reliable on clay or chalk, where trails and slopes become slippery. Be careful on the corners, especially if there are exposed tree roots — they can really trip you up. Approach them more slowly than you would in dry conditions and be ready to stand up if either one of your wheels suddenly spins. The wetter it is, the better the grip, not vice versa.

On double-track, the line to choose varies from puddly tire tracks at the sides to the grassy center hump.

You get better with experience at making the right decision. As a rule of thumb, go for surface that you can see, and when conditions are really bad, even tiny pieces of grass can hold the tire for a second or two. You'll also see that wet conditions are the ones when most damage is done to the trail, so for the sake of future riding generations, decide when it's better to give up traction and less resistance and go for the harder, ready-churned track, which is already beyond repair, than to mark up the virgin edges. You'll get a nice eyeful of mud as the tires start to clean themselves at higher speeds.

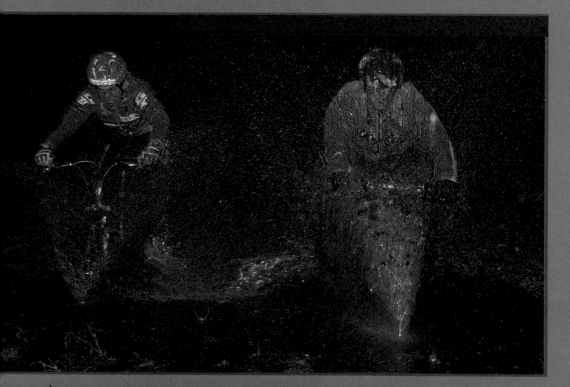

Watch out for water

On ski slopes and exposed meadows, keep an eye open for raised or dug irrigation ditches. These little things are a good place for experienced riders to show off their bunny-hops and for beginners to practice.

The ditch diverts rain and meltwater from

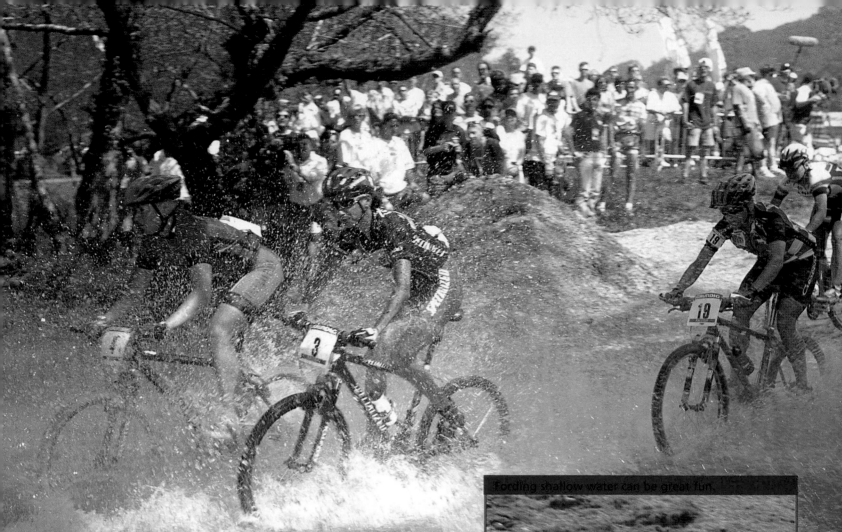

World Cup competitors get wet in Devon, England.

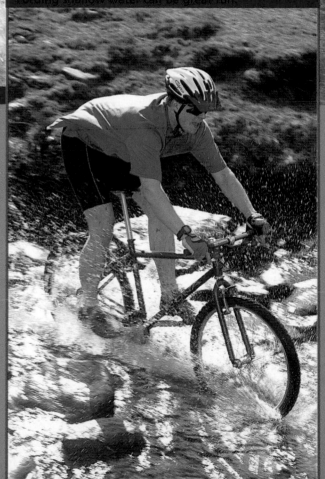

Fording shallow water can be great fun.

the trails. Without the ditches the trails would erode because they form perfect escape routes for flowing water.

As far as grip is concerned, clear running water is a good cleaner, so you may get more grip in a stream on a track on greaseless rock, than at its slimy edges, even if your feet do get wet.

Streams and river-crossings

Crossing rivers that are too deep to ford is one of the few times when being off the bike can help. Think of yourself as one leg of a tripod with the wheels forming the other two legs. Put the bike in the river, hold onto the handlebar and saddle and step on to your first foothold. Move the bike a little further, first one wheel then the other, then yourself on to the next foothold. The bike may get wet but you stay dry.

You can ride through a big puddle or shallow stream if you don't mind the drama and the waterworks. But you'll need to be going fast; use your judgement to avoid touching down and getting a wet foot if the water is deeper than 6in (120mm). If that's the case, the bottom could be loose and slippery, but the water may slow you right down to a stop. In freezing temperatures, ride through slowly to keep the spray to a minimum.

so you want to race

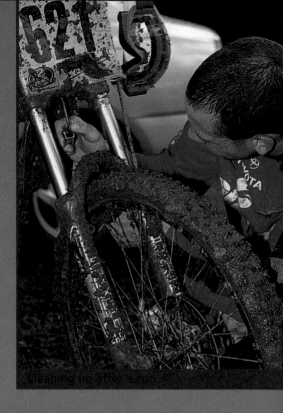

Cleaning up after a run

Your first race

After you've got your condition, stamina and confidence in shape, you may feel ready to start competing. There are certain procedures and tips that are useful to remember before you race. After a few events, these things will become habitual. Always remember to have fun and — good luck!

RACE GEAR LIST

Helmet — compulsory

WARM-UP GEAR
Jacket, spare jersey, tights

RACE GEAR
Jersey, shorts
Race shoes and socks
Gloves or mitts
Bottle(s)
Pump and tools
Towel and cleaning water
Food — bananas & cookies
Water or another drink
like juice or
an energy drink
Complete set of clothes to
change into, including wet
and cold weather gear
Race number and licence
if necessary

Entering a race

Choose an event that isn't too far from your home, or perhaps combine the race with a weekend of mountain biking and camping. Ideally, being a green sport, you'd want to get there by bike or train, but in cool temperatures a car provides shelter and allows you to carry more clothing to wear after the event. Scour the specialist press or contact local clubs for dates and venues of events. Enter beforehand if you can. The more important the event, the more likely there is to be an entry deadline, although local races may take entries at the start line.

■ **On the day** — make a mental plan of when to sign-in, warm-up, and the start time. Leave nothing to the last minute — allow for changes of times to be made on the day, due to weather or accidents.

■ **Signing-in** — even if you've entered in advance you still need to sign-in to pick up your number and pins or zip ties.

Riding against others brings out the best in you.

■ **Pre-ride the course** — in cross-country events, ride the circuit once or twice beforehand to practice the tricky bits and enjoy yourself. In downhill races try to do the run as many times as possible.

PREPARING THE BIKE

Follow the principles of the pre-ride check (see p. 36). Never fix major parts the day or the morning before the race in case they don't work properly, or you've brought the wrong tools.

Allow new cables to bed-in before a race. This is particularly important for the gear cables — mis-changes can lose you places and temper. Set the tire pressure between 35–55psi, to suit the softness or hardness of the surface.

In case of flats during the race, carry a spare tube, tire levers and a gas cartridge inflator. Take a chain tool too. Practice fixing flats at home. The pros aim to fix them in two minutes.

RULES

Mountain bike racing was once noted for its absence of rules, but now they increase year by year. The main one is that there should be no outside assistance — the mountain bike racer must be mechanically self-sufficient throughout the race. This encourages riders to learn to fix their own machines, and creates an open and level playing field between those who have spare machines and those who do not.

In cross-country, several categories may race at the same time, so riders show each other mutual respect. Overtaking riders should announce when they are "coming through". Slower riders should hang back and let the leaders go down ahead over difficult descents.

Riders are largely trusted to choose the appropriate category, although some ranking systems do exist to move riders up and down. Racing licences are optional but recommended for committed racers.

EATING AND DRINKING

Carbo-loading is essential for XC races over 90 minutes long and for an afternoon downhill or dual slalom competition. For most riders, it's sufficient to eat a high-carbohydrate meal the evening before and again for breakfast. Don't skip breakfast. Don't eat for 2 hours before a race. In cross-country, start nibbling dried fruit or pieces of energy bar 45 minutes into a race, and keep nibbling till the finish.

As always, water is essential. Sip water for a few hours beforehand and drink small amounts frequently throughout the race or event. You can exchange empty bottles with full ones from supporters. If it's hot, take plenty of cold water to keep you hydrated.

ON THE CROSS-COUNTRY START LINE

If you're serious about your finishing position, arrive early on the start line. Pick a middle ring, middle sprocket gear to start in. The pack will set off at a very fast pace as riders race to the point where the wide opening track narrows down.

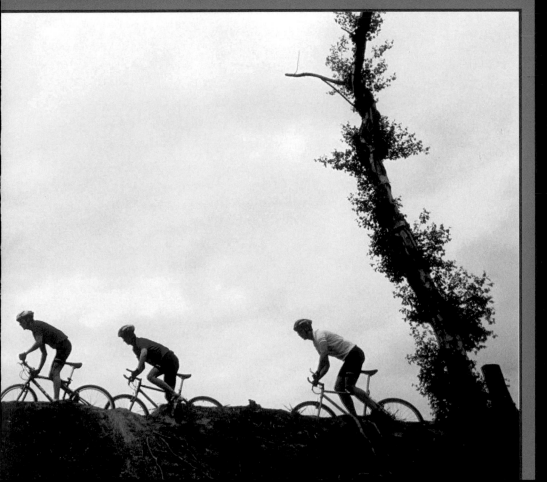

HOW TO BE WORLD CHAMPION

■ **Start to race in your teens.**
■ **Train full time from around 18–20 years old.**
■ **Have ambition, tenacity, patience — neither too much nor too little ego.**
■ **Stay in shape, have a good power to weight ratio and handling skill.**
■ **Enlist support from family, friends and partner.**
■ **Have a healthy diet.**

downhilling, dual and cross-country

Downhilling

Flying down descents is the best part about mountain biking — a piece of adrenalin-filled escapism open to anyone with the guts to do it. No wonder downhill racing's become exclusive with its own stars and technology.

Among the winners are current young gun Greg Minnaar of South Africa and American veteran Myles Rockwell, also the extraordinary Anne-Caroline Chausson of France. Chausson has gone down in history as the winner of the most titles in international mountain biking and shows no signs of letting up. Just off the top is the phenomenon Nicolas Vouilloz, who dominated men's downhilling, winning the majority of World Cup and World Championship titles for eight years. Another top dog is Britain's big blond Steve Peat.

There are always packs of other riders just a tenth of a second off their times. Most mountain biking countries have local and national downhill events. These allow amateurs to improve their skill and nerve, so that they can climb steadily in the rankings.

Downhill runs are short, anaerobic bursts — the longest lasts about 7 minutes — and the effort can bring riders gasping to their knees once over the line. Crashing is an occupational hazard. Spaceage jackets with bizarre spine protection, Kevlar chest, knee and elbow pads, and full face helmets are the flesh and brain savers, and allow

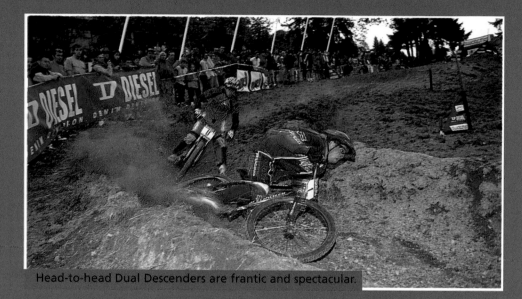
Head-to-head Dual Descenders are frantic and spectacular.

you to get up and fight another day.

Dual & Four-Cross

The most flamboyant MTB race discipline takes the form of two or four riders in a head-to-head knockout down a short course of berms and jumps. Renowned for crashes, barging and concussion, the unmissable event is accompanied by yelling commentators and pumping music.

Cross-country

XC is the other main branch of competitive mountain biking. An individual endurance challenge, it can be taken lightly or seriously. A thrilling self-awareness comes out of pushing yourself harder than usual and, while racing is a natural way to lose weight and get in shape, it's also a great way to make friends. The people, drawn together by

a love for bikes, excitement and the land, are unusually friendly. Many X-country racers have no background in any other endurance sport, and a minority weren't even athletic before picking the sport up.

The aim is to get yourself and the bike to the finish in one piece, preferably in the top half of the field. After a crunching, bustling mass start, the bunch will thin out over the length of the race, with riders moving up and down places according to whether they went too fast at the beginning or they are warming up. As with all mountain biking, crashing is an occupational hazard, so be prepared for impressive scars, even though the cuts aren't usually more than skin-deep.

There are categories for men and women, for ten years of age and up, that account for existing ability. A good goal for a beginner is to finish a "Fun/Novice" race asting 30–50 minutes in their first year. Then build up to "Sports", where races last between 45 minutes and two hours. Many amateurs are happy to never go further, but those with the time, freedom, skill and competitive ambition may rise gradually over a couple of years to the "Expert" category. This is for committed amateurs and top former juniors, where equipment sponsorship deals are sometimes available. At the top, in "Elite", the races last between two–three hours. It's generally made up of full-time cyclists, usually with sponsorship and may even feature a world champion or two.

Miniature circuits are organized for kids at many of the larger events, with large juvenile (14–16) and junior (16–18) categories for the oldest. The men's "Veteran" and "Master" categories, which race for 45–90 minutes, are large and highly competitive at the front. Although the numbers are smaller, women's racing is well established and more acknowledged than in road racing, with a number of professional riders.

Professional salaries on par with full-time road racers are limited to a very few riders. Despite its physical demands, cross-

country is less televisable, and is less attractive to outside sponsorship money than downhilling and dual slalom.

Sponsorship

To most mountain bikers getting paid to ride, whether in cash or equipment, is a dream deal. One of the motivating forces for a young amateur is the idea of being given one of the best bikes and being required to do nothing but ride it long and well. The social kudos attached to being a sponsored rider is unrivaled, too. Although the majority of mortals never see more than the club name next to theirs on the race results, most racers will admit to fantasizing about a sponsorship with Cannondale, Giant, Global Racing, Gary Fisher or Foes.

Top money-makers in mountain bike racing can be counted on the fingers of four hands. As is similar in most other fringe sports, in MTB the five big international bike companies compete for a tiny pool of this and next season's winners. If you get on the podium year after year, like Missy Giove and Steve Peat, and bring plenty of fans into the deal, you can expect to make up to six fig-

ures. If you fall outside the top ten, but are still a national champion, you may get travel, a bike, and a simple support salary. Outside the top 50, and if you're under 20, you're looking at national youth development schemes, and national bike distributors for your lunch ticket. Sometimes support comes from local outfits unconnected to the sport. Top Italian downhiller Corrado Herin was a fireman in real life. The fire department let him draw his full-time salary and take time off to train and compete, considering it an honour to have him in their ranks. The philanthropic Italian attitude to sport is unfortunately rare. The only comparison is support given by the military and the police, where men and women are encouraged to be physically active and competitive. Now that's a career tip.

The place for beginner racers is the local bike shop, or local companies or employers or any outfit they may have a blood or friendly connection with. Bike clubs may have connections, or already receive club sponsorship that you can draw on, but that'll probably amount to a van to races and a discount on parts and clothing. The point is that mountain biking is a thickly concentrated bike sport that remains small in size and funds. Mainstream commercial sponsors like BMW, Volvo, Chrysler or Ralph Lauren, crop up now and then, and fizz out after a few years. The sport boomed financially around 1994–98, at the time of the first Olympic cross-country race in Atlanta, but that's mainly trickled away. Now, the sport mostly funds itself. Some racers turn to specialist manufacturing or retailing, where they subsequently make just enough money to be able to give a gifted pal a ride.

Elite racers are mostly full-time sponsored mountain bikers.

World Cup racing and Olympics

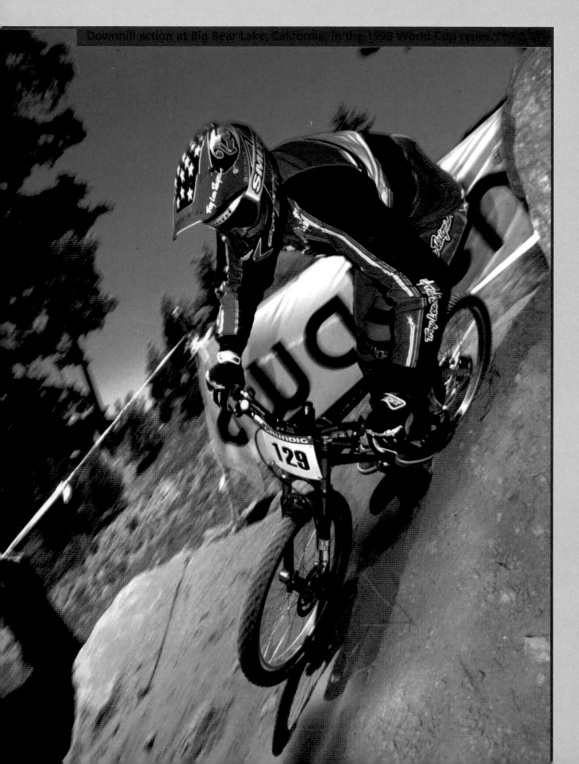

Downhill action at Big Bear Lake, California, in the 1998 World Cup series.

World Cup

It's tough at the top. A dozen times a year you have to pack your bike and take off to the Rocky Mountains, the French or Swiss Alps, the Spanish Sierra Nevada or the Scottish Highlands to thrash your steed on the best courses in the world. All in the name of physical excellence and contributing to the essence of mountain bike cool. Oh yes, it's hard all right.

The pinnacles of the racing world are the UCI World Cup downhill, cross-country and dual series. Featuring anything between four and ten events during the summer months, they attract 200 of the very best bikers in the world to mountain venues that may host other sports like skiing or biathlon. The site of the 2002 Winter Olympic downhill skiing events, at Deer Valley near Salt Lake City, Utah, has been used several times for MTB World Cup events.

Leading nations include the USA, France, Italy, Canada and the Netherlands. France excels across all the disciplines, while America has traditionally been number one or two in downhilling but flounders in cross-country, particularly in the men's line-up. One reason why is that the European road-racing nations have completed their adaptation to off-road sport. The French in particular have all the cycling knowledge and a superb country in which to practice.

Events at World Cups are effective rather than destructive. The X-country races aren't long: men ride for two hours, women (for no substantiated reason) for one-and-a-half, which is shorter by half-an-hour to an hour than elite domestic races. The main difference is the amount of climbing involved. Courses are composed of two to four circuits of a loop, often in a figure eight pattern so that spectators can see riders as often as possible. A loop can have, for example, 500ft of climbing, so riders will climb and descend the equivalent of a full mountain height and back in total. Courses can be pretty grim, technically — especially if there's a rainstorm thrown in. Elite riders have an amazing ability to pick a line at top speed, and can descend as well as downhillers without the jumps. And they aren't even fazed by wet, cold or deep all-consuming mud.

Where domestic racing is no match for World Cup events is downhilling. Knowing they're designed for guys and girls who can drop chutes and take gaps like isn't human, the course builders put lines down mountains that water would think twice about following. One of the toughest is Mont Sainte Anne in Quebec, Canada. The slopes of this ski resort are covered in alternating vertical strips of runs and pine trees. The course begins high out of the ski lift down a run, drops into the first dark bouldery pine stand, bursts back out into the sun with a 20ft jump, sprints then brakes hard around gravel flats, and dives into the trees again, to ride virtually blind for the first few sec-onds. At an average run of six minutes, Mont Sainte Anne is also fierce in endurance terms. Riders tumble from their bikes at the bottom, clutching their swollen arms, which burn from hanging on for their lives. Then they come back for more.

The funkiest and least serious of the three disciplines is dual slalom. Practiced by downhillers and cross-over BMXers, a pair of riders go head-to-head down a 30-second course of banks, moguls, table-tops and camel-humps. Great for spectators, TV and loud music, it imitates sports like snow-boarding and skateboarding and produces spectacular somersaulting crashes and plenty of gravel rash.

The UCI World Cup competitions are series, the winners being the hero and shero who rack up the most points overall, in all the rounds. More emphasis is placed on the annual one-off World Championship event, where everything's decided in one race held at the end of the season.

The Olympics

Cross-country made its Olympic debut at Atlanta, the 100th anniversary games, on a hot and humid course unfortunately noted for its dullness. The inaugural gold medals were won by Paola Pezzo of Italy and Bart Brentjens of the Netherlands, who both rode away on their own. In 2000, the Sydney Olympics made up for it with a course designed by the World Cup dual slalom builder. This time, spectators and riders were treated to dramatic technical twists designed for tight racing. Paola Pezzo won again and the French wonder Miguel Martinez took his first gold. Controversially, downhilling continues to be excluded from the Olympics, on the pretext that another cycle sport would have to be dropped to make room. Downhillers carry on anyway.

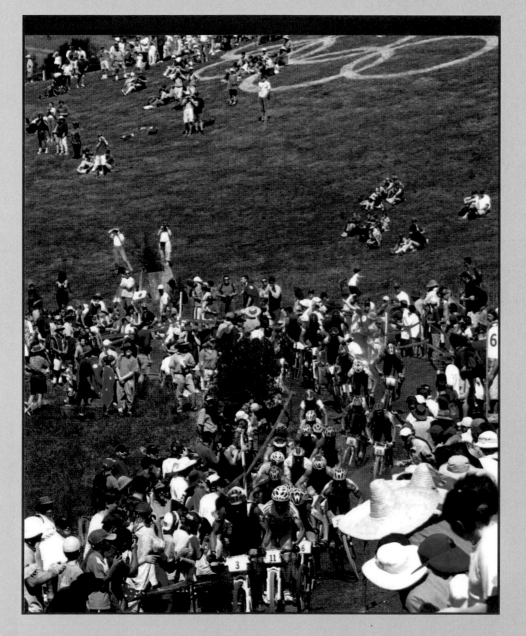

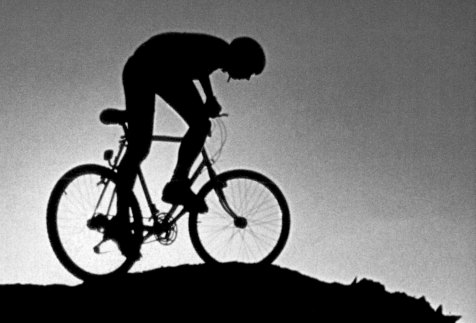

des

On a bike, as Greg Yeoman, who completed one of the first MTB crossings of Russia, sums up, "You have everything around you — the sights, the sounds, the smells of flowers and trees. It's not just a moving display witnessed from the window of a car, train or plane. And you can stop anywhere you want to."

Travelers have tales of being offered pennies for their bikes, and of welders able to manage tricky frame repairs in the most unlikely corners of the world. Bike tourists enjoy a status somewhere between hero and freak. The sight of an approaching bike helps win the trust of local people, who are often more welcoming to strangers when they pass through under their own power.

On the downside, you're exposed to unpredictable traffic and are at the mercy of the terrain and bad weather. It's all part of the improvization. The bike traveler must sit back in the saddle and let experience and self-knowledge unroll like the trail in front of them. If you're leaving Western culture, the bike fades into the background and becomes an essential part of the backstage rig while the land and the cultures come to the forefront.

Most of the planet is mapped for mountain bikes. Numerous tour companies, usually small, friendly and competent, run tours to most of the rugged destinations you could name. It's not the case that these tours are a soft option, but they're simpler than independent travel and suit those cyclists who are limited to two weeks of vacation a year.

This chapter celebrates contrasting routes through the planet's more mountain bike-worthy areas. The tour begins with a remarkable journey that involved cycling over 8,000 miles (13,000km) across the full width of the former Soviet Union, from Moscow to Vladivostok. What follows is the Sawtooth Mountains of Idaho, where great trails mix with log cabins and good food below the Rockies. Then we travel the relatively short distance to Moab, in Utah, to enjoy the outrageously bikable red gorges and pinnacles of Canyonlands National Park and the Slickrock trail. In the French Alps, in the shadow of magnificent Mont Blanc, graded tourist mountain bike trails offer a pure bike blow-out. And finally, this trip takes us to Morocco, where rock tracks and peasant villages dot the foothills of the high Atlas mountains.

Before you start packing, here are some names to look out for in the bookshop, who may provide both ideas and inspiration. Historically, accounts of cycling journeys start in 1886 with *Round the World on a Bicycle*, an account of the first world circumnavigation on a penny-farthing by Thomas Stevens. Walter Stolle ended up living on his bike from 1959 to 1976, as he covered 400,000 miles (640,000km) through 159 countries. Other names to look out for are Dervla Murphy, Josie Dew and Bettina Selby.

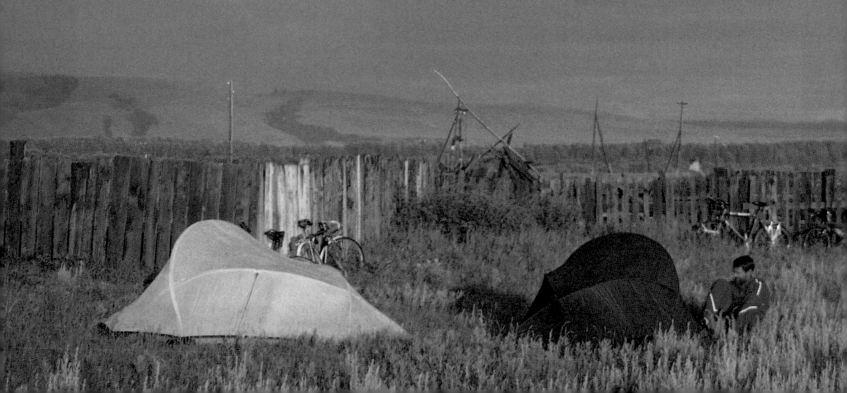

THE Trans-Siberian Tour

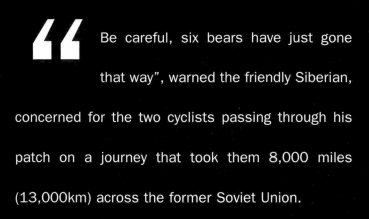

" Be careful, six bears have just gone that way", warned the friendly Siberian, concerned for the two cyclists passing through his patch on a journey that took them 8,000 miles (13,000km) across the former Soviet Union.

"We saw paw prints, but never actually the beasts", says the British biologist Greg Yeoman, about one of their countless brushes with adventure on the trans-continental trip. It took Yeoman and his fellow traveler, Australian fitness instructor Kate Leeming, 5 months to pedal along the only road across a country that begins in Europe and finishes at the Sea of Japan, and includes large stretches of land that until recently were closed to Russians, let alone Westerners. Contrary to the image of dour Soviet existence, this is a land inhabited by warm, resourceful people. It was this hospitality that boosted the couple's determination to overcome daily difficulties — including walking 100 miles (160km) along the Siberian railway track itself.

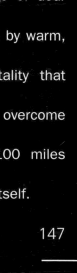

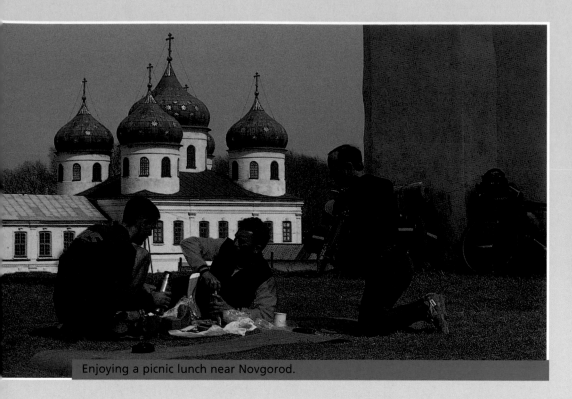

Enjoying a picnic lunch near Novgorod.

FACTS AND FIGURES
Dates — May 1 to
September 30, 1993.
153 days or 722 hours,
30 minutes in the saddle.
Total distance traveled —
8,304 miles (13,286km)
Daily average — 73 miles
(117km), 6 hours 24 minutes
in the saddle.

Kate and Greg's trip lasted a whole season during which the leaves budded, came out and fell off. "You become used to the daily pedaling, just as you become used to a 9–5pm. We did several days of more than 100 miles (160km). 50 miles (80km) felt like a short day," says Greg. The couple's timing was impressive, "We arrived in Vladivostok 12 hours behind schedule."

Cycling for a cause

Greg and Kate's trip raised US$4,000 for Childrens' Aid International. April 1996 was the 10th anniversary of the Chernobyl accident and this American charity helps the disaster's youngest victims, many of whom have thyroid cancer. Greg found that under-standing of the cause and effect of radiation is low.

"One area had a very high number of sick children, but the local people said it could not be related to an 'old' nuclear acci-dent, which occurred 36 years earlier," he said. "The money raised has provided a valuable English–Russian computerized translation system, and also helped to establish summer camps in Byelorussia.

This is so that children can enjoy cheap holidays in non-contaminated areas, without the sometimes disastrous culture shock of sending them to other countries. The advice and close co-operation of the local people is actively sought for these projects."

The cyclists

■ Greg Yeoman, a British biologist and occasional cyclist, had done a little cycle-touring in Europe, but was interested in traveling across the former Soviet Union.

■ An Australian fitness instructor who lives in the UK, Kate Leeming decided to add the Baltic–Pacific odyssey to 10,000 miles (16,000km) of cycling in Europe.

The bicycle karma

Greg sums up his philoso-phy like this: "Cycling is a non-threatening way of traveling, so people trust

you. It is also the best way to see the coun-try which you are visiting, because you can ride all the way into the heart of the cities and all the way out into the countryside. You have everything around you, the sights, the sounds, the smells of flowers and trees. It's not just a moving display witnessed from the window of a car, train or plane. And you can stop anywhere you want to."

The Russian escorts

Although the days are gone when foreigners had to be accompanied by officials on every step of their visit to the Soviet Union, Greg and Kate knew they couldn't do the trip unsupported. They needed help with the

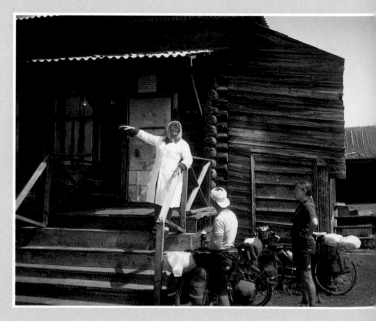

Trans-Siberian

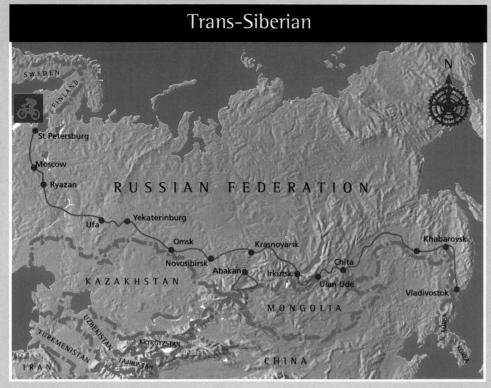

carried for 8,000miles (13,000km), without the right tools for it. Also I carried a pair of new boots for thousands of miles, in anticipation of the final section of the route where there is virtually no track. Before that I was using a pair of old touring shoes, which night after night I glued back together. When these finally gave up ... I put on the new boots — and within a few days one lost an eyelet. They weren't very good."

language, with customs, to get food and for security. Getting a visa is no problem, but it's still necessary to have some form of invitation. So they invited and paid members of a Russian cycling club to escort them eastward. Five cyclists helped during the journey: Vladimir, George, Yuri, Eugene and Sasha. Greg and Yuri had little language in common, but both happened to be biologists and managed to discuss the flora using its Latin nomenclature.

Before they set off the travelers established a base HQ, at the office of Centre Pole, an expedition-organizing company run by Polar explorer Misha Malakhov at the westerly town of Ryazan. From here, supplies and funds were sent out with each new escort. They also kept a spare bike there in case the Russians should need it.

Where they stayed

The couple found they could rely on villagers to put them up.

"The hospitality was fantastic," says

Greg. "Many times we spent the night in people's houses, rather than camping. On arrival we would find out where the mayor of a village lived. They would always be thrilled to put us up and to enjoy a communal photo. Or we would arrive at a village and cycle around, asking people for hot water or milk, and hope to be offered shelter."

EQUIPMENT

- 3 Scott Windrivers
- 1 Specialized Stumpjumper
- Karrimor panniers
- North Face tents
- North Face waterproofs
- Sleeping bags
- Russian gas stove

Judging what to take and what to risk leaving behind is one of the skills of traveling.

"In all we carried about 66lb (30kg) of equipment, which was far too much," says Greg. "We should have taken more first aid, but we could easily have left behind some clothes, and the new bottom bracket I

DISTANCES TRAVELED (Accumulated Mileage)

St Petersburg, May 1, 1993
The journey begins

Moscow, May 7
501 miles (802km)

Yekaterinburg, June 2
2,139 miles (3,422km)

Krasnoyarsk, July 13
4,528 miles (7,245km)

Irkutsk, July 28
5,249 miles (8,398km)

Chita, August 16
6,010 miles (9,616km)

Blagoveshensk, September 13
7,304 miles (11,686km)

Vladivostok, September 29
8,304 miles (13,286km)
The journey reaches its end.

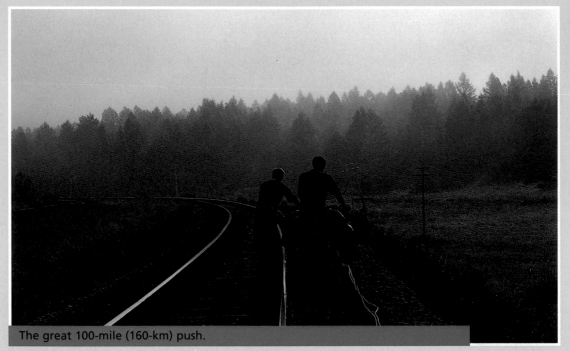

The great 100-mile (160-km) push.

Mechanical hitches

No trip of such length and daring could be trouble free, and this one suffered several setbacks.

- 20 flat tires.
- 6 broken spokes.
- 1 broken saddle, which was easily fixed.
- 11 worn-out tires, replaced with ones brought out by the next new escort.
- 1 broken chain.
- 2 broken computers.
- 1 broken water bottle cage.
- Greg's steel pannier rack, chosen because it could be re-welded, broke seven times and was twice rebuilt. Kate's alloy Blackburn rack did not break the whole trip.
- Kate broke a rib when she slipped off the bike where the road was just mud track. She rode on it for the remaining 3 months of the trip — luckily, it healed.
- 78 days into the trip one rear rim split with wear. The wheel from the spare at HQ was sent and luckily it fit. The lesson learned is to start a trip of this length with new, slightly worn-in wheels.

Crossing the Steppes

Crossing the Russian Steppes involved a two-week 1,100-mile (1,760-km) pedal along a stretch of flat road heading for a flat horizon. Greg and Kate found the challenge was to distract from the saddle soreness they suffered because of never shifting position, the way you would normally as the road rises and falls. In these dreary days Kate actually worked out the total number of pedalstrokes they would make on the journey.

Pushing along the railway

The last third of the trip was the most difficult. Here the road, which is the only way across Russia and yet is unpaved throughout much of its length, runs for hundreds of miles parallel to the Trans-Siberian railway. During the winter the hard-packed snow makes it easily passable for vehicles. During the summer, being mud track, it progressively deteriorates and eventually becomes impassable, and completely choked with plants.

"First the tarmac stops, and then the dirt track stops," explains Greg. "In places we were down to following single-track. When that finally disappeared we had no choice but to climb on to the ballast of the railway track itself and get walking. We covered 100 miles (160km) of the railway on foot, pushing the bikes the whole way, after failing to invent a way of keeping the wheels on the rails."

The Trans-Siberian trains are a summertime lifeline — the only connection then between the east and west of the country.

"We could hear the trains early enough to get out of the way, although if we were between the lines it was nerve-racking standing for minutes between these monsters as they thundered by in each direction. The wheels finish above head-height, they are very long and carry all sorts of cargo; cars, lumber, foodstuffs, coal. The drivers whistled at us, and must have carried the news of our journey down the line, for people seemed to expect our arrival."

Unforgettable cuisine

Food while you are traveling by bike is so very important — it's what fuels the trip, but Kate and Greg enjoyed few culinary delights on their trip. They made picnics of bread, cucumbers, nuts and raisins, but most of what was available was appalling. Greg says he will never forget the worst thing they ate — garlic sandwiches.

"There is little fresh fruit or vegetables — and what there is costs a lot of money, but we did enjoy the seasonal food. The people know how to make the most of the wild harvest. When mushrooms came into season the woods we passed were crawling with people, bags in hands, collecting as many as they could find. That went some way toward enlivening our staple nightly diet of Russian packet soup, which we bulked out with rice, then pasta, then rice... Fresh carrots, presented to us by a hospitable local towards the end of the trip, were a delicacy and our first in four months. Luckily we rode through Siberia as the wild salmon season began." After the solitude of the wilderness they hoped that towns along the way would bring relief.

"The towns were about two weeks apart," says Greg, "and we wanted to get some rest at them, but re-supplying and tracking down food in the different shops was just as tiring as traveling. And because of a currency crisis [in Russia] the price of bread rose by approximately ten times during the five-month period of the trip."

NAVIGATION

"Further, straight on," was the persistently incorrect response to most of the travelers' enquiries about the way. Sense of direction,

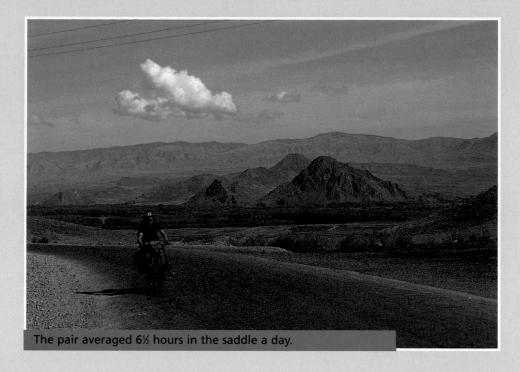

The pair averaged 6½ hours in the saddle a day.

they concluded, thousands of miles and many misdirections later, is not a strong national characteristic. The journey had started as it meant to go on, explains Greg.

"We were on the outskirts of St Petersburg, our starting point, on our way to Moscow, when we came across a vast roundabout. Vladimir, our first escort, ignored the big sign for Moscow, claiming he knew a better route. However, within the

first 15 minutes of the trip we were hopelessly lost."

Wisely, rather than relying on local help, the pair furnished themselves with declassified American military maps. However, these can be dated, and won't always provide much more help.

"Even they were hopelessly wrong about the status and location of the road in places," says Greg.

Cycling through idyllic Sayan in July.

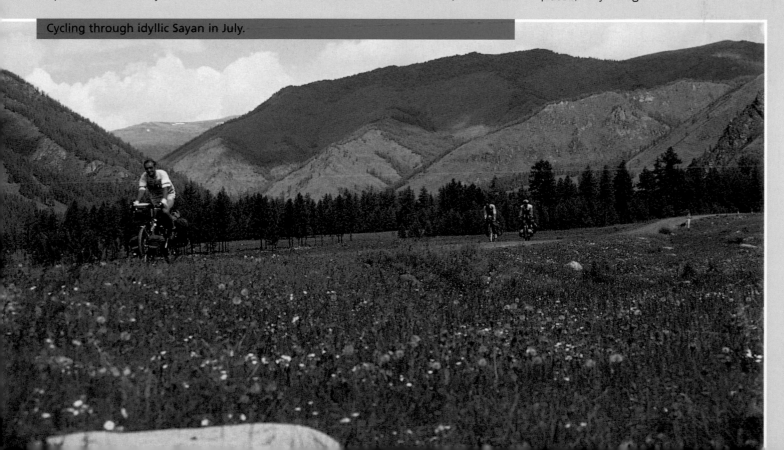

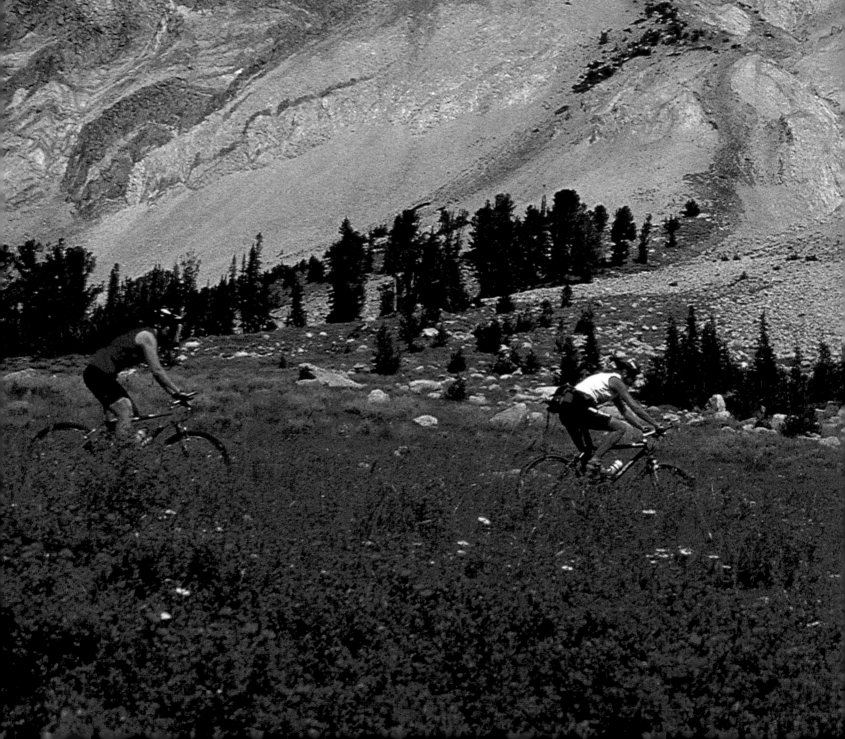

Riding Sawtooth in the Idaho Rockies

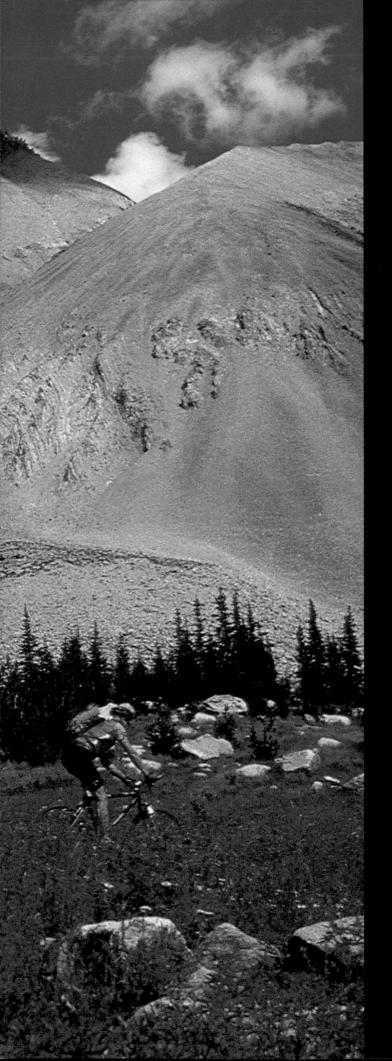

throughout their 1,500-mile march from the borders of Mexico to the Yukon of Canada, the Rocky Mountains are rich in chart-topping off-road destinations.

Head up to Idaho, and you'll find one of the very best Rocky destinations, the Sawtooth National Recreational Area, which has spectacular rides graded from family to hardcore.

This large and magnificent national park spans four mountain ranges, the Sawtooth, Boulder, White Cloud and Smoky. More than 40 peaks in the park top out above 10,000ft (3,280m) and four of Idaho's major rivers rise within the NRA. More than 300 mountain lakes sparkle in the sun and freeze in the winter. Trails run up, down and around the mountains, serving the interests of the US Forest Service, anglers, horseback riders, whitewater rafters and even llama trekkers.

Just to the south, equally good trails are to be found around the Ketchum and Sun Valley area, where the stars go to ski.

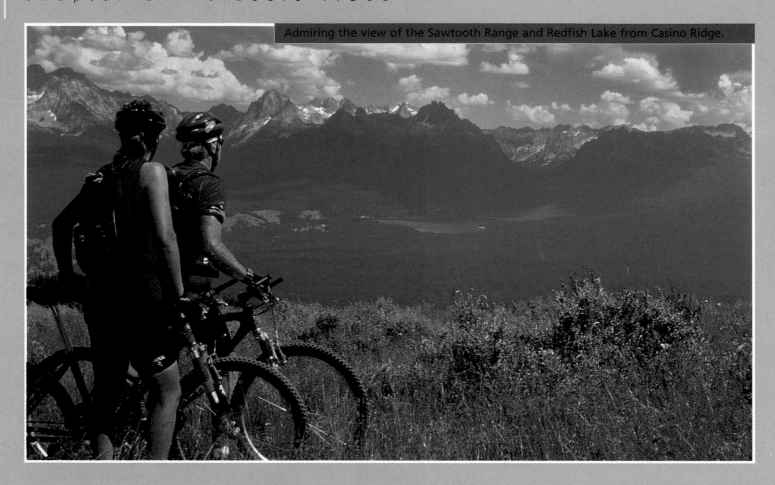
Admiring the view of the Sawtooth Range and Redfish Lake from Casino Ridge.

Stanley and the trails of Sawtooth

In Sawtooth's 25 by 25 mile area, the best place to base yourself is the small old mining and ranching town of Stanley, which sits at an altitude of 6,300ft (1,920m) surrounded by spectacular scenery. This is wild northern territory, settled in the mid-19th century by prospectors and trappers. It's snow-free only between June and August, but locals know they can get snowed on every month of the year. Stanley's year-round population is barely 1,000 people and despite the Sawtooth NRA's popularity with outdoor tourists, the town remains pretty much off the beaten track.

Today most visitors come in those high summer months, when chances are the trails will be clear and the sun hot on your back. Most accommodation is in modern log cabins, and there are campsites at Stanley, Obsidian and Sawtooth City. Stanley may be small, but its isolation is cause for an airport (Stanley Air, ph 208–774–2276).

The Sawtooth NRA Visitor Center in Stanley is good for details and maps (ph 208–727–5000), and the NRA Ranger Station (ph 208–774–3000). It's four miles south of Stanley, on Highway 75.

Please note that mountain biking is not permitted in the Sawtooth Wilderness area around the peaks themselves. If you want to explore here, put on your walking boots.

THE NIP & TUCK TRAIL

For starters, one of the most fun and least strenuous dirt road rides heads away from Stanley through the big rolling cattle pastures of the southern portion of the Stanley basin in a 17-mile loop. Named the Nip & Tuck trail (no one knows why) you ride on what was the main route northwest before the construction of modern Highway 21. Come springtime, the trail enjoys colorful wild flower displays of shooting stars, mules ears and geraniums, with lupin coming into bloom in early summer. There are stunning views of the Sawtooth mountains and a chance to spot elk grazing in the meadows.

Park in Stanley, ride down Highway 75 to Lower Stanley, then go left (north) and continue for 10 miles to Highway 21 near Stanley Lake. It's a further six miles back to Stanley along Highway 21. Arm yourself with the forestry map first.

An easy extension of the route is the Valley Creek ride, going north along the old road after the Stanley Creek turn-off.

THE FISHER/WILLIAMS CREEK LOOP

One of the most popular mountain bike

rides in the Sawtooths, the Fisher/Williams Creek ride is an 18-mile loop that takes two to three hours and isn't so technical, but isn't for beginners either.

The route climbs nice and easy up 1,500ft (457m) on an old dirt road up Fisher Creek and peaks at 8,280ft (2,524m). Then comes the reward, a beautiful smooth singletrack descent down Williams Creek. The trail is popular with hikers and horseriders, so you can't let yourself go completely. The rangers here say you can stop in half the distance you can see, so slow down for corners. What's around it, who knows!

Ride the loop counter-clockwise. The trail lies 10 miles south of Stanley, off Highway 75. Park at the Williams Creek trailhead and ride down Highway 75 to the Fisher Creek road, or park right at Fisher Creek road. The route is signposted fairly well, but you should also carry the forestry map.

THE CASINO CREEK LOOP

For hardcore-istas only, the high remote Casino Creek loop is a great Sawtooth challenge. In 20 miles the ride climbs 4,000ft (1,219m) up one creek, tops out at the main 10,000-ft (3,048-m) ridge for amazing views of the Sawtooth and White Cloud peaks, and drops way back down another creek.

The tracks are rough, technically and aerobically, and you deserve a beer in the bar that night, according to riders who have the experience behind them. A fair number of riders and hikers tackle Casino Creek, but not too many. The route is not well signed (take your own forest map) because it climbs high into the mountains.

Head north from Stanley four miles along Highway 75 for the start. Get details and maps from the Sawtooth ranger station (see page 154).

Rafting in Idaho

Idaho has some of the world's best whitewater rafting. The Middle Fork Salmon River, northwest of Stanley, is ranked as one of the world's top 10 whitewater rivers. You can run its 100 rapids in 100 miles (167km) in approximately six days. Combined with the Main Fork Salmon River, you've get 11 to 12 days of thrilling boating in a dramatic, beautiful mountain area.

Winter sports

Cross-country skiing is big in Sawtooth, with over 120 miles (200km) of trails that have been specially groomed to challenge all levels of ability. Snowmobilers have their pick of over 60 miles (100km) of trails in the Stanley and Stanley Lake areas and elsewhere, and then there's ice skating on the frozen beaver ponds of the Big Wood River.

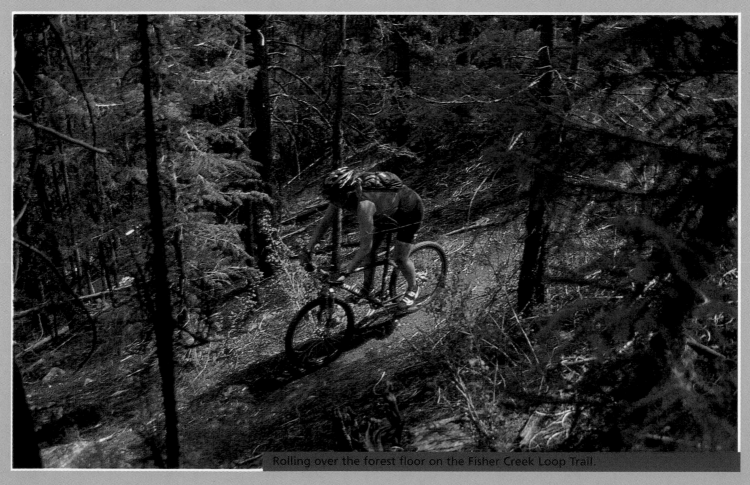

Rolling over the forest floor on the Fisher Creek Loop Trail.

Trails around Ketchum & Sun Valley

60 miles (100km) south of Stanley, seven miles beyond the edge of the Sawtooth NRA lies the town of Ketchum, serving America's original luxury ski resort, Sun Valley. Marilyn Monroe skied here, and in 1961 Ernest Hemingway ended his life in Ketchum with a single shot. The lobby at the grand old Sun Valley Lodge displays photos of the rich and famous taking to the slopes.

Groomed mountain bike trails here are well known like those in nearby Sawtooth, with another advantage being that they have fewer hikers and horseriders.

Ketchum itself is geared up for visitors all year round with abundant accommodation and over 80 places to eat. You can rent bikes and guides from two mountain bike companies; Sun Summit Ski and Cycle (ph 208–726–0707) and the Trail Quest Mountain Bike School (ph 208–726–7401).

Good Dirt II, The Mountain Bike Guide is the authoritative local MTB trail book covering Sun Valley. Written by Greg Roberts it's published by Pinon Trading LLC, PO Box 600, Hailey, ID 83333, email mcbob@ sunvalley.net.

For information on the area, maps, details and contacts get in touch with the Ketchum Ranger District office (ph 208–622–5037).

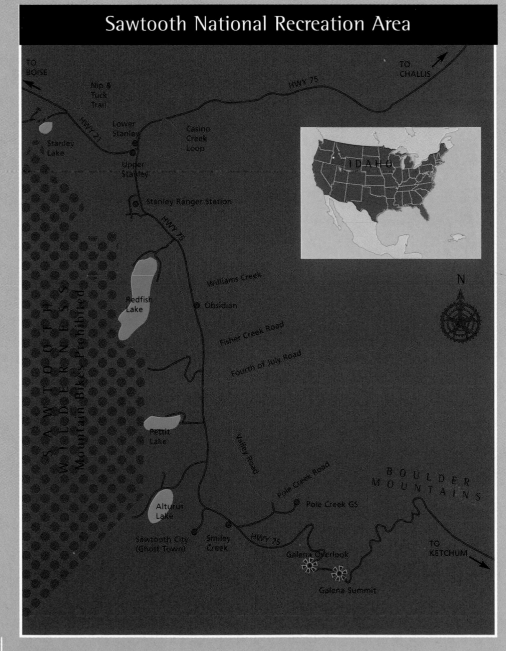

ADAM'S GULCH TRAIL

Just right for beginners, Adam's Gulch trail starts one mile immediately north of Ketchum. The easy 5.5-mile (9.2-km) loop runs round a sunny canyon, and has four other trails linking up to it.

SHADY SIDE LANES LOOP

This special, easy ride bounces along a section of singletrack through Aspen groves. The five-mile Shady Side Lanes loop has a little moderate climbing, but just as stimulating is flashing through these tall graceful trees in slanting sunlight — watch those handlebars.

This ride also has great views, and a very smooth downhill that you can ride all the way along. It's an outing that's very popular with families.

THE GREENHORN TRAIL SYSTEM

One of those things that America does so well is building networks like the Greenhorn trails. From the Greenhorn trailhead you get not one ride, but a choice of three main loops with any number of variations. You could ride all day without covering the same track twice. Some sections are serious lung-busters, not as tough as Sawtooth's Casino loop, but they still give a really good workout and "some of the best downhill you can imagine" according to a local recreation manager.

Recommended is the Imperial Gulch loop, which comes down Mahoney Creek.

Weather and the seasons

High up in the Idaho Rockies, the summer season is short. Even the bottom of the Sawtooth NRA valleys sit above 6000ft (1,829m). The trails, snowbound most of the year, open up about mid-June, or as late as 4 July and stay clear until September.

One insider tip is to visit this area in September — if you're not interested in winter activities. All the tourists are gone, and so are the bugs. You get an off-season rate at the hotel and, though the nights are getting colder at this time of year, the days are almost always warm. Sure, you may get a snowstorm, but at least you'll have the trails to yourself.

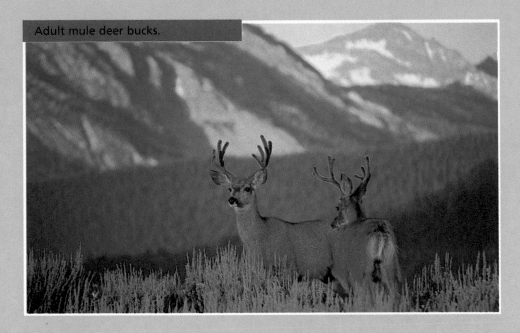

Adult mule deer bucks.

Wildlife

Idaho's mountains are home to masses of wildlife, including a variety of large mammals. You may see black bears, beavers and mountain lions.

The bears, which are smaller and less aggressive than grizzlies, are rarely a threat, but they'll steal your food at night if you don't take care to store it properly. Wolves, coyotes and mountain goats, also lots of Rocky Mountain elk (see the Nip & Tuck trail) are local fauna. You might also spot mule deer. Don't try arguing with any of these animals (even if they are eating your supplies!). Respect all the animals and plants that make the trail so fascinating.

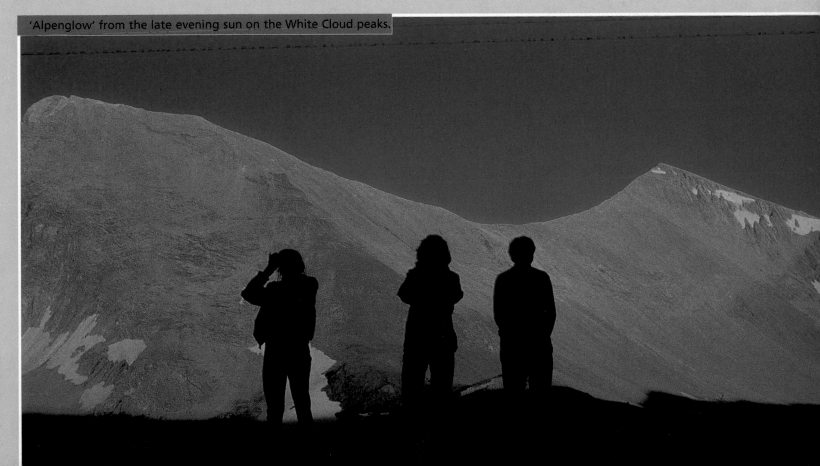

'Alpenglow' from the late evening sun on the White Cloud peaks.

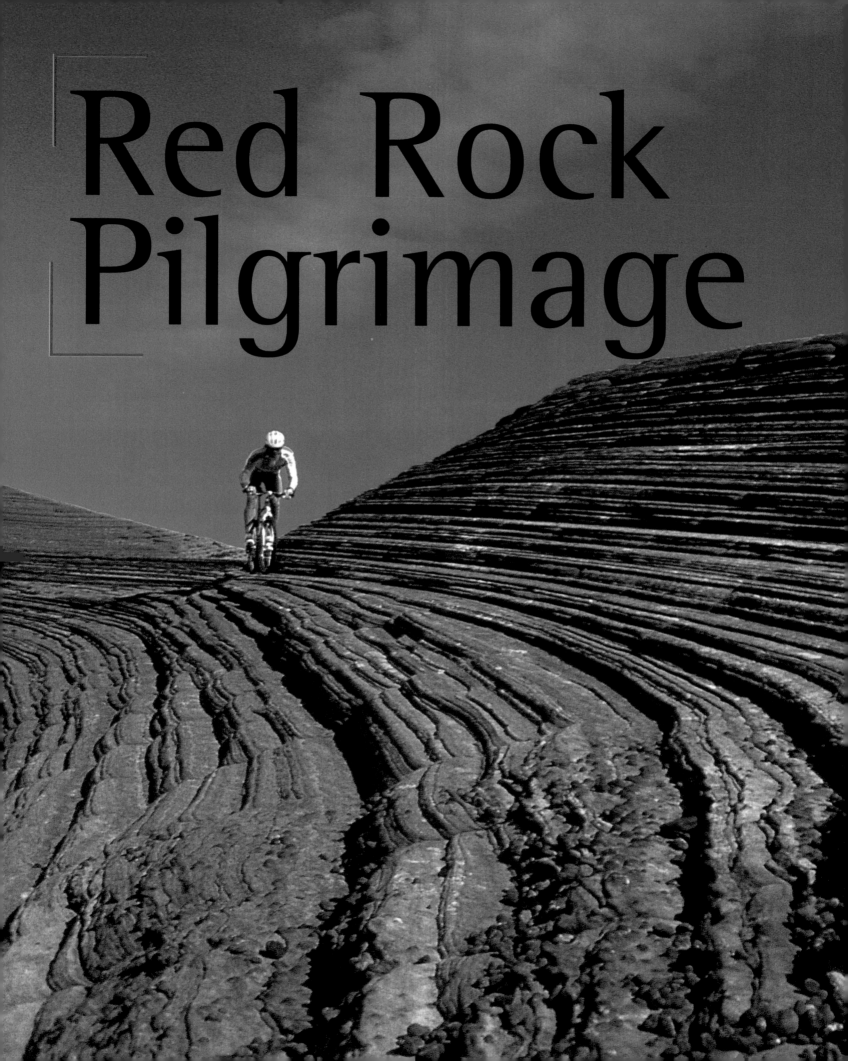

Red Rock Pilgrimage

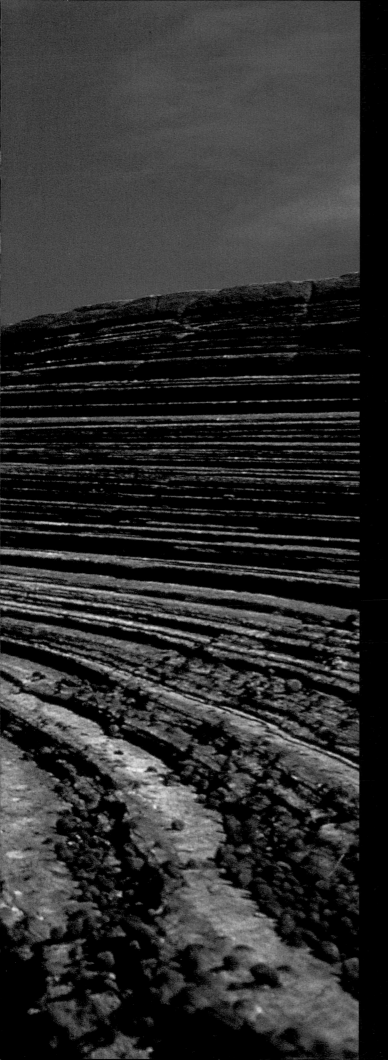

for a reminder that the real world will always be stranger than any virtual experience, go and ride the primitive, bare red rock of Moab in Utah. Its most famous mountain bike trips, the Slickrock Loop and the White Rim Tour in nearby Canyonlands National Park, draw cyclists from all over the world into an area of breathtaking sandstone formations that are supremely bikeworthy.

Situated on a high, empty plateau above the canyons of the Colorado River, the surface of the bulging rock has been eroded to its slick surface by wind and water, resulting in miraculous tire-gripping properties. This means that you can stay in the saddle on the steep slopes of the natural half-pipes long after the grade should have forced you off. The eeriness, heat and drama of these desert trails and the bike-loving atmosphere of Moab, an old uranium-mining settlement, attracts thousands of fat-tire pilgrims. This is without doubt one of the world's most exciting biking destinations.

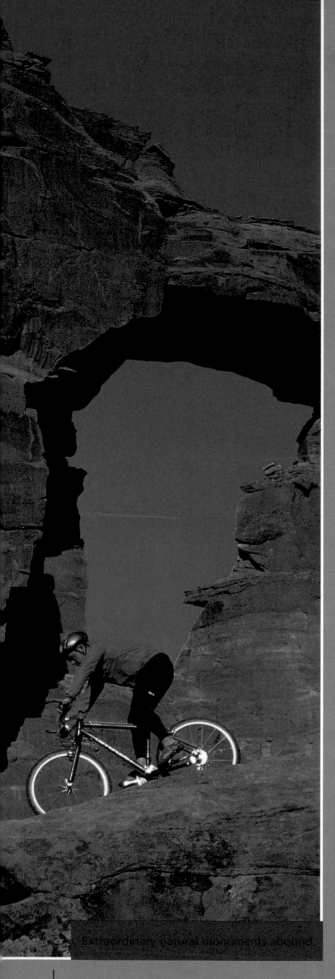

Extraordinary natural monuments abound.

The natural world — a crash course for bikers

Putting rubber to the extraordinary rock spires, arches and canyons of the high altitude desert of Utah, means putting all former off-road experience into storage and letting your imagination run wild.

Forget the details etched into your consciousness by long hours anywhere else in the saddle, this weird, wonderful landscape delivers a unique sensory experience. There's sight — the air seems to be colored red as you gaze at the soaring heights and plummeting depths of majestic sandstone canyons. There's feel — the tires on the smooth rock, sticky, yet bone dry, found across the area. The sound, on a still day, is of timeless silence. Even when it comes to smell, the hot, red rock exudes a sweet, pungent odor.

There's virtually no vegetation to pollinate the air, to shelter behind or to headbutt — only rock. There's no mud, none of that rich, brown life-giving humus that many mountain bikers know too well. Instead, in the cracks and crannies of the overbearing rock there's just a little sand and dust. In this fragile environment, damage takes decades to repair. The 50-year-old tracks of the uranium prospectors who graded the trails in the name of American nuclear capacity are still at the beginning of nature's slow recycling process.

No water, only rock ...

There's not much water, other than the tomato soup-colored flow of the Colorado River on its way from the Rockies to the watercourses of Los Angeles and the Gulf of California. With summertime temperatures averaging between 80–100°F (25–40°C), the priority is water-preservation, not waterproofing. This is desert with an average annual rainfall of 10in (250mm), where the US Department of the Interior insists you drink 8 pints (4.5 litres) of water a day.

The rain that does fall comes at the end of the summer, and in the early fall, when thunderstorms carry a risk of being struck by lightning and flash floods on the parched sandstone can fill up a creek or gully within seconds.

Bearing in mind the delicate ecology that tries to survive in this high, bare habitat, bikers are requested to leave their "cool" behind, and to see themselves as crusaders who protect a delicate and barely perceptible eco-system. Life finds a toehold in the most unlikely places — an apparently infertile grit is held in place and protected from the elements by what's called a cryptobiotic crust. Far from barren, the crust is an ecological niche, a mixture of lichen, algae, fungi and cyanobacteria that forms a living seal against the sand being blown or washed away. This is where the seeds of the high desert are waiting for the rainstorms. Nature's sign above these precarious plant nurseries says, "do not disturb".

The First People

Ancient and more recent Anasazi Indian wall art peppers the area. Many of the sites are easily visited by the bike, and are a feature on the bike tours organized by Moab's five licensed companies. Scenes of people hunting and living are shown in petroglyphs (etchings) and pictographs (paintings) on walls of many of the canyons of the area. They date back to a time when this advanced society was growing corn and hunting Bighorn sheep in the area, and before that too, to more primitive societies. Petroglyphs exist on the paved road from Moab to the White Rim trail and are found at other points like Newspaper Rock. One of the most famous is the Harvest Scene pictograph in the Maze, the south-west portion of the Canyonlands park that has a veritable labyrinth of canyons.

Having viewed this evidence that the ancients expressed themselves in color and form in similar ways as we do today, it becomes understandable that there's a

movement to rename Columbus Day "Indigenous Peoples Day".

Loose your juice on the Slickrock Trail

Claimed to be "the world's most popular trail" Moab Slickrock features prominently in mountain bike folklore. Described as a giant, natural skateboard park, it has spectacular scenery and fabulous riding. Bikes get a big welcome in the town of Moab a couple of miles back on Highway 191, with its established bike shops and hospitality.

The 12-mile (19-km) circuit, hovering between 4,000–5,000ft (1,220–1,500m) altitude, was first laid out in 1969 by local motorcyclists — the outback miners who knew the country like the back of their hands. Mountain bikers stumbled across the trail in the 1980s.

And what about riding the trail? Nothing is straight, or flat, but it is elevated. Every time you pop up out of a gulch you can see way into the distance across lines of red rock humps formed from petrified sand dunes. In the distant east are the snowy foothills of the Rocky Mountains, and to the

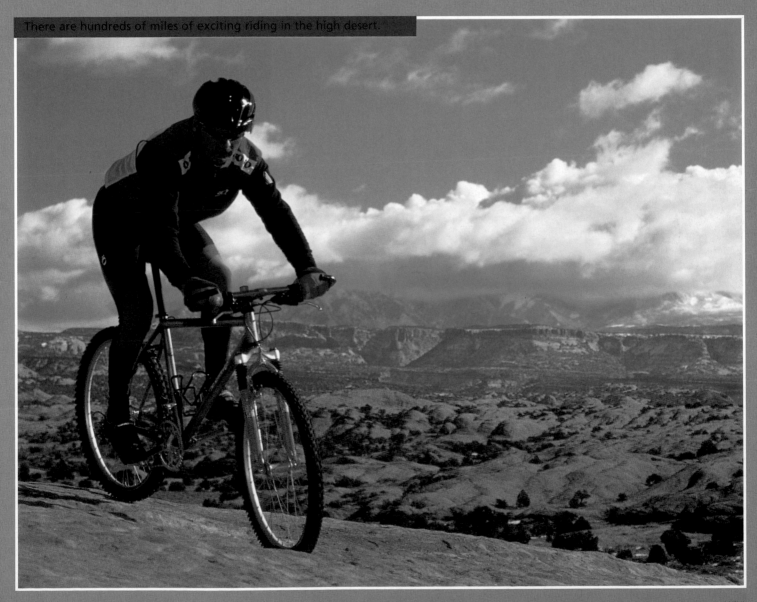

There are hundreds of miles of exciting riding in the high desert.

Slickrock Bike Trail, Moab

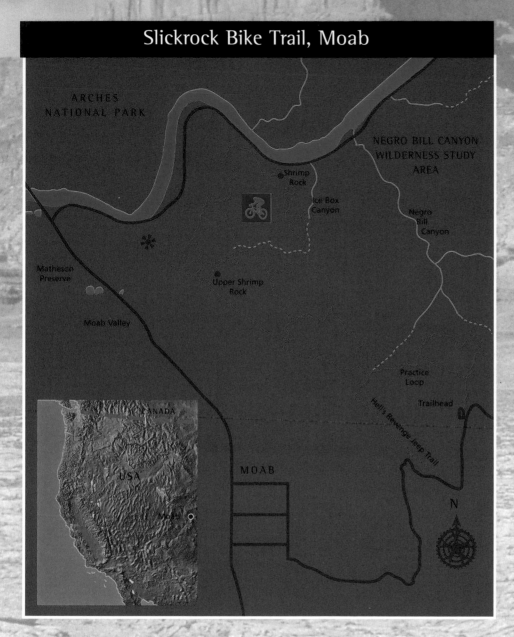

ARCHES
NATIONAL PARK

NEGRO BILL CANYON
WILDERNESS STUDY
AREA

Shrimp
Rock

Ice Box
Canyon

Negro
Bill
Canyon

Matheson
Preserve

Upper Shrimp
Rock

Moab Valley

Practice
Loop

Trailhead

Hell's Revenge Jeep Trail

CANADA

USA

Moab

MOAB

N

mapped tracks in Canyonlands and even into Colorado. Slickrock takes between 90 minutes and 8 hours to ride, depending on ability and stops to take in the view.

Sweat and skill

Every piece of the trail has been christened and given a two-figure sweat and skill grading. For example, one section called "Interval Straining'" has a 2/8 grading, meaning 2/10 for technical difficulty and 8/10 for effort. Another climb, "Staircase" rates 8/8, which means it's both mentally and physically hard. "Loose the Juice" is a sweet drop marked 3/5 and then there's the aptly-named "Baby Bottom Bowl". The viewpoints include "Natural Selection" at the far end of the trail which overlooks the Colorado river gorge towards Arches Park, some of whose jewels can be seen.

Heading for a fall

The words "Danger (stop or die)" appear a couple of times on the trail and need no explanation. Falling down cliff edges and getting lost are two good reasons to stick to the trail, and you're advised not to ride alone. For regulars — Slickrock is the backyard of the citizens of Moab — new spurs and sections of trail were added in 1989, and are distinguished with dots, as opposed to dashes. One bisects the loop via the Black Hole, where caution is advised.

Autumn and spring are the best times to go to Utah. There's no water up on the Trail plateau, not even at the parking lot. In the cooking summer temperatures you should carry as many as three water-bottles, and drink before you're thirsty. Wear full sunburn protection and good sun-shades. If riding in a party, make sure everyone is keeping up and can cope. Wintertime might mean snow.

north is the awesome Arches National Park, named after its hundreds of natural red rock arches and holes.

White dashes, like road markings, show you the way to go, over huge rock "pillows" and slopes. Extreme slopes become ridable both up and down, sometimes over perfectly smooth rock and other times across the close-contoured lines of strata. There are wonderful, easy swooping downhills and half-pipes, and also uphill grades which will test any rider to their limit. Riding the loop

is, for many riders, a feat in itself, and despite its easy surface, Slickrock begins with a 2.5 mile (4km) practice loop, as the rest of the trail is designated as technically difficult. But that shouldn't put off beginners; you can easily walk with the bike anywhere that you can't ride, as long as you stay on the marked trail.

Experienced riders won't believe what's hit them. They can use the Slickrock Trail as a warm-up for longer, more varied tours, like the White Rim trail and any of another dozen

Blazing rubber on the White Rim Trail

With the relatively busy Slickrock Trail under your belt, nearby Canyonlands National Park offers remoter adventure.

There's the 100 mile (160km) White Rim Trail, an epic circuit with four days of riding and camping. The route runs along what is the seat of a massive white sandstone bench. Below are the 1,700ft (518km) walls of the Colorado and Green river gorges. Above it is the "back" of the seat, an extraordinary upper plateau called the "Island in the Sky" with its highest point at 6,000ft (1,828m).

Overwhelming vistas of sky and rock make this canyon country trip a must-see. You can either ride it on your own, in which case you have to stay in the official simple campsites (firewood needs to be brought in, and garbage must be taken out) or have someone else take care of everything by joining one of the guided bike trips.

DOWNTOWN MOAB

A little town with a big name, Moab is home to several cult bike shops and the center of information on guided bike tours in the area as well as where to stay.

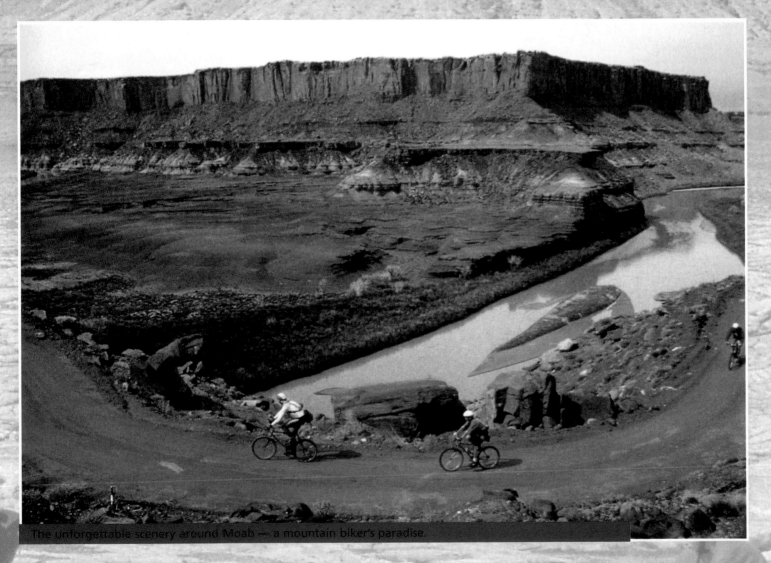

The unforgettable scenery around Moab — a mountain biker's paradise.

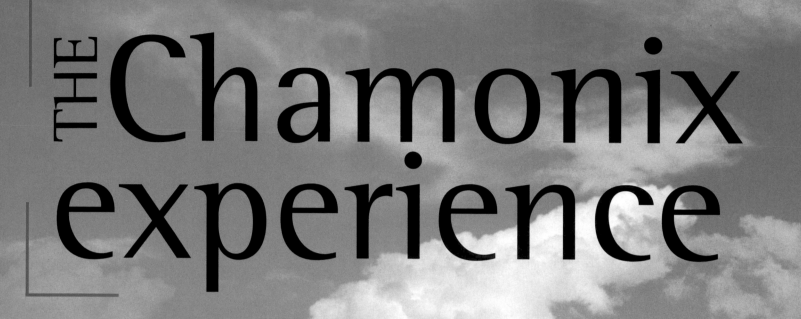

THE Chamonix experience

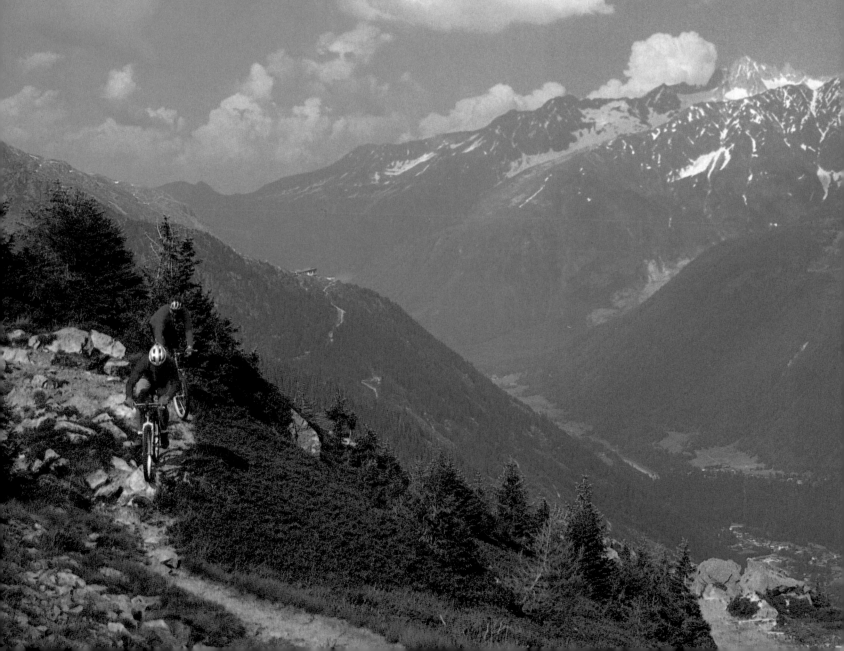

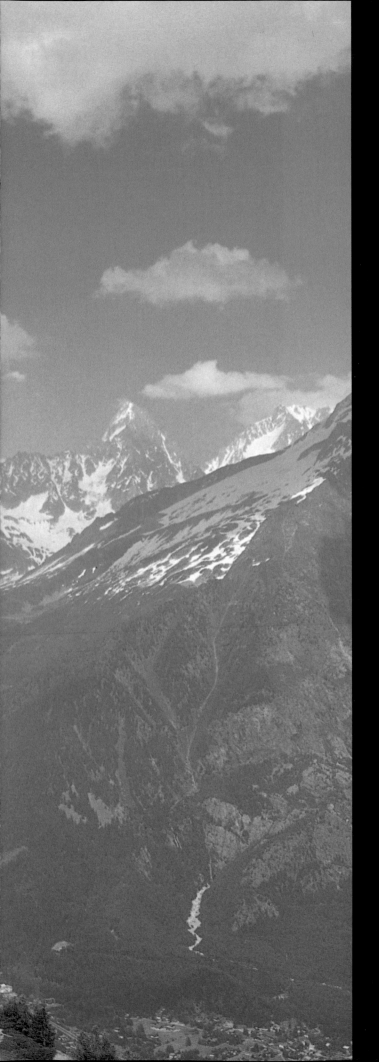

the mountain resort of Chamonix, directly below Mont Blanc in the French Alps, is famous in all walks of alpine sport. The place is revered in mountaineering for its concentration of glaciers and sharp, soaring peaks and in skiing for its high-quality slopes. So, naturally, it's also become a superb summertime mountain bike destination. Halfway between the world of the exposed climber above, and the tourist below, a cyclist can test his bike's "mountain" pedigree on an abundance of great tracks that pass along the mountainsides, through beautiful valleys and over high passes, using the spectacular cable-car network to link trails and mountain cafés.

Chamonix has some sign-posted local mountain bike trails. These are color-graded like the ski slopes and are mostly suitable for gentle rides, beginners or as a warm-up for more strenuous rides. For more experienced cyclists, specialty tour companies offer more adventurous trips.

Chamonix history

Chamonix has always been a fashionable winter resort. At the end of the 19th century, the town hosted one of the first ever package tours, run by Thomas Cook, and the first Winter Olympics in 1924. As well as being a mountaineering base, busy ski resort and hard-core hiking center, it has developed a reputation as a location for extreme stunts such as ultimate skiing.

Chamonix — peaks and glaciers

The town's main attraction is the highest Alpine peak, Mont Blanc, which, at 15,771ft (4807m), looms directly above it. The valley also features no fewer than six major glaciers, the most famous of which, the Mer de Glace, sits just 650ft (200m) away from the town boundary, as well as more than 20 smaller ones. Lying in an alpine corner where France, Switzerland and Italy meet, just an hour's drive from Geneva airport, Chamonix is also the location of the northern entrance of the 8 mile (12km) Mont Blanc tunnel, which provides a link between France and Italy. The closest open-air border crossing is the 8100ft (2469m) Grand St Bernard Pass between Switzerland and Italy, 50 miles (80km) to the east.

The uniquely spectacular character of the European Alps over some of the world's other higher mountain ranges is the absolutely breathtaking height difference between the valleys and the mountain tops. The beautiful snowy Monts, Dents and Aiguilles dwarf smudges of civilization below. Chamonix itself sits at a height of 3,360ft (1035m), a full 12,260ft (3772m) drop below the tip of Mont Blanc, which measures only 6 miles (10km) away from the town center on the map.

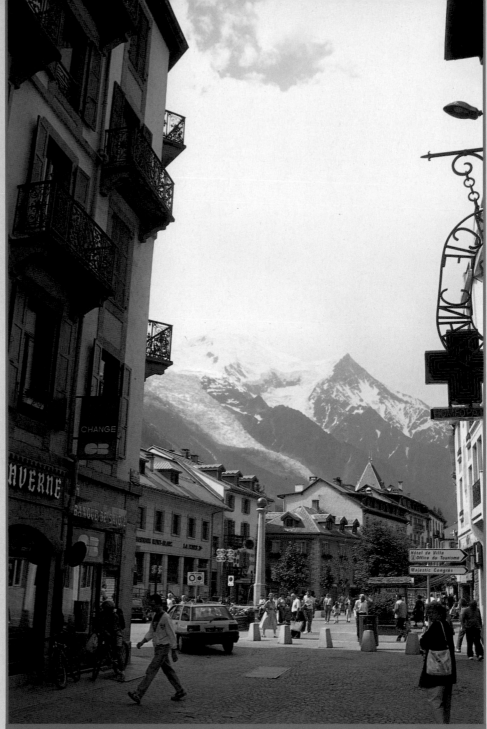

With expensive stores and dozens of cafés, Chamonix is a magnet for mountain bikers.

Mountain biking in the Mont Blanc area

Chamonix is a good place to get a taste of biking the Alps, where you can ride in three countries in as many days, without even seeing a border crossing. Like many of the alpine ski resorts the town switches between summer and winter sports. The mountain biking season lasts from May to September, with visitors attracted by the fact that the town is geared around vacationers, with plenty of restaurants and clothing stores. You can arrange accommodation on your own and follow your own routes, or use the services of an MTB tour company, which also offers full-board chalet accommodation.

The tourist board has produced a starter map showing several easy sign-posted routes — using the symbol of a triangle with two circles to the left. The guided tours take bikers of all standards on more adventurous routes, lasting anywhere between one and seven days, over some of the area's hundreds of miles of tracks.

One ride guided by Mont Blanc Mountain Biking (a specialty cycling tour operator — see acknowledgements for details) uses the cable car to climb up to 6000ft (1850m), for a pure descent of 4050ft (1250m) back down into the valley — the height, their brochure points out, of Ben Nevis, the United Kingdom's highest peak. Another ride has a 3250ft (1000m) climb up to a mountaintop café.

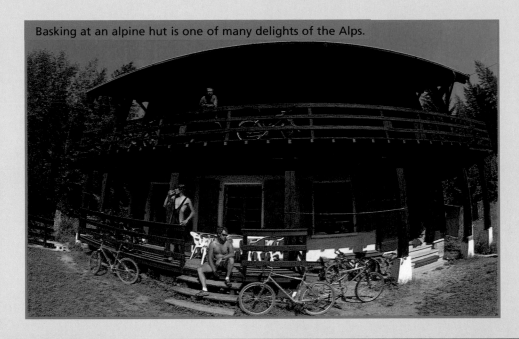

Basking at an alpine hut is one of many delights of the Alps.

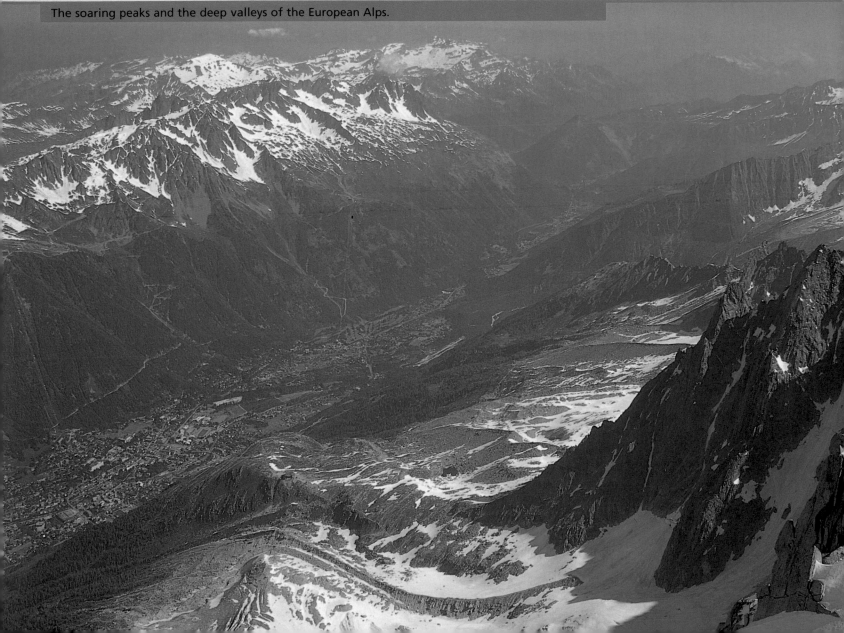

The soaring peaks and the deep valleys of the European Alps.

The Tour du Mont Blanc

The classic MTB route of the area is the 5-day circumnavigation of the Mont Blanc massif. The trip takes in four passes above 6500ft (2000m), meaning lots of climbing and descending, and is only suitable for fit bikers who are either already experienced, or who are on the fast-track to MTB wisdom. Staying in shape and in alpine huts, the trip is an unusual one.

Supported 7-day tour

You spend seven days in the saddle. In the Mont Blanc area, the accommodation is at inns up in the high mountain villages, with the luxury of full baggage support.

Sample rides

18-MILE INTERMEDIATE RIDE

Starting from the Foyer de Ski de Fond on the main road, follow the tourist office map along the trail marked No. 1. Follow this until you reach the "Pont de Corrua". From here follow the signs for Lavancher (route No. 5). When you arrive in Lavancher descend on the road. A hairpin right, a hairpin left, then look out for the MTB trail sign on the right (route No. 7). Take this trail (Petit Balcon Nord) to Argentiere. Follow the Petit Balcon to Le Tour (good luck on the "Le Planet" climb!) Go to the cable car station and take the lift to Charamillion. Once out of the cable car, ride towards the Col Des Possettes (6500ft/2000m). Over the Col

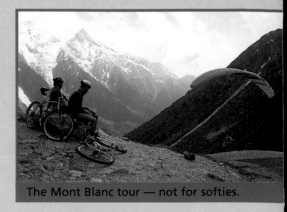

The Mont Blanc tour — not for softies.

des Possettes, ride downhill toward Vallorcine. The track is a logging trail and is quite fast and stony, but great fun.

Once you've got your breath back in Vallorcine, ride in the direction of Le Buet on the trail on the left side of the valley. Go through Le Buet and follow the trail until it meets the road on the Col des Montets. Join the road and pass the Col des Montets. Start the descent after the Col but after about a quarter mile (500m), take a left to

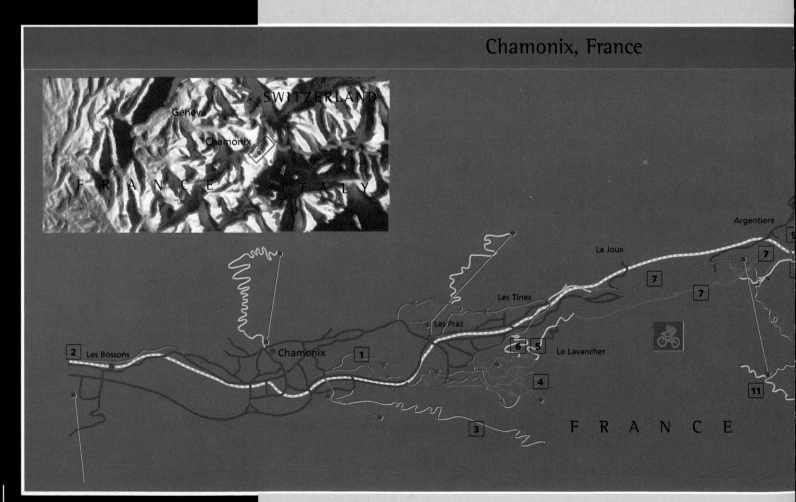

a hamlet called Trelechamp. Take the gravel track through Trelechamp and just before it meets the road again take a little single-track to the left, for some great hairpins. Go through Argentiere on the road but just before the railway bridge, take a right and pick up a trail called the "Petit Balcon Sud". You'll arrive at "Paradis des Praz" where you can get back to Chamonix via the details in ride 1 on the Tourist Office Map.

24-MILE HARD RIDE VIA THE "CORKSCREW"

This is a tough one. Pick up the road out of Chamonix to Les Gaillands. At the climbing wall in Les Gaillands pick up the trail leading to Les Bossons. Using signs and your map go to Les Bossons, Les Montquarts, Les Roches to the train station in Les Houches

(Gare SNCF). Cross the main road and ride to the Bellevue cable car station in Les Houches and take the cable car to the top.

When you get out of the cable car, descend to Col de Voza. Follow the trail that leads to "Prarion", but not all the way. After four hairpins take the trail on the left to La Charme. Follow this trail for at least 2½ miles (4km). You arrive at a T-junction where you will see an asphalt road descending to the left and a trail going right. Take the right and follow the trail for about ⅔ mile (1km) until you reach a small hamlet called Montfort. There's a left turn that's tricky to find, but you will if you're careful. This is the start of the legendary "corkscrew", a trail known only to a handful of the local MTBers. This brings you out on to the main road connecting Le Fayet and St Gervais. Descend to Le Fayet.

Take the D43 road toward Chedde. When you arrive at Chedde by the hang-glider landing field, you see a sign left, "Servoz par D13". Take this road and after the first sharp left hairpin you'll see a trail on the right marked "Chemin du Butteaux". This 15-minute climb will bring you to the D13 road to Servoz. Go through Servoz on the road, following road signs to Chamonix. When you meet the main road (Route

Blanche) head towards Chamonix. After only about ½ mile (700m), you'll see a right turn-off that appears to go nowhere. Take this but don't follow the road to the house. Go straight on following a trail under the railway bridge and on to Les Houches. Go through Les Houches and you'll come to the Bellevue cable car that you took earlier. From here you go back to Chamonix via Taconnaz, Les Bossons and Les Gaillands on the road. Or, you can return along the trail you rode in the morning.

CLOTHING

These are high mountains where the weather can change drastically, and quickly. During the winter the slopes are snow-bound, and in the spring and autumn you should take clothing for cold wind and snow or rain. If you're going high, remember that the temperature drops 1.8 degrees for every 300ft (100m) climbed, and that the air can be much cooler than the sunshine might suggest. By contrast, summer is warm, and carrying drinking water is the priority. Most of the rides in the Chamonix valley pass alpine drainage pipes that have a constant supply of running spring water that's safe to drink.

echamp

ontroc

Planet

10

9

8

Le Tour

Key

Cable Car

N

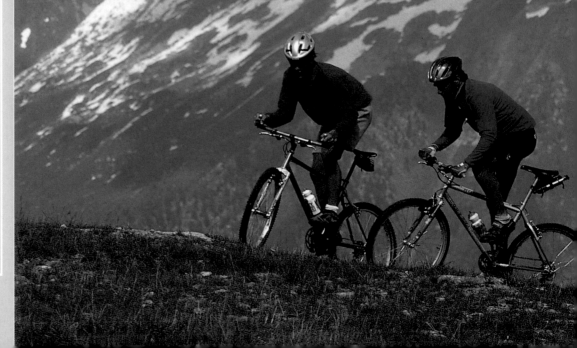

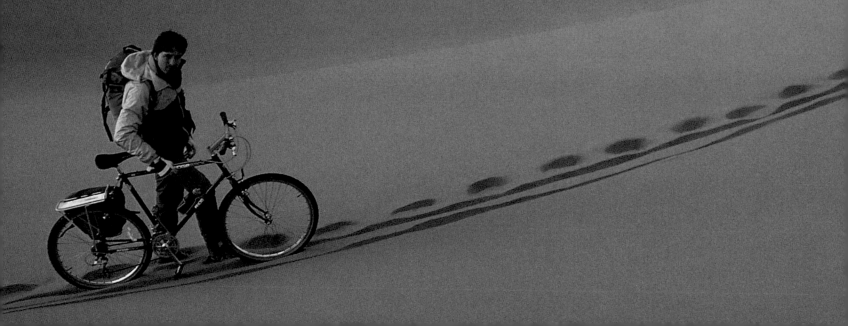

mountain biking in
Morocco

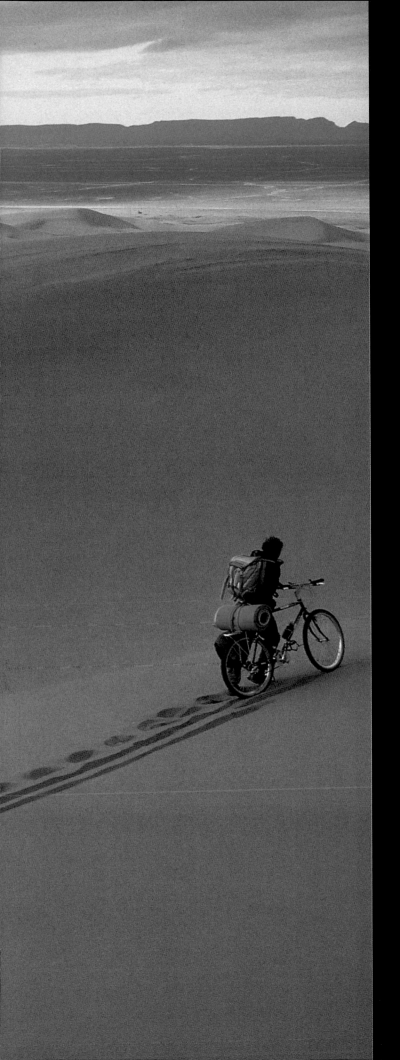

t racks formed over thousands of years by the Berber people and their animals, linking fortified villages through gorges and over barren mountains which shimmer with the heat from the Sahara below. That's the riding that draws mountain bikers to the High Atlas range in Morocco.

The Atlas mountains have become one of the favorite destinations among the sort of wanderlusting mountain bikers who enjoy experiencing other cultures as much as they enjoy the views, effort and highs of an athletic adventure.

Morocco is well-served by flights from Europe, speaks French and cooks a mean, colorful cuisine, which makes a visit here relatively practical and accessible. Alternatively, specialty mountain bike tour companies offer a selection of supported trips that also take in the beauty of the Atlas range. This means that all you need to do is push the pedals and enjoy the sights and smells.

"The mountains that time forgot" is the description used by Moroccan tour guides who do business in the High Atlas. The sentiment is one of cultural rather than geographical accuracy. The ancient and remote Berber villages, which carve out a living from the high, dramatic slopes of the Atlas range are way above the reaches of power and indoor plumbing. But they are not beyond the reach of the knobbly tire and a determined rider — as long as she or he is happy with the idea of living simply while exploring the rich network of tracks.

The Atlas mountains are made up of four roughly parallel ranges that form the southern edge of the Mediterranean bowl. All together the four ranges, the Anti Atlas, High Atlas and Mid Atlas in Morocco and the Algerian Atlas run for 1400 miles (2,250km), from the Atlantic coast almost to Tunisia. Much of the guided mountain biking takes place in the 200 mile (320km) High Atlas range, which rises well over 12,000 feet in places, with some in the Anti Atlas to the south as well. The highest point is Mount Toubkal at 13,665ft (4165m) — the fourth highest peak in Africa.

Despite being a neighbor of the Saharan desert and having "Africa" in its address, the ice-capped High Atlas range is an example of how dependent temperature is on altitude. Although warm during the day most of the year, the sun deserts the steep upper valleys early in the day, and night-time frost is common. So travelers cannot pack as lightly as they might expect. Recommended equipment includes a three-season sleeping bag and long johns.

When Nick Crane and his colleagues made their end-to-end trip in 1989, they traveled in the age-old explorers' tradition —

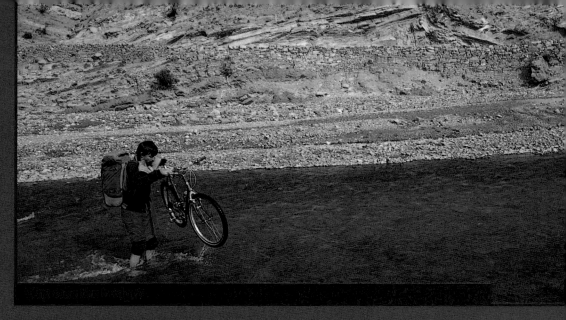

to see whether the range was at all navigable by MTB. It is, and since then the area has become a destination for more far-sighted mountain bikers, keen to experience the Arab and Berber cultures and itching for hundreds of miles of rock and dung trails. For Europeans, Morocco is relatively close — just 5 hours flight from the UK — with a choice of travel options courtesy of the boom in "roughing-it" travel and young, enthusiastic tour companies.

Visiting the High Atlas on your own is quite possible if you're confident outside Western culture, or if you'd like to become so, and tough enough either to camp or to seek simple shelter with the people on a day-to-day basis. After flying either to Agadir at the western tip, or to Marrakech, the former Berber capital, inland to the north of the range, the mountains are a day's ride away, or less if you travel by bus. From there you're free to roam, using hiking maps, your nose and local knowledge.

The alternative, for people who want the riding and culture without the unpredictability that comes with being self-sufficient, is an all-inclusive tour. On these, experienced guides and a support team take care of the routes, travel, food, camping and logistics.

The mountain biking scores highly in this land, where the rock is the color of oxidized copper. The number of trails is huge in what is a 200 mile (320km) mountain range. You never get to the end of them. These are working tracks; unpaved, extremely rough under-tire but well packed down by thousands of years of hooves and feet. Barring the mule trains and tourist Landrovers, there are very few vehicles — another reason for the "forgotten by time" tag. As long as you don't disturb the local people or the animals they depend on to survive, you can enjoy a rare biking treat — unfettered riding according to your energy, ability to stay in one piece and the hours of daylight.

The tracks run through the valleys and along the mountainsides, linking village to pasture, village to village, and village to town. The lower valleys are fertile but goat-nibbled, but the upper plains are barren with tough desert scrub and trees are the only greenery. Up there, above the rain-clouds, the water source is melt-water fed springs. Mud, the biker will be glad to know, plays no role in MTBing Moroccan-style.

The mud and stone settlements are built of the same material as the surrounding rock and are so well camouflaged that from a distance they melt into the background. The more significant villages are dominated by crumbling fortresses, or kasbahs, which are worth a detour and which feature on the itineraries of the tour companies. Another Atlas specialty is the dozens of spectacular gorges; deep, still clefts, maybe with a stream at the bottom, but more likely a dried-up stream-bed.

There's no problem finding food in the foothills, but the higher the altitude and more remote the hamlet, the fewer supplies there may be, particularly during the Muslim month of fasting, Ramadan. Highly recommended is *tagine*, a delicious meat and vegetable stew and staple of the Moroccan diet. Berber hospitality, like in most untouristed cultures, is warm and friendly, and the Berber people are no strangers to Westerners, apart from those who live in extremely remote hamlets.

MTB tours are organized and take place all year round, except in July when the heat is too intense. These tours are suitable for anyone of any age, as long as you are in moderately good shape. The trips involve several hours of biking a day, usually between 20–30 miles (30–50km), and vary between a tour of "the valley of a thousand kasbahs" and a special winter-sun trip, which is 70% downhill — a Landrover does all the uphill work for you.

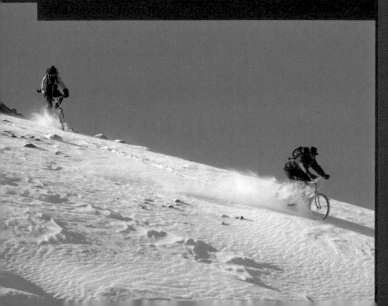

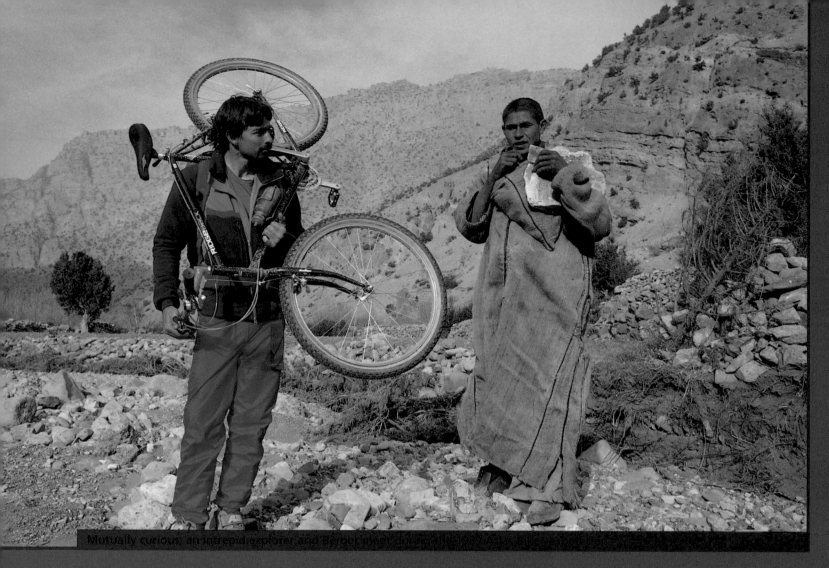

Mutually curious: an intrepid explorer and Berber meet during the 1989 Atlas Biker expedition.

Atlas Biker Route — Sahara to the Sea

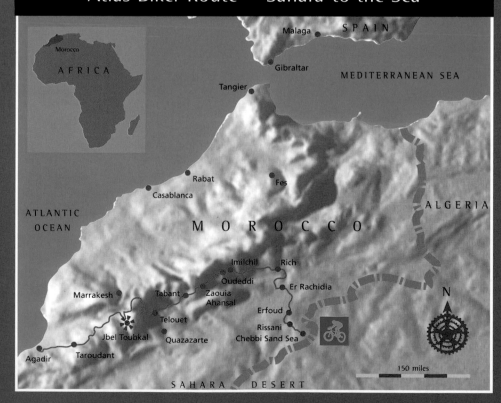

Morocco

AFRICA

SPAIN
Malaga
Gibraltar
MEDITERRANEAN SEA
Tangier

ATLANTIC OCEAN

Rabat
Casablanca
Fes

MOROCCO

ALGERIA

Imilchil   Rich
Oudeddi
Marrakesh   Tabant   Zaouia   Er Rachidia
Ahansal
Telouet   Erfoud
Jbel Toubkal   Rissani
Quazazarte   Chebbi Sand Sea
Agadir   Taroudant

N

150 miles

SAHARA   DESERT

Highlights of the Atlas range

■ **Ait Benhaddou** — a pretty, fortified village used for location filming of the epic movies *Lawrence of Arabia* and *Jesus of Nazareth*, this makes it a tourist trap.

■ **The Cascades d'Ouzoud** — a 100ft (35m) waterfall in a fertile cauldron.

■ **The Dades Gorge** — one of the most impressive in the area.

■ **The Tizi**, or passes, for memorable climbing and descending:

■ **Tizi n'Tazzazert** — 7000ft (2200m)

■ **Tizi n'Tichka** — 7350ft (2260m), on the road from Marrakech on the north side, to Ouarzazate on the south side.

■ **Tizi n'Ouano** — 10,700ft (3300m), near Imilchil towards the eastern end of the Atlas range.

174

NICK CRANE'S ATLAS TRAVERSE

What first drew mountain biking attention to the High Atlas was adventurer Nick Crane's "Atlas Biker" trip in 1989. Inspired by traveler Wilfred Thesiger, he and Matt Dickinson successfully completed a 750 mile (1200km) continuous MTB traverse of the range from the Sahara to the Atlantic Ocean, conquering the icebound summit of Mount Toubkal at 13,665ft (4165m) on the way. The purpose was to see if the mountains were navigable by MTB using the most direct route possible from east to west. The pair stuck to the high route, even when it meant carrying the bikes for hours, and using difficult, often dangerous tracks over outcroppings and along the sides of steep gorges, to save losing altitude going around them. Their bikes, rigid Ridgeback 501s, were not sophisticated by current standards, but they proved that it's not necessary to have a supercharged bike to perform a supercharged feat — you just have to be crazy enough.

The trip was filmed so the bikers had the advantage of vehicle support, but rode every inch of the trek themselves. The film was broadcast on TV in the UK in June 1989 as a half-hour programme, "Blazing Pedals". No less than 6 million people tuned in, which unexpectedly brought Nick closer than any other mountain biker to household name status and put High Atlas mountain biking firmly on the map.

Starting at the east end of the range on top of the highest dunes in Morocco at the Chebbi sand sea, the trekkers averaged 38 miles (60km) every day, before finishing at the Atlantic in Agadir, three bruised and bumped weeks later. Their elevation averaged between 3,250 and 8,125ft (1000–2,500m) with a high diversion up Mount Toubkal.

Conditions were often tricky, as the men froze at night and boiled during the day. The bikers split off from the Landrovers whenever their cross-country route became undrive-able, which usually meant slow progress. For example, the 45 barely mapped miles to the Berber sanctuary of Zaioua Ahansal ended up taking them three days, delayed by several factors. They had to do their own filming and carry the equipment themselves in backpacks wrapped up in sleeping bags. Chris Bradley, a third rider, went over the handlebars, damaged his knee and had to hobble painfully on it for the next two days before quitting the biking attempt. Also, the map that these highly experienced men were using was a 1:100,000 general map of North Africa, and the directions given to them by the rare goatherd or whoever crossed their path, were flawed.

The ascent of the peak Djebel Toubkal took two days, most of which was spent carrying the bikes through steep, deep snow and ice. But the trek had to be done to maintain the image that cyclists and explorers do it only for the heroism and eccentricity.

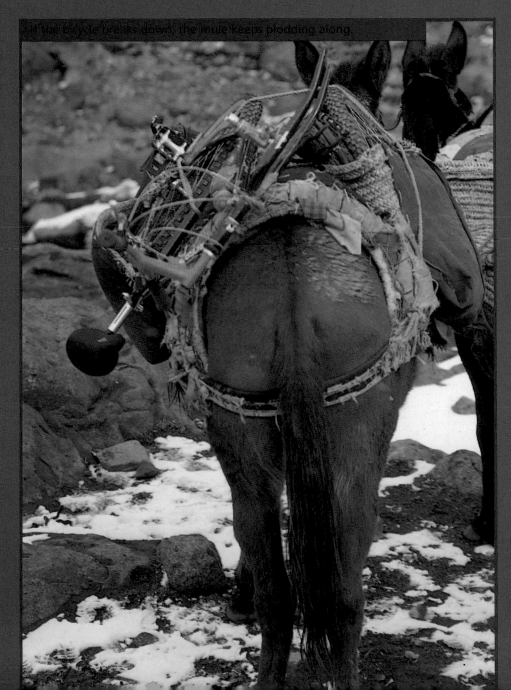

If the bicycle breaks down, the mule keeps plodding along.

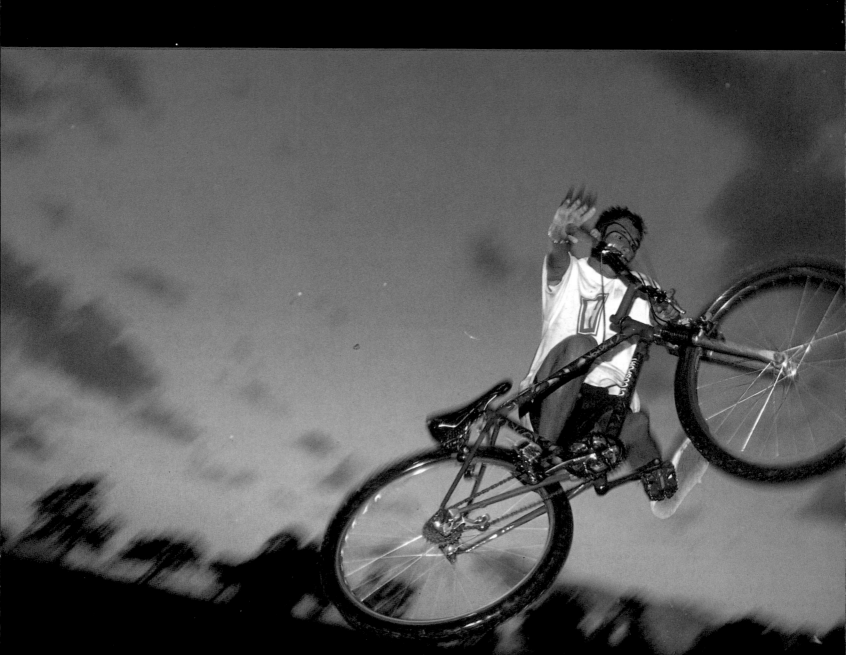

chapter four stunt

riding

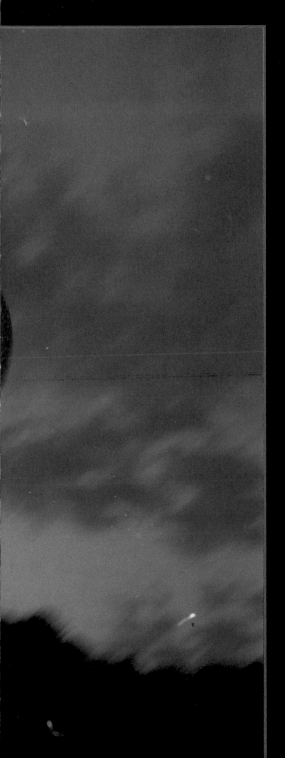

representing the circus ring of mountain biking, trick riding is a highly skilled and spectacular branch of the sport. Here it's acceptable for full-grown women and men to fool around on bikes and perform feats beyond the comprehension of most mountain bikers — how ever many times they've circum-navigated the world or how ever many gold medals clutter up the mantelpiece.

These are acrobats doing the things on bikes that you are supposed to grow out of in your teens — grown men and women behaving badly, and who should know better, but who are desperate to explore to the limits that they and their bike are capable of, and give the onlookers the thrill of watching. The list of tricks is always growing, as new riders choreograph their own repertoires. Stunt riding is an individual thing. Look at Hans Rey, the king of the MTB entertainers, giving the graffitied wall on California's Venice Beach a glancing blow from his wheels, six feet up, or jumping from car roof to car roof in an LA traffic jam as part of a Swatch promotion, or giving a feisty young woman lying on her back a front-wheel kiss in the middle of London's Piccadilly Circus.

In Britain, the mysteriously named "Switzerland Squeaker" was a trick unique to Jez Avery, who could balance on his front wheel while the rear one was whisked away by his lovely assistant, Paul — just one in a bag of improvised, personalized tricks.

Everyone likes to develop their bike-handling skills, and stunt riding is a way of improving your overall off-road control. There's also a sense of intense satisfaction when you start getting a trick right after practicing it over and over again, whether it's your first bunny-hop or lengthy wheelie, track-stand at the stoplight. Trick riding is a great equalizer for MTB riders who are never going to be particularly fast or have the levels of endurance needed to shine in the cross-country pack. Check your equipment and ride with care, because if you land awkwardly and bend the fork, or wrap the frame around a tree, the manufacturer won't sympathize.

This chapter features some great examples of flamboyant MTB riding to enter-tain and inspire. See trials competitions, which are rare despite their great crowd appeal and the ballet-like balance displayed by the professionals. Riders hop around obstacle stations made up of cars, logpiles or boulders as cleanly as possible. There's no world series in trials, which is too bad, considering the talent that's come over from BMXing since the manufacturers got busy with 26in-wheel street bikes. And then, get ready to duck as the air bandits get jumping and lake leaping. There's also a piece on 24-hour racing. No stunts, but insanity just the same!

A word of warning — many of the tricks shown here are done by professional riders with years of practice and should not be attempted by inexperienced riders.

mountain bike trials

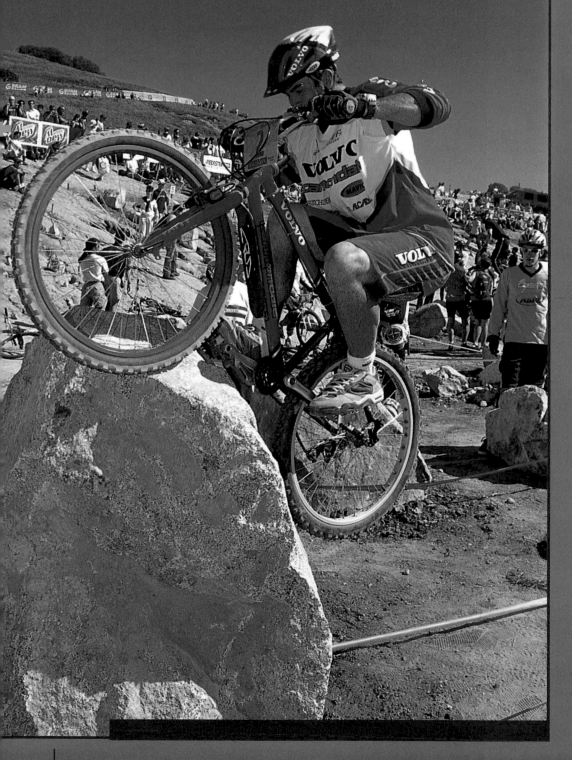

Almost a part of the biking underground, trials competitions are not too common, but very popular with bikers who have the light touch. They're the competitive expression of the self-testing that all bikers, particularly urban cowboys, practice when they do track-stands at red lights, or wheelies, when they hop crates or ride see-saws. Most competitions have ability and/or age groups, so anyone can give it a shot, although teenage boys seem to do it best. A world championship was once held in the '90s, but was more just a sideshow for the downhill and cross-country championships. The situation undervalues the incredible skill of the riders and the visual appeal of this branch of mountain biking.

So what is it? The trials course has a number of different obstacle stations, each obstacle being more or less within sight of the next. No two trials arenas are alike. The obstacles vary from carefully constructed works of art to natural features, like those found in a forest. Forests have huge trials opportunities; you can try to get over fallen logs, or hop 180° round a tree-trunk on a slope, or see who can hop highest up a slope sideways.

Elite courses are extremely difficult, designed so that only experts stand a chance of finishing. The favorites are head-high log-piles, that might take the competitor up to 5 minutes of continual hopping to complete. Other creative obstacles include burnt-out wrecks, where you have to jump up

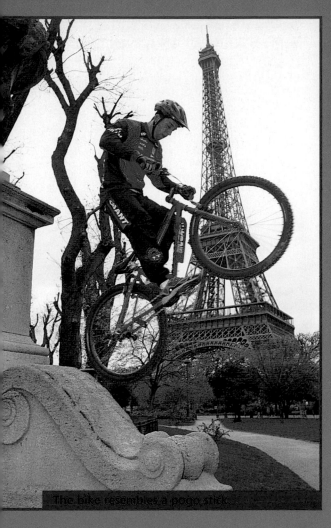

The bike resembles a pogo stick.

it right. The reward is successfully clearing an obstacle, and a big cheer goes up as the tension is released. There's frustration when you make a mistake, followed by a ripple of sympathetic applause. Many of them dream of one day toppling professional stunt rider Hans "No Way" Rey, who's famous for saying: "just don't say 'no way'" as he performs another impossible trick. A man who can hypnotize his bike, Rey relocated from his native Austria to the USA to hone his MTB skills after starting out in BMX. Rey has pulled off stunts such as riding *up* the cascade of the Dunn River Falls in Jamaica, holding a front wheel end in the face of some unamused guards outside Buckingham Palace, and launching off the roof of his house into the swimming pool.

Like downhilling and dual slalom, MTB trials have grown from BMX, where the smaller bikes are more malleable but the bigger you grow, the more oversized you look on one.

You can use your rigid mountain bike for trialing — but a badly timed jump or hop can mean the end of your front fork; remember that the damage won't be covered by the warranty. To increase the clearance above the ground, experts use just the small front chainring, and trials frames are built around a high 12-inch-plus bottom bracket. All-purpose MTB riders, whose bikes are

used for both cross-country and downhilling, might just add a chain-guard to stop the big ring from losing its teeth on the obstacles.

Of all MTB disciplines, trials is the one that improves most with practice. Timing and balance are the key qualities, as well as upper body strength. Some techniques you can practice are continuous hopping with turning, lifting the front wheel under perfect control to mount an obstacle, and pivoting on the front wheel to change direction. Check out your local trails for obstacles, or build your own progressively more difficult versions, and always wear a helmet, and elbow and knee pads. Trials are great for sharpening off-road skills and are lots of fun, but don't attempt them until you know what you're doing.

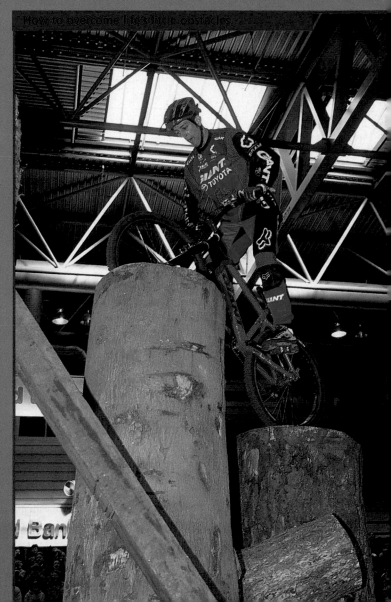

How to overcome life's little obstacles.

into the back of a rusting van, and come out through one of the rear doors.

Each station has its own dedicated marshall to do the scoring. You tackle the stations in whatever order you want. The aim is to get through the station without putting down your foot, which is known as a "dab". Every dab scores one penalty point on your scorecard, and the winner at the end of the event is the one who has the lowest score, maybe even a clear round. You've blown the section if you dab three times, or even worse if you put down both feet, which scores five penalty points. Expert riders will use tactical dabs when they find themselves in an impossible spot, which is better than total failure.

The atmosphere is calm and controlled, because the spectators concentrate on the riders and the riders concentrate on getting

the reebok dual eliminator

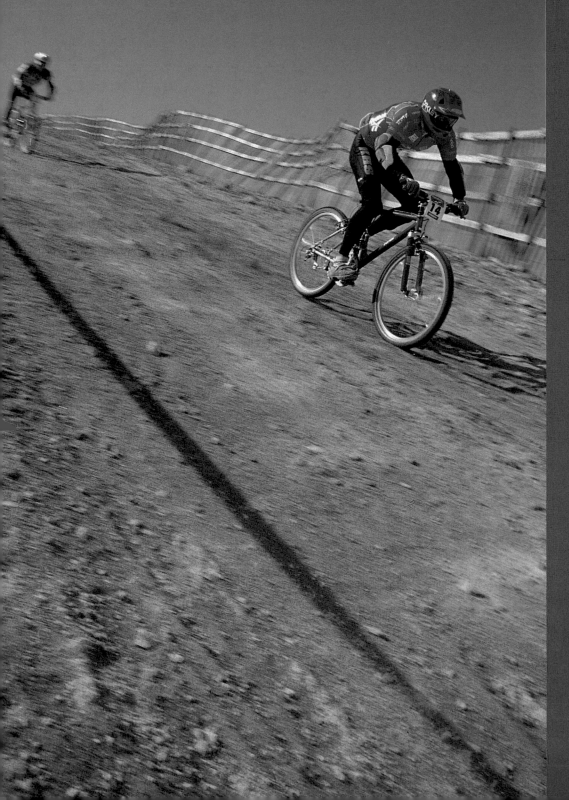

California 1992. The sunshine state and the birthplace of mountain biking. A new event, the Reebok Dual Eliminator, is born which, like the 1970s' Repack Downhill, will set new levels for off-road adrenalin and media coverage. The course and the nail-biting format draw speeds that rival the Tour de France swooping down the Alps.

Commissioned by ESPN, with $5,000 prize purse for the winner in both women's and men's categories, the Reebok has gone down in history as the mother of downhill duels. Unlikely to be surpassed in scale or speed, it has remained an unforgettable triumph for the un-Eliminated: Missy Giove and Dave Cullinan in 1992; Kim Sonier and Myles Rockwell in 1993, Regina Stiefl and Jürgen Benecke in 1994 and in 1995 Myles Rockwell and Giovanna Bonazzi.

Mammoth Mountain

The Dual Eliminator was run on the slopes of Mammoth Mountain — a high-altitude ski resort. The course, which began at a height of 10,000ft (3,000m), was already notorious as the home of the "Kamikaze Downhill", an open national championship event. Any competitor in the Kamikaze, hurling their body out of ski-gates down the track with Californian magma rocketing out from under the wheels knew they were riding for their lives — a fact celebrated on a video made of the event, which captured in gruesome detail the sliding crashes.

Devoid of technical trials the course was a wide, plain piste that curved around the mountain and descended a total of 2,050ft (630m) over 3.5 miles (5.6km). The surface was gravel with small rocks and a couple of dustbowl corners. The top half of the course extended over huge drops and was above the vegetation line. It was very exposed, with the Californian sun glaring down summer and winter, and surrounded by a fabulous vista of peaks covered with snow.

With so few obstacles to slow the riders down, the Kamikaze speedometers told a scary story. The course speed record had gradually risen in these events past 45–50mph (72–80km/h), as technology introduced full suspension bikes and life-preserving body armour. The speeds were unheard of on any other mountain bike course, even on the notorious European runs designed and hammered by riders born and bred in the traditions of Alpine downhill skiing.

The Reebok went one step further. From the first year, the involvement of ESPN and Reebok as sponsors threw fuel on the fire. The organizers, facing the task of making the event televisable, announced a new format for the competition. The Dual Eliminator would be an invitational pairs knock-out. While the Kamikaze event was just one rider against the clock, the Eliminator was a head-to-head, which meant unwelcome consequences if either duellist lost control too close to the other or to the edge.

The first year, the fastest downhillers in the world, 32 men and eight women, were selected. Each pair had two tries, the difference between riders' total run times deciding who went into the next round. The final was decided the same way and, with the exception of some small changes, that was the original format.

The action that first time in 1992 was watched by hundreds of spectators as the pairs shot by a total of 76 times in about five hours. As they completed each run, there was no time for the riders to contemplate how good it felt to be alive. As one commentator put it, they had to stay, "smiling brightly for ... the television soundbites".

The men's finalists managed to complete an exhausting total of ten runs; the women finalists achieved six. To save time and keep the pace going, a helicopter picked up the riders who had qualified for the next round and choppered them back to the top of Mammoth Mountain — shaving ten minutes off the gondola's uphill run.

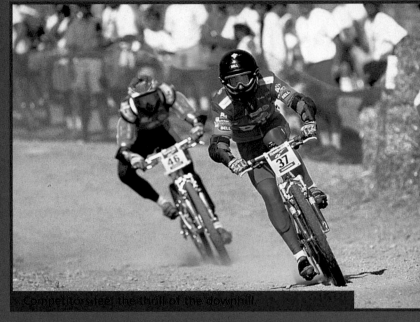
Competitors feel the thrill of the downhill.

Faster and faster

The Dual Eliminator was always a showcase for the latest downhill bikes. There full suspension and chain tensioners became universal for the first time, and booming disc wheels and single chainrings as big as 60T made their inaugural appearance. The first year, the fastest time was less than 5 minutes, with an average speed over 30mph (48km/h). Top speeds eventually reached 55mph (88km/h) or even higher, it was rumoured, as the world's fastest and most colorful mountain bikers opened throttle.

In the first year, excitement and curiosity overcame doubts about the recklessness of elbowing for dusty corners at 45mph (72km/h). Although no-one was ever badly hurt, John Tomac, the king of US racing, declined invitations to compete in any more Dual Eliminator races. The event itself was finally eliminated in the mid-Nineties, largely because of fears about safety. 1996 was the last year in which it took place.

The Dual Eliminator pushed riders frighteningly close to downhilling limits — limits still being challenged worldwide today.

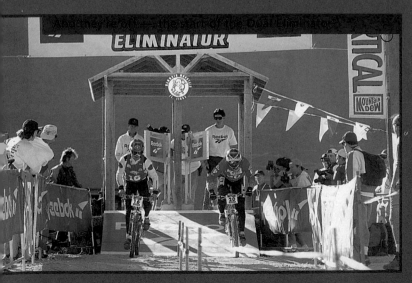
And they're off — the start of the Dual Eliminator.

24-hour racing

Mountain biking is incredibly versatile. You can ride 30–second slalom sprints in ski resorts or you can take four to six weeks exploring the Continental Divide from Mexico to Canada. Having tested those limits of the spectrum, another way to have a good time on an MTB has caught on in a big way — racing for the duration of one revolution of the planet, the 24-hour race.

Starting at noon on a Saturday, solo riders set off on a long circuit and continue through dusk, then dawn, and noon the next day. Then they collapse, claiming, in one rider's case, that he believed the only comparison was childbirth. Most people form a four-person team instead, and take turns to ride the circuit, exchanging a baton before catching some sleep while their pals take over.

Inspired in the US in the early '90s by the 24-Hours of Canaan (pronounced ka-nane) event in West Virginia, the sport has gained popularity with both specialists and general riders. Team riders are amazed at the camaraderie prompted by dragging yourself out of a sleeping bag in the middle of the night for the sake of your squad. Soloists belong to the fringe element symbolized by the renowned John Stamstad (see box).

24-hour events take place only a few times a year — they take a lot of organizing as well as riding — but have become annual events in people's calendars. There's the 24-Hours of Moab in Utah and the 24-Hours of the Donner Pass in the California Sierras, while Canaan has evolved into the 24-Hours

of Snowshoe. A series of 12 events, the 24-Hours of Adrenalin tours different venues in Canada, while Britain has Sleepless in the Saddle and the 24-Hour Red Bull Mountain Mayhem. Where the first Canaan had a 35-team entry, events now cater for up to 530

teams and are wildly over-booked with hundreds of folks turned away at registration.

The line-up now includes elite professional teams, who at first turned their noses up at 24-Hour racing in favor of the World Cup circuit. Now there are plans to develop

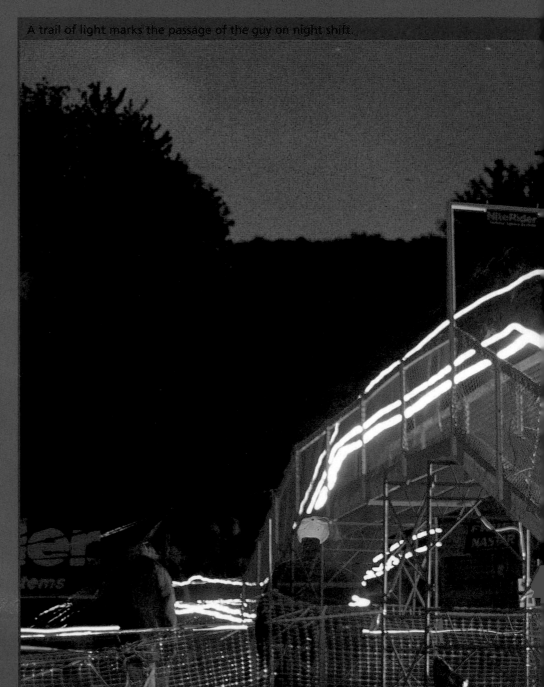

A trail of light marks the passage of the guy on night shift.

a world series sanctioned by the UCI, cycling's international body. Probably as astonishing as Stamstad's pioneering achievement is the sight of a professional hurtling over technical terrain at night at the same speed as in daylight.

Tips for 24s

■ Teams need to get to know each other well. Ride together beforehand, to build up the familiarity and friendship needed to endure the tough hours and to stay competitive, not stay asleep!

■ Ride at night as much as you can. Some teams, who've bumped into trees and had their lights fail, prepare for a 24 with a weekly night ride starting six months in advance. You need to learn about the limitations of your lights and batteries, about recharging and shine times. Carry a back-up light of good quality.

■ For eating and drinking, make everything as easy and idiot-proof as possible. Don't cook at 5am. Open packages or heat up pre-prepared favorite meals like pasta. Remember lots of fluid and milk for hot drinks and cereals.

■ Bring all the cycle clothing you own. If conditions are wet, you'll need a complete change for every lap, and warm sitting-around and waiting-on-the-line wear.

■ Have a minimum of two support crew, ideally one at camp, and one at the start/finish, to get riders to the line, or to bed down for a few hours. Get the hand-over right. Successful teams have no mechanical breakdowns, no light failures and no missed handovers, even if they aren't the fastest.

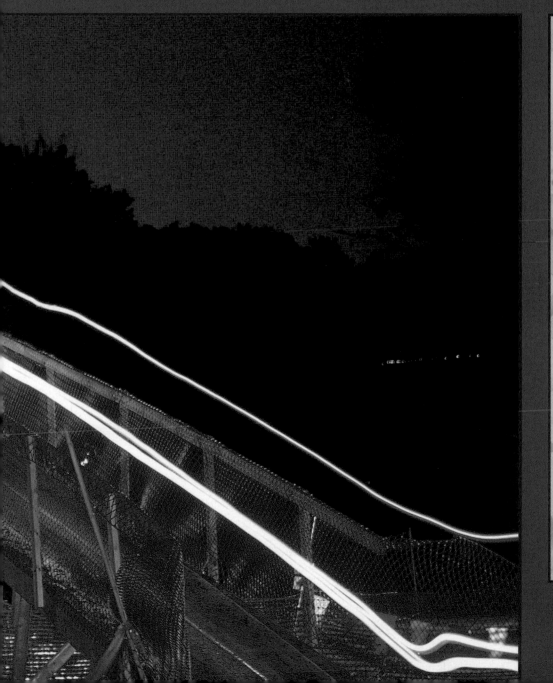

JOHN STAMSTAD, I PRESUME

Athlete John Stamstad was the first solo rider to take part in the 24-Hours of Canaan — before, in fact, there was a solo category. A renowned ultra-endurance competitor, Stamstad made his name by winning the Race Across America (RAAM), riding non-stop from coast-to-coast. To get a Canaan entry, he filled out a team form with a quartet of personal variations — John Stamstad, Mister Stamstad, JJ Stamstad, Stamstad Jnr, etc.

At registration, the stunned organizers couldn't turn him away, and Stamstad went on to ride something like 20 times around a 13-mile lap with a height gain/loss of 1700ft each time, totaling around 300 miles and 34,000ft. Trivia buffs may like to know that he used to train in the winter by running up and down multi-storey parking lots. And he survived on water and Goo, a perfectly-packaged energy gel.

big-time air

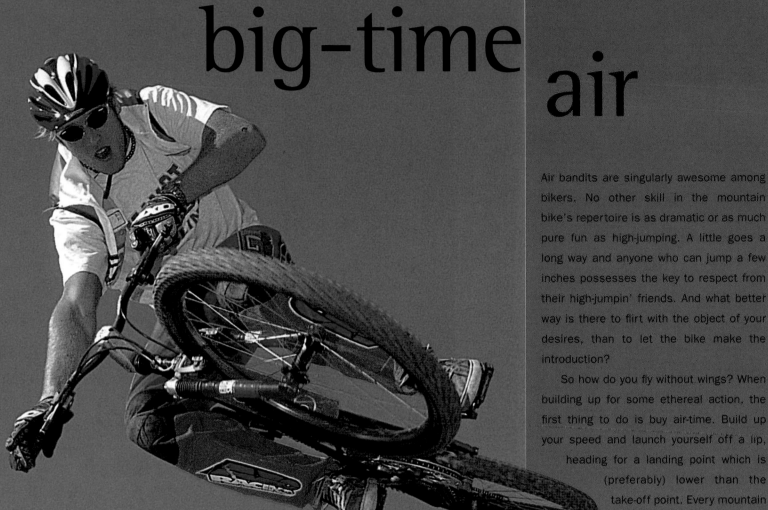

Air bandits are singularly awesome among bikers. No other skill in the mountain bike's repertoire is as dramatic or as much pure fun as high-jumping. A little goes a long way and anyone who can jump a few inches possesses the key to respect from their high-jumpin' friends. And what better way is there to flirt with the object of your desires, than to let the bike make the introduction?

So how do you fly without wings? When building up for some ethereal action, the first thing to do is buy air-time. Build up your speed and launch yourself off a lip, heading for a landing point which is (preferably) lower than the take-off point. Every mountain biker should be able to take air on any old off-road track, using even little ripples and momentum. Then there are proper launch pads, for example the bumps and flat-tops, abundant on BMX tracks, which have long run-offs. Or, as in trials, check out the local abandoned quarry (make sure that it's safe!) or forest for bomb-holes and drops.

The bigger the lip, the closer the sky, so start low and work up to greater height. Approach the launch-pad fast, and either let momentum drive you upward, or help it by pulling up on the pedals on take-off. Rule number one is to land with the front and back wheels level.

Once you're airborne, it's time to start styling. Most bikers who can jump grew up

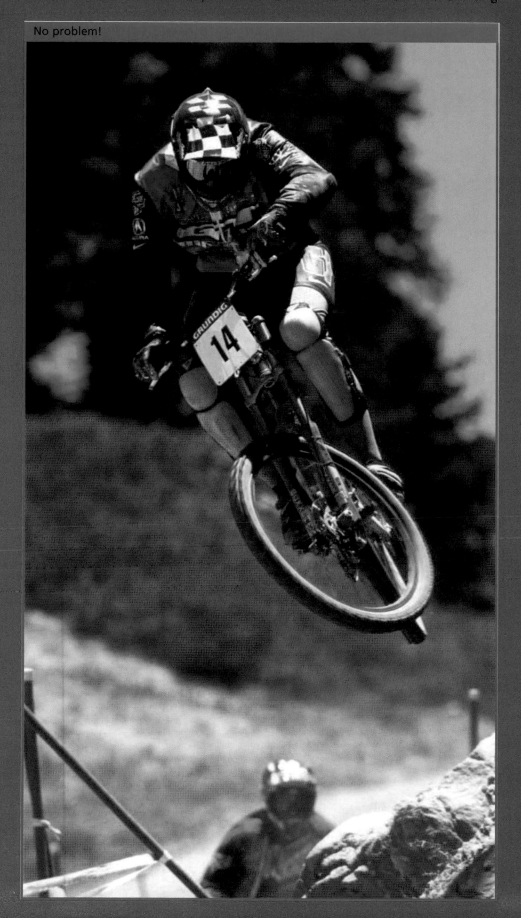

No problem!

in BMX, and have applied the tricks to the faster, but less maneuverable mountain bike, and you can see the crossover in airborne positions. Try the "pointer", where you point at your desirable individual, or the camera or the spectators with one hand, or cross it over your heart as you pray for deliverance.

There's the "cross-up", where you steer the wheel around an invisible corner in the air until the brake levers go plink on the top tube, then try to get pointing straight ahead again before touch-down. The "table-top" is a bigger version of the cross-up, where you pull the whole bike up flat in the air ahead of you, perpendicular to the trail, and then re-align in time for landing. Sticking one or both legs out is only part of the most outrageous position, the fabled "nothing" where nothing is in contact with the bike, arms, legs or butt. Catching the bike again is the trick, or getting a big mattress in place quickly.

Wear the gear. A helmet, plus elbow and knee-pads will take the brunt of a bad landing, as will the bike, which can't be protected the way you can. Apart from a stack of new pairs of forks, the best equipment is a pair of shorts with waterproof lining, and, if you're a beginner, a pair of clip-in pedals. They make it much easier to boost the bike's upward motion.

Great jumpers get high wearing platform shoes and no-clip pedals. Maybe their co-ordination is better simply because the air up there is cleaner. Take it easy, bike birds.

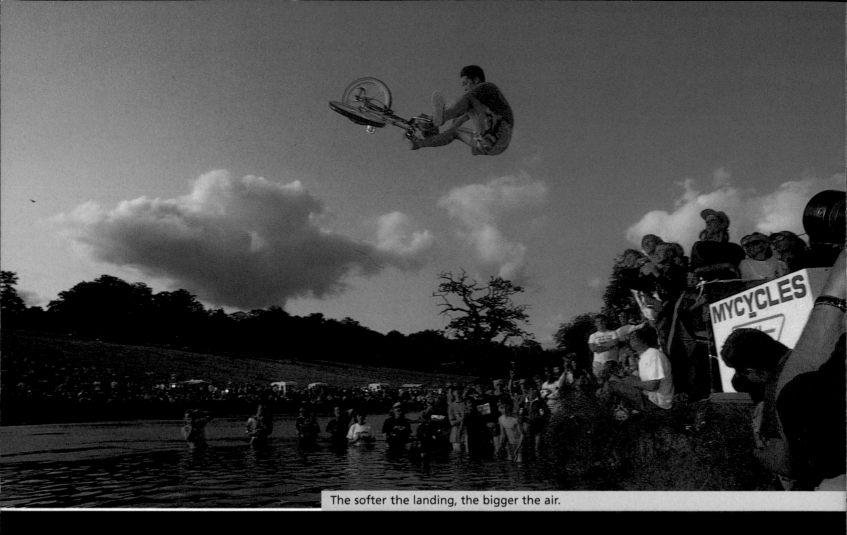

The softer the landing, the bigger the air.

making a splash

A few years back, the trigger for the UK's annual lake-leaping spectacle at the Malverns Classic festival was spontaneity. A handful of splash-loving bikers, a ramp, a waist-deep landscaped pond and some rapidly withdrawing ducks was all it took. Like a Broadway musical number, hurling your bike and body into water off a ramp shouldn't look rehearsed, but there is inevitably some forethought involved. Although these guys could build jump ramps in their sleep, what they weren't used to was the soft, wet and, for once, warm, landing. They saw Malvern's muddy waters, felt the 95°F (35°C) heat, remembered their ramp-ant BMX education and got launching.

First there were two, then three, then five. The multi-colored crowds gathered to join in the outburst of fun and the discovery of another crazy new bike thing. Forget off-road, the MTB could now go off-land, confirming its legendary versatility. Guys and a single girl who wanted to give it a try tentatively peered into the murky shallows, observed the guy who had just bobbed back up grinning, his arms held high in triumph, flinging his hair out of his eyes, and very much not drowned. One by one, intrepid bikers committed themselves to the Malvern baptism and took their place a short distance back from the ramp until 20 bikers had jumped.

The crowd loved it. Each sprint on the ramp was accompanied by a roar of cheers. The cheerleader, and likely ring-leader of the affair, was hidden under the ramp, like a prompter at the theater, supporting the plywood with his back, as he got the crowd going.

The styles ranged wildly from the high trajectory short-distance splashdown, to the low trajectory, long-distance splash-down. Lots of favorite jumping styles were on display, like table-tops and cross-ups, neither of which really left enough time to get rid of the bike before hitting the water. But what are a few more bruises when the sun is shining?

For lake leaping in shallow waters the main safety rule is to let go of the bike — even better to push it away forcibly — the second you leave the ramp. The two of you can then go your separate ways. The worst leap was where one of the guys, apparently scared stiff, held firmly on to the bike, hands on the handlebars, bum on the seat and feet on the pedals, all the way into the water.

The best leap that first year was a single front somersault with unbelievable height, maybe 20ft (6m) into the air. The guy threw the bike aside while he tumbled about in the ether and eventually hit the water near the far bank after what seemed to be a full 20 minutes in the air.

In those heady days the Malverns Classic festivals were some of the biggest summer events in Britain. There were attempts to recapture the spontaneity of the initial lake-leaping bonanza, but, everyone agreed that, by making the watersport official — it was subsequently

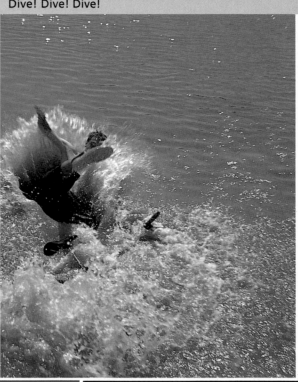

Dive! Dive! Dive!

Rule number 1 — rapidly let go of the bike.

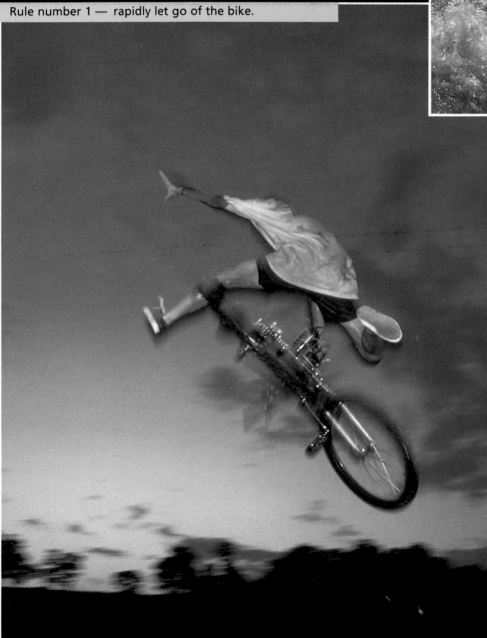

included on the event timetable — the spirit of the moment was somehow lost.

A group of British bikers based in the Lake District have since claimed to have pre-empted that occasion — in the chilly and much deeper waters of Lake Windermere. No ramp needed here, just a jetty or a quayside, a lifebelt and a mug of cocoa. In winter if you're submerged in the waters of the northern lakes for more than a minute or so, the chill can quickly lead to hypothermia. Another wild and crazy crew has since exploited the waterski jump ramp at Britain's national water sports centre for a bit of their own big leaping.

Of course, you can drown playing around in water hanging on to things that sink like stones. So, don't do it unless you can find shallow water to jump or fall into (and not just by yourself!) or have a fully qualified lifeboat crew keep an eye on you.

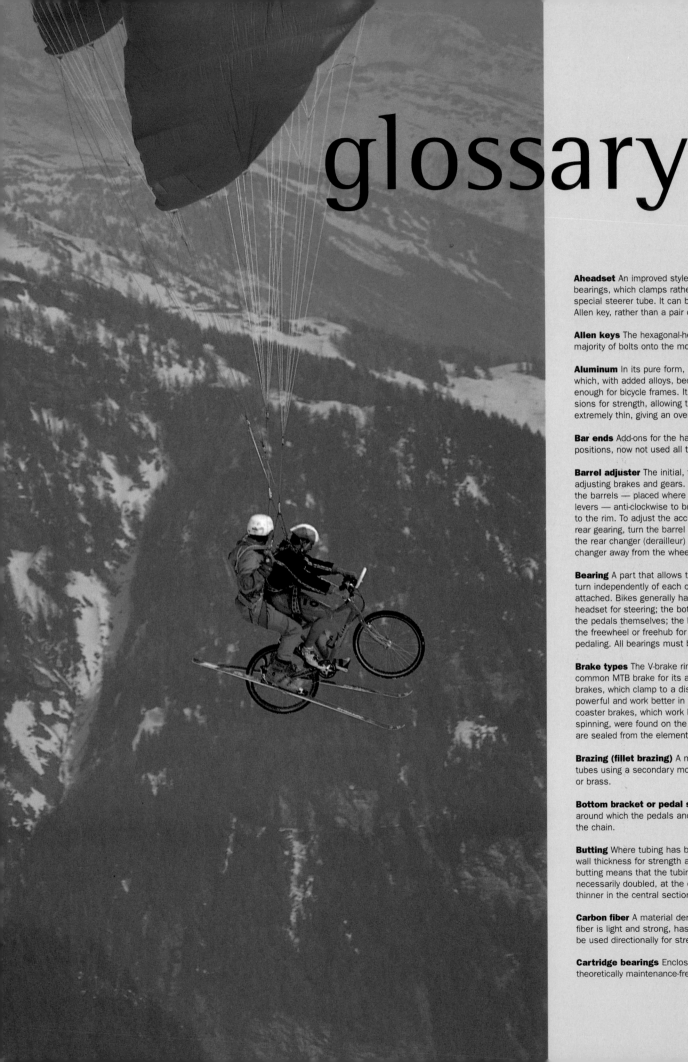

glossary

Aheadset An improved style of headset steering bearings, which clamps rather than screws on to the special steerer tube. It can be adjusted using a single Allen key, rather than a pair of bulky headset wrenches.

Allen keys The hexagonal-head tools that screw the majority of bolts onto the mountain bike.

Aluminum In its pure form, a soft, light material, which, with added alloys, becomes strong and stiff enough for bicycle frames. It is used in oversize dimensions for strength, allowing the tube walls to be made extremely thin, giving an overall weight advantage.

Bar ends Add-ons for the handlebars to give more hand positions, now not used all that much.

Barrel adjuster The initial, tool-free method of adjusting brakes and gears. To adjust the brakes, turn the barrels — placed where the cables come out of the levers — anti-clockwise to bring the brake pads closer to the rim. To adjust the accuracy of the indexing in the rear gearing, turn the barrel — where the cable exits the rear changer (derailleur) — clockwise to pull the changer away from the wheel.

Bearing A part that allows two pieces of the bike to turn independently of each other, while remaining firmly attached. Bikes generally have five sets of bearings; the headset for steering; the bottom bracket for pedaling; in the pedals themselves; the hubs (the wheels) and in the freewheel or freehub for freewheeling and back-pedaling. All bearings must be maintained.

Brake types The V-brake rim brake is the most common MTB brake for its accessibility, although disc brakes, which clamp to a disc at the hub, are more powerful and work better in wet weather. Old-time coaster brakes, which work by stopping the pedals from spinning, were found on the early clunkers. Hub brakes are sealed from the elements but have never caught on.

Brazing (fillet brazing) A method of joining steel tubes using a secondary molten material, like silver or brass.

Bottom bracket or pedal spindle The axle bearing around which the pedals and cranks turn to operate the chain.

Butting Where tubing has been made with a variable wall thickness for strength and lighter weight. Double butting means that the tubing is thicker, but not necessarily doubled, at the ends near the joins, and thinner in the central section.

Carbon fiber A material derived from crude oil, carbon fiber is light and strong, has a grain like timber and can be used directionally for strength and light weight.

Cartridge bearings Enclosed bearing units that are theoretically maintenance-free (see bearings).

Chainrings On cross-country MTBs, the triple front gear rings; on downhill bikes, a single front gear ring. Chains wear together with chainrings, so change the chain frequently to save money on replacing the rings.

Chainset The cranks, crank spider (to which the chainrings attach) and the chainrings.

Chain stay The tubing that runs from the rear hub to the bottom of the seat tube at the bottom bracket. Usually around 16–17in (405–430mm) long. A shorter chain stay gives better grip at the rear of the bike when climbing, but is more difficult to control downhill.

CNC (computer numerically controlled) Cut or carved from a thick piece of material, usually aluminum, by a robot blade or laser directed by computer.

Componentry One of the two main parts of a bicycle, the other being the frame. You can either choose an almost complete set of componentry (groupset) from one manufacturer, or mix-and-match your choice of parts to include those from specialists, according to budget and performance.

Crank A simple part with a pedal at one end and the bottom bracket at the other.

Cromoly (chromium-molybdenum) A steel alloy that varies in price and performance from basic to top class.

Derailleur The French word for de-railer, or front and rear gear changers.

Down tube The strongest tube in the frame, running diagonally from the head tube to the bottom bracket.

Dropouts The slots at the back of the frame and bottom of the fork into which the wheels slip and are secured. In road riding, horizontal dropouts allow you to set the front and rear position of the wheel, but MTBs almost universally have easier, pre-set vertical dropouts.

End-stop screw The tiny Phillips screws on the front and rear changers that set how far the changers can move. These are adjusted to prevent the chain falling off on either side.

Fork Holds the front wheel on; forks are manufactured with or without suspension.

Frame materials The skeletal structure of an MTB can be made from steel, aluminum, titanium, carbon-fiber or magnesium.

Gear ratio The relationship between the number of teeth in the chainring (front) and sprocket (rear) engaged. If equal, the gear ratio is 1:1 — the rear wheel turns at the same speed as the pedals. On fast ground, if the chainring has 48 teeth and the sprocket 24, the ratio is 2:1 — the rear wheel turns at double the speed of the pedals, twice for every pedal revolution.

Gear shifter types Three main versions include SRAM TwistShifters where the whole handgrip turns, underbar (Shimano Rapidfire) levers and overbar thumb levers.

Groupset A set of compatible componentry from one maker, like Shimano or Campagnolo, found on the majority of shop bikes. Groupsets are made at different prices and quality.

Gussets Individual reinforcing plates placed at tube junctions, particularly the head tube.

Headset The steering bearing.

Head tube The short length of tubing that forms the front apex of the frame.

Hi-tensile steel The grade of steel below cromoly, found either in part or in full on cheaper bikes.

Hub The bearings on which the wheels turn.

Indexing (index shifting) Pre-set "click-click" gears.

Jockey wheel The two wheels in the rear changer that align the chain across the sprockets.

Kevlar A branded, highly-resistant carbon material layered in tires to prevent flats.

Lubricant The grease, oils and lubes that keep a bike turning and prolong its life. All moving surfaces should be kept lubed, so lubrication is an essential part of pre- and post-ride maintenance.

Lugging (lugwork) Reinforcing sleeves that may be used in the brazing process in making steel frames. On aluminum frames, the tubing may be bonded inside aluminum lugs at low temperatures.

Main triangle The front half of a regular diamond-shaped frame, containing the top, seat, head and down tubes. On cheaper steel bikes, often the rear triangle, or the secondary tubes in the front triangle, such as the seat tube, will be made of high-tensile rather than cromoly steel.

Microdrive The original SunTour name for close MTB gearing (smaller chainrings and sprockets) that has the same ratios as former wider gearing with less bulk, more clearance and, in theory, more wear. Shimano followed suit, and this is now standard.

Play The looseness that needs to be eliminated in bearings and brake cables.

Quick release Securing levers for the wheels and seat post.

Rear triangle In a conventionally-shaped diamond frame, the back tubes, the chain and seat stays. They may be of a lower grade steel on cheaper bikes.

Rim The structural outer edge of the wheel, the rim is made of aluminum alloy, and provides the braking surface, hooks the tire and tube in place, and anchors the spokes. Its size is measured in millimetres according to the diameter of the inside edge that holds the bead of the tire. The average for an MTB is 559mm.

Seat cluster The tube junction of the seat tubes and the seat stays at the saddle. It's often reinforced when using a long seat post with lugging, a gusset or butting.

Seat stay The double tubes that run from the rear hub to the seat cluster below the saddle. The two configurations are "wishbone" — where the stays come together above the wheel and a single tube connects them to the seat cluster — and the standard "dual" — where the two tubes run all the way to the seat cluster, usually with a reinforcing bridge for rigidity.

Seat tube The central vertical tube that runs from the bottom of the bike at the bottom bracket to the seat post.

Single-butting No butting, where a tube has the same wall thickness throughout its length (see also butting).

Single-track Where the trail is only wide enough for a single bike, or person, or horse. Great fun.

SPD pedals (Shimano pedaling dynamics) The standard clip-in pedal (and compatible shoe cleat and shoe) is also made under licence by other manufacturers. Essential for cross-country racing, not used in downhill or stunt riding though helpful for touring, but clogs up in bad mud.

Spokes The tensioned wires in the wheel that spread the load and keep the rim circular under compression from the ground. Butted spokes are thinner in the middle than at the edge.

Spoke nipple The little nut used to put tension into the spokes with a spoke key.

Sprockets The seven, eight or nine rear gear cogs.

Standover height Measured from the ground to the top of the top tube where you would stand over it. It is the key measurement in getting the right size mountain bike, and should be 2–3in (50–75mm) shorter than your inside leg measurement.

Stem The section that attaches the handlebars to the head tube.

Straddle cable The brake wire that bridges the two arms. In older cantilever brakes it should hold the arms at 45° at rest. V-brakes do away with a single straddle cable, by running the main cable all the way to one brake arm and having a shorter wire for the other arm.

Suspension Allows either the front or both wheels to move independently of the frame and rider for better control and higher speeds. For comfort, secondary suspension in the seat post or stem is also available.

Titanium An abundant element, used extensively in the aerospace industry. It is lighter than steel, stronger than aluminum and expensive to work with.

Toeclips and straps Simple, effective, versatile way of keeping the feet attached to the pedals that has been superseded even for touring by clip-in SPDs.

Top tube The horizontal tube that connects the head tube with the seat cluster.

Tungsten Inert Gas (TIG) welding A method of welding steel and aluminum tubing without oxygen or a secondary welding material.

Tire pressures MTB tires should be run at 35–55psi, according to the softness of the ground — this information will be written on the sidewall of the tire. Lower pressure means better grip; higher pressure mean less comfort — no problem if the bike has suspension.

Tire types MTB tires are 26in (650mm) in diameter, with a variety of patterns, from slick for pavement, to spiky for deep mud. They come in different widths, averaging 1.95in, with a minimum 1.5in allowable in MTB racing. There is a lot of talk about tires for different conditions — dry, wet, muddy — with the fundamental requirement that they're knobby and wide.

Valves The most popular American type is the thick Shraeder. Less common is the thin Presta, also found on car tires, which needs a wider-drilled hole in the rim.

Wheel size Everyone calls the standard MTB wheel a 26 inch (650mm) wheel, referring to the size of the tire (the outside diameter). However, according to the standard metric Système Internationale (SI), wheels are actually measured in millimetres, using the diameter of the inside edge of the rim where the tire beading sits. This is generally 559mm (22in).

index

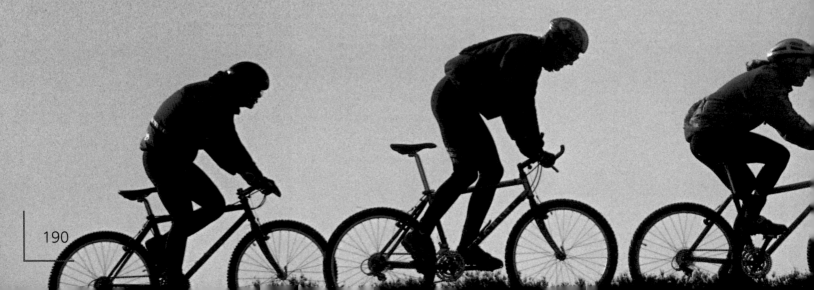

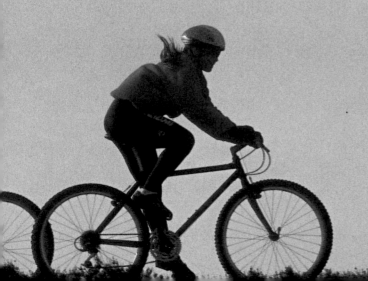
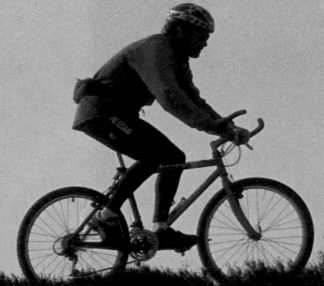

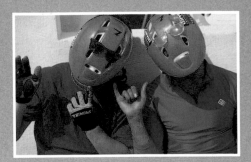

further reading

Nick Crane, *Atlas Biker — Mountain Biking in Morocco*,
The Oxford Illustrated Press, 1990

Judy Ridgeway, *Food for Sport*,
Boxtree, 1994

Bicycling Science,
The MIT Press, 1993

Douglas Hayduk, *Bicycle Metallurgy for the Cyclist*,
Johnson Publishing Co, 1987

Edmund R Burke, *Cycling Health and Physiology*,
Vitesse Press, 1992

acknowledgments

With thanks to the following for their help:
Mel Allwood of Brixton Cycles, London, for her expertise, and Brixton Cycles for loaning equipment; Chipps Chippendale for information on 24-hour racing; *Exodus MTB Travel* for their help with the section on Morocco; Carole Bauer-Romanik, curator of the Mountain Bike Hall of Fame; Crested Butte, Colorado, for information on the history of mountain biking; Rim Tours, Moab, Utah, for their help with the Slickrock section; Ed Cannady, recreation manager of the Sawtooth NRA for details of rides and conditions; Mont Blanc Mountain Biking, for help with the Chamonix section; Colin Palmer, *CTC Off-Road*, for all his good work; Richard Hemington, *Specialized UK*, for UK reminiscences; Geoff Apps, Cleland MTBs for his tales; Trek, Foes / Hotlines UK, Rocky Mountain, Orange Mountain Bikes, Santa Cruz Bikes, 24Seven, Dickon Hepworth of Stif, Mike Cotty of Cannondale, for bike photos and specifications; Madison for Shimano information.

picture credits

The publishers would like to thank the following sources for their kind permission to reproduce the pictures in this book:

Actionsnaps/Dave Stewart 180cl, 181bl, 186tc; **Jules Bellier** 6, 43, 57c, 62; **Bliss/M.Fearon** 12br, 14, 41c, 58r, 66, 77, 85, 91br, 91bl, 93br, 101tr, 102, 103bl, 106, 110c, 132tr, 138, 160tl, 161bl, 162, 163, 181tr, 185tc; **Buzz Pictures** 4-5, 68, 138-9, 142; **Ed Cannady** 152-3, 154, 155, 157tr, 157b; **Cannondale** 81, 81r; **Chipps Chippendale** 140, 179tl, 182-3; **Nick Crane** 170, 172cl, 173tr, 173bl, 174tc, 175tr; **Nicky Crowther** 158; **C. Hultner/MTB Action**.78; **David Epperson** 8tc, 9bl, 10tr, 11tr, 86, 133bc; **Foes/ Hotlines UK** 26; **Image Bank/JKelly** 158; **Madison** 10bl, 27, 74; **Phil O'Connor** 143; **Orange Mountain Bikes** 83; **Pace Cycles** 80br, 80bl; **Rocky Mountain** 83l; **Santa Cruz Bikes** 29; **Schwinn Cycles** 11bl; **Science Photo Library** 20,21; **Stockfile/S.Behr** 11tr, 12tl, 13tl, 16, 20, 21, 25, 28, 34c, 60c, 64, 65, 66, 67, 70, 72, 73tr, 76, 79, 85, 88, 90, 92bl, 93tl, 100, 104tl, 105tl, 105br, 109c, 110 tcr, 111br, 112cr, 113r, 114tc, 116, 117tl, 117l, 118, 121bl, 121tr, 123tr, 124br, 125tc, 126, 128bc, 129r, 129tl, 130, 134tc, 135cr, 135bl, 136bl, 137tc, 137br, 138tr, 141b, 164, 166tl, 167bc, 167tr, 168tr, 169, 178, 179br, 184cl, 185br, 187cl, 187tr, 190; **Trek** 24 82; **24Seven** 73b, 74br, 75; **Dave Yates** 13; **Greg Yeoman** 38l, 146, 148tr, 148tl, 150tl, 151tr, 151bc.

Every effort has been made to acknowledge correctly and contact the source and/or copyright holder of each picture, and Carlton Books Limited apologizes for any unintentional errors or omissions which will be corrected in future editions of this book.

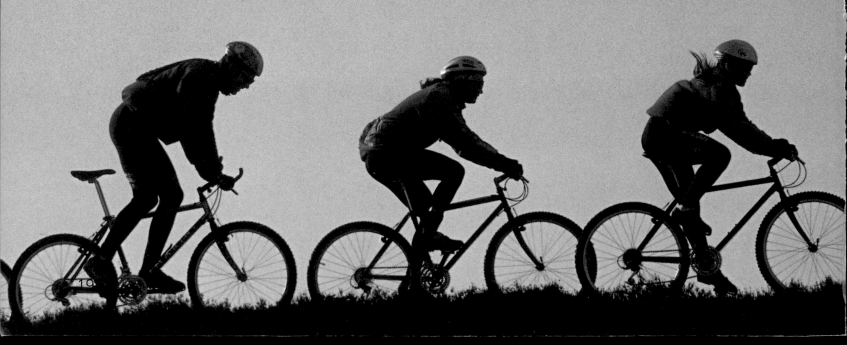